Obstetric and Gynecologic Care

in Physical Therapy

SECOND EDITION

Obstetric and Gynecologic Care

in Physical Therapy

SECOND EDITION

REBECCA G. STEPHENSON, BS, PT

Senior Clinical Therapist, Dedham Medical Associates
Dedham, Massachusetts
Medical Writer, RGS Physical Therapy
Medfield, Massachusetts

LINDA J. O'CONNOR, MS, PT

Physical Therapist, Easter Seal Bay Area
Oakland, California

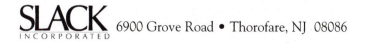

SLACK 6900 Grove Road • Thorofare, NJ 08086
INCORPORATED

Publisher: John H. Bond
Editorial Director: Amy E. Drummond
Assistant Editor: Lauren Biddle Plummer
Cover Illustration: Lisa Blackshear

The procedures and practices described in this book should be implemented in a manner consistent with the professional standards set for the circumstances that apply in each specific situation. Every effort has been made to confirm the accuracy of the information presented and to correctly relate generally accepted practices. The author, editor, and publisher cannot accept responsibility for errors or exclusions or for the outcome of the application of the material presented herein. There is no expressed or implied warranty of this book or information imparted by it.

Care has been taken to ensure that drug selection, dosages, and treatments are in accordance with currently accepted/recommended practice. Due to continuing research, changes in government policy and regulations, and various effects of drug reactions and interactions, it is recommended that the reader review all materials and literature provided for each drug, especially those that are new or not frequently used.

Any review or mention of specific companies or products is not intended as an endorsement by the author or the publisher.

The work SLACK publishes is peer reviewed. Prior to publication, recognized leaders in the field, educators, and clinicians provide important feedback on the concepts and content that we publish. We welcome feedback on this work.

Stephenson, Rebecca G. (Rebecca J. Gourley)
    Obstetrics and Gynecologic Care in Physical Therapy/ Rebecca G. Stephenson, Linda J. O'Connor--2nd ed.
        p.; cm.
    Includes bibliographical references and index.
    ISBN 1-55642-415-9 (alk. paper)
    1. Obstetrics. 2. Gynecology. 3. Physical Therapy. 4. Exercise for women--physiological aspects. I. Stephenson, Rebecca G. II. O'Connor, Linda J. Obstetric and gynecological care in physical therapy. III. Title.
    [DNLM: 1. Obsterics. 2. Physical Therapy--Pregnancy. 3. Physical Therapy--methods. 4. Womens' Health. WQ 200 S837o2000]
    RG129.P45 O18 2000
    618--dc21   99-059223

Printed in Canada

Published by: SLACK Incorporated
            6900 Grove Road
            Thorofare, NJ 08086-9447 USA
            Telephone: 856-848-1000
            Fax: 856-853-5991
            World Wide Web: http://www.slackinc.com

Contact SLACK Incorporated for more information about other books in this field or about the availability of our books from distributors outside the United States.

Last digit is print number: 10   9   8   7   6   5   4   3   2   1

DEDICATIONS

Second Edition

To all the physical therapists who so lovingly treat women and make their lives better.

Rebecca G. Stephenson, BS, PT

To our dedicated students and fellow practitioners who made this second edition possible.

Linda J. O'Connor, MS, PT

First Edition

To Jared and David for their love, patience, support, and confidence that allowed me the freedom to undertake and complete this project; and to the memory of Steve Rose, whose zest for life, enthusiasm for physical therapy, and drive to pursue a vision, live on as an inspiration for all in physical therapy.

Rebecca G. Stephenson, BS, PT

To my husband John for his evenings spent alone; to my three children—John, Scott, and Lisa—for letting me use the computer; and to the many physical therapists and physical therapy students who expressed the need and desire to perpetuate a new field of practice.

Linda J. O'Connor, MS, PT

CONTENTS

Dedications v
Acknowledgments xi
About the Authors..xiii
Prefaces xv

Section 1: Foundation for Physical Therapy Practice in Women's Health

Chapter 1   Women's Health Care in Physical Therapy 3
           Yesterday and Today
           Historical Insights in Obstetrics and Gynecology
           Women's Health Physical Therapy: Development of Practice
           Current Role of the Physical Therapy Practitioner in Women's Health
           Marketing Physical Therapy Services
           Certifications, Specializations, and Instructing Educational Classes
           Internships
           Research Needs
           Self-Assessment Review
               Answers
           References

Chapter 2   Anatomical Considerations...15
           Historical Insights in Female Nomenclature
           General Female Anatomy
               The Female Breast
               The Female Abdomen
               The Female Pelvis
                   The Bony Pelvis
                   Biomechanics of the Female Pelvis
           Obstetric Concerns
                   Pelvic Axes, Position, Obstetric Diameters, and Shape
                   Abnormal Bony Pelvis
                   Mechanical Impact of the Fetus on Anatomic Relations
                       Influence of Fetal Weight on Blood Supply
                       Influence of Fetal Weight and Postural Changes
                   Hormonal Impact of Pregnancy on Anatomic Relations
           Gynecologic Concerns
                   Contents of the Pelvic Cavity
                   Muscles of the Pelvis and Pelvic Floor/Diaphram
                   The Perineum/External Genitalia
               Self-Assessment Review
               Answers
           References

Section 2: Role of Physical Therapy in Gynecologic Care

Chapter 3   Physical Therapy and the Female Client: Evaluation and Treatment 37
           Practice Issues
               Restrictions and Cautionary Note
           Taking and Interpreting a History
           Pelvic Floor Examination
           Female Reproductive System
               Normal Menstrual Cycle
               Abnormal Menstrual Cycles
               Painful Menstrual Cycles
                   Premenstrual Syndrome
                   Dysmenorrhea
           Pelvic Pain: Acute and Chronic
           Urinary Disorders
           Pelvic Floor Training
               Initial Training
               Position
           Breast Rehabilitation
           The Aging Female

　　　　Anatomical and Physiological Changes
　　　　Menopause
　　　　Psychological Changes
　　　　Cardiovascular and Other Systemic Changes
　　　　Osteoporosis, Falls, and Fractures
　　Case Studies
　　　　Client with Genuine Stress Incontinence
　　　　Client with Vulvar Vestibulitis
　　　　Client with Osteoporosis
　　Self-Assessment Review
　　　　Answers
　　References

Section 3: Role of Physical Therapy in Obstetric Care
Chapter 4　　Maternal Physiology 87
　　Reproductive Changes
　　Renal Changes
　　Cardiovascular Changes
　　Neurologic Changes
　　Gastrointestinal Changes
　　Breast Changes
　　Weight Gain
　　Metabolic Changes
　　Respiratory Changes
　　Endocrine Changes
　　Dermatologic Changes
　　Multiple Pregnancies
　　Exercise
　　　　Maternal Responses to Exercise
　　　　Fetal Response to Maternal Exercise
　　　　Placental Responses to Maternal Exercise
　　　　Effect of Exercise on Pregnancy Outcome
　　The Physical Therapist as an Instructor
　　Early Pregnancy Classes
　　　　Teaching Relaxation: Why it is Important
　　　　Teaching About Emotional Changes
　　　　Teaching Fetal and Maternal Changes
　　　　Teaching Nutrition
　　　　Teaching Pelvic Floor Toning
　　　　Teaching Body Mechanics and Center of Gravity
　　　　Teaching About Partner's Role
　　　　Teaching Exercises
　　Self-Assessment Review
　　　　Answers
　　References

Chapter 5　　Maternal Disorders and Diseases 133
　　Death and Mortality Rates
　　Cardiac Diseases and Disorders
　　Pregnancy-Induced Hypertension
　　Vascular Disease
　　Endocrine Disease
　　Renal Disease
　　Respiratory Disorders
　　Infectious, Gastrointestinal, and Dermatologic Diseases and Disorders
　　Reproductive Tract Disorders
　　Neurologic Diseases and Disorders
　　Musculoskeletal Disorders
　　Self-Assessment Review
　　　　Answers
　　References

Chapter 6　　Physical Therapy Care in High-Risk Pregnancies 161
　　General Considerations for High-Risk Pregnancies

The Role of Physical Therapy in High-Risk Pregnancies
Teen Pregnancy
Pregnant Women with Disabilities or Chronic Illness
    Pregnant Women with Cardiac Diseases
    Pregnancy-Induced Hypertension
    Pregnant Women with Respiratory Disease
    Pregnant Women with Arthritis
    Pregnant Women after Transplant
    Pregnant Women with Multiple Sclerosis
    Pregnant Women with Spinal Cord Injuries
Self-Assessment Review
    Answers
References

Chapter 7   Evaluation and Treatment of Maternal Musculoskeletal Disorders 175
Contraindications
    Avoid
Musculoskeletal Evaluation
    Posture
    Muscle Testing
        Adapted Manual Muscle Test Positions
Treatment of Selected Musculoskeletal Conditions
    Neck and Upper Back Strain
    Temporomandibular Joint
    Thoracic Outlet
    Carpal Tunnel Syndrome
    De Quervain's Disease
    Diastasis Recti Abdominis
    Costal Rib Pain
    Sacroiliac Joint Pain
        Posterior Innominate
        Anterior Innominate
    Symphysis Pubis
    Low Back
    Piriformis
    Coccyx
    Knee and Patella Dysfunction
    Nerve Palsies
    Muscle, Tendon Injuries
Case Studies
Pregnant Client with Back Pain Relating to Posture Changes
Pregnant Client with a Herniated Disc
Pregnant Client with Low Back Strain
Self-Assessment Review
    Answers
References

Chapter 8   Care of the Fetus: Preconception to Birth 205
Preconception Concerns and Genetic Counseling
Teratogens and Environmental Hazards
Conception
Fetal Growth
Fetal Development
Fetal Physiology
Fetal and Neonatal Assessment
Self-Assessment Review
    Answers
References

Chapter 9   Physical Therapy Care During Labor 223
Late Pregnancy: Prodrome to Labor
Normal Labor
Complicated Labor
Maternal Position and State

          Pain Mechanisms and Relief
          Self-Assessment Review
            Answers
          References

Chapter 10 Physical Therapy Care During Delivery 241
          Second Stage of Labor
          Third Stage of Labor
          Alternative Birth
          Pain Management for Delivery
          Positions for Delivery
          Complicated Deliveries
            Forceps
            Cesarean
            Vaginal Births After Cesarean
            Multifetal Birth
          Repair of the Perineum
          Injuries Involving Uterine Support
            Retrodisplacement of the Uterus
          Injury to the Pelvic Joints
          Genital Fistulas
          Childbirth Preparation Classes
          Self-Assessment Review
            Answers
          References

Chapter 11 Physical Therapy and Post-Partum Care.................................265
          Anatomical and Physiological Changes Post-Partum
            The Uterus
            The Perineum
            Urinary Tract
            Gastrointestinal Tract
            Circulation
            Musculoskeletal
            Diastasis Recti Abdominis
            Emotional Adjustments
            Lactation
          Exercise
          Post-Cesarean Delivery
          The First Six Weeks at Home
            Going Home
            Sexuality
            Post-Partum Checkup
          Post-Partum Case Study
            Exam
          Instructing Post-Partum Classes
            Post-Natal Exercise Program
            Post-Cesarean Exercise Program
          Self-Assessment Review
            Answers
          References

Conclusion 283

Appendix A: Suggested Reading by Topic 285

Appendix B: Product Information and Resources 291

Appendix C: Suggestions for Use of the *Guide to Physical Therapist Practice* 303

Glossary 307

Index..317

Acknowledgments

Second Edition

I am grateful to my friend and coach, Toni Stone, founder and director of *WonderWorks Studio*, who helped me define the scope of this second edition, nudged me in the process, and coached me monthly to hold the vision of the possibility of an expanded edition. She offered seasonal workshops in Vermont where I worked on the book uninterrupted. Special thanks to Linda O'Connor, my co-author, for agreeing to take this project on again and do what it takes to bring this to completion. Many thanks to those who extended their friendship and support: Linda White for her excellent computer problem-solving skills that were always available and given in such a friendly manner, Sara Mastronardi for her enthusiastic library and computer research, David for all the ways that he continues to support me professionally and personally, Jeremy for understanding my time away from him, David P. Simmons, M.D. and Dot Aronson for foreign language translation. I acknowledge Candice Schacter, PhD, for her consultation, writings, and research on survivors of childhood sexual abuse that added another layer of understanding for the physical therapist working with women, and Lynne Assad, PT, friend and colleague, who enthusiastically read important chapters from a clinical vantage point, offering valuable suggestions, and Suki Kuck for medical illustrations. And to all my supporters at SLACK Incorporated: John Bond, Publisher, who always validated this project, Amy Drummond, Editorial Director, who first came to me with the idea for a second edition and never faltered with her support or commitment to me, Debra Christy and Lauren Biddle Plummer, who took such loving care of the book in production, the artists for the book's cover, and to all the anonymous reviewers who contributed much with their critique of this second edition.

Rebecca G. Stephenson, BS, PT

First Edition

The authors wish to thank Jane Frahm, Z. Annette Iglarsh, and Linda M. Pipp for their participation in interviews; Barbara Savi for her assistance in manuscript preparation; David P. Simmons, M.D., for his support and help with library privileges; Melanie Wallace for acting as our model; and the Section on Obstetrics and Gynecology of the American Physical Therapy Association for providing background material on the development of this practice.

ABOUT THE AUTHORS

Rebecca G. Stephenson, BS, PT, received her physical therapy degree from Boston University in 1974. She is also a certified childbirth educator and medical writer, member of the American Physical Therapy Association and its Section on Women's Health, and of the American Medical Writers Association.

She has practiced in diverse environments including rehabilitation, outpatient clinics, school settings, nursing homes, a residential care facility, and private practice. She has taught early pregnancy classes and currently lectures nationally on topics of women's health. As a medical writer, Rebecca co-authored the first edition of *Obstetric and Gynecologic Care in Physical Therapy*, has been a journal abstractor of the *Physical Therapy Journal*, a past book editor for the *Journal of Obstetric and Gynecologic Physical Therapy* (currently the *Journal of the Section on Women's Health of the American Physical Therapy Association*), and is now a products editor for the *Journal of the Section on Women's Health*. She has written for print- and web-based publications.

She created the video *Back Care in Pregnancy* and has been a consultant for other video productions. She was secretary for the Section on Women's Health and is currently secretary for the International Organization of Physical Therapists in Women's Health, a sub-group of the World Confederation of Physical Therapy. Rebecca was awarded the Section on Women's Health of the American Physical Therapy Association highest honor, the Elizabeth Nobel award, for contributions to the field of women's health. She practices women's health and adult and pediatric rehabilitation as senior clinical therapist in the outpatient clinic at Dedham Medical Associates and in private practice in Medfield, Massachusetts.

Linda J. O'Connor, MS, PT, received her physical therapy degree from the University of California, San Francisco, in 1974. Since then she has practiced in a variety of settings, including obstetric and gynecology clinics, private homes, skilled nursing facilities, school districts, residential care facilities, hospitals, and outpatient facilities. She has taught childbirth education, mother-infant exercise, and early pregnancy classes for over 15 years, intertwining teaching with independent contracting and private practice in pediatrics, geriatrics, and women's health care. As part of her interest in women's health care, Linda was editor of the *Bulletin of the Section of Obstetrics and Gynecology of the American Physical Therapy Association* (later the *Journal of Obstetric and Gynecologic Physical Therapy*) and the *Journal of the Section on Women's Health of the American Physical Therapy Association* for 15 years. The role of editor, combined with an interest in journalism and writing, led to the completion of her master's degree in mass communications in 1990. While working on her master's degree, Linda co-authored the first edition of *Obstetric and Gynecologic Care in Physical Therapy*, reviewed manuscripts and books for the journal *Physical Therapy*, and had several articles published in parenting, nursing, and childbirth education publications. She also worked on a variety of media projects while working as a medical writer for a major pharmaceutical firm. Linda currently practices in pediatric home health, adult and pediatric outpatient and community care for Easter Seals Bay Area, and in pediatrics through various school districts.

PREFACES

Second Edition
It is now 10 years since the original publication of *Obstetric and Gynecologic Care in Physical Therapy*. The practice of OB/GYN physical therapy has changed in some ways and not in others. The Section on Obstetrics and Gynecology of the American Physical Therapy Association (APTA) changed its name to the Section on Women's Health of the APTA to reflect the expansion of the practice and to encourage more interest in the field. Although the basic field of practice has not significantly changed, practitioners have become increasingly involved with nonobstetric issues, and a variety of treatment techniques have been proposed for various diagnoses. This text adheres to its original intent—as an introduction to the field for students and clinicians unfamiliar with obstetrics and gynecology practice, as well as a resource that can be used to initiate practice in the field. Chapters have been expanded, consolidated, and updated, and new sections and chapters have been added to reflect progress in the field. Physical therapists are making their mark in the care of the female patient, in all phases of her life. The establishment of physical therapists in this role in health care serves to benefit countless women and their families who thought their problems were unresolvable.

First Edition
Pregnancy is not a pathologic condition, and a pregnant woman does not become a physical therapy client simply because she is pregnant. However, pregnancy does impose normal physiologic changes. The pregnant woman's ability to adapt to these changes will determine her need for services. Physical therapists have discovered that not every pregnant woman must suffer from posturally-induced backache, numb hands and arms, aching legs, pelvic joint pain, or the long-term effects of disease, injury, or traumatic event. Indeed, the effects of childbirth and of some gynecologic conditions can cause disorders years later. Many of the symptoms of these disorders, however, can be relieved to some extent and even prevented by therapeutic instruction during the childbearing years.

The flexible nature of physical therapy allows the practitioner to develop intimate, one-to-one relationships with patients. This potential relationship and an understanding of kinesiology, physiology, and family dynamics make physical therapists uniquely qualified to build upon an already solid knowledge base and modify techniques for the pregnant woman. But when considering the health of the fetus, in addition to the altered effects of standard therapy techniques during pregnancy, evaluation and treatment become complicated.

How, then, does a physical therapist learn about changes that occur during pregnancy and the implications these changes may have for future health? Physical therapy curricula, in general, lack adequate instruction in obstetrics and gynecology. Those who later become involved in the field must acquire that specialized knowledge through extensive reading, on-the-job training, and more recently, through continuing education courses offered regionally by the Section on Obstetrics and Gynecology of the American Physical Therapy Association (later changed to Section on Women's Health). Most of the other literature and educational courses, though, are presented from a physician's or nurse's viewpoint and lack that critical link to physical therapy. Physical therapists have written books on perinatal exercise and childbirth techniques, but so far none have presented a comprehensive overview of the field for the physical therapy student or clinician with no background in obstetrics and gynecology. As even the specialized field of obstetric and gynecologic physical therapy branches into subspecialties (early pregnancy education, perinatal exercise, supportive care for labor and delivery, pain management post-Cesarean, remediation of musculoskeletal disorders of pregnancy and the post-partum, development of programs for high-risk pregnancy patients, and treatment of gynecologic conditions), the need for a single basic reference becomes crucial for practitioners.

This volume attempts to answer that need by providing current literature reviews, examination of controversial evaluation and treatment methods, and exposure to current practices. For physical therapy students and perennial students, many of the chapters include self-assessment reviews. At the end of the book are appendices for suggested readings and product information related to this field of practice. Through an awareness of the many facets of obstetric and gynecologic practice, physical therapists can expand their services for the female client and improve their value to the medical community.

Section 1

Foundation for Physical Therapy Practice in Women's Health

Chapter

Women's Health Care in Physical Therapy

YESTERDAY AND TODAY

In the early days of practice in the field of women's health, the American physical therapist had little choice but to enter the field through childbirth education or treatment of incontinence. Over the past 20 years, physical therapy assessment and treatment has matured, with practitioners using their basic skills in musculoskeletal and neuromuscular care to treat a number of women's complaints that have previously been considered untreatable. Yet, physical therapists are not fully accepted as medically necessary personnel in the treatment of obstetric and gynecologic (OB/GYN) problems by other health team members and third party payers. To gain a firm background in the field, it is recommended that physical therapists become acquainted with all aspects of OB/GYN care, including its evolution in physical therapy.

HISTORICAL INSIGHTS IN OBSTETRICS AND GYNECOLOGY

Highlights in the history of OB/GYN are included in this text for the simple reason that obstetrics, like some other medical specialties, is a field in which practices tend to become popular, fade away, then become popular again in a slightly modified form. Therefore, the physical therapist who is aware of basic evolution of the practice, as well as the cyclic trends in OB/GYN, may provide clients with insightful advice and recommendations. For instance, obstetric care was provided by women until physicians, who were predominantly male, assumed the responsibility. It is believed, however, that early male "midwives" were ridiculed and embarrassed by physicians and patients alike. Male-designed inventions of tools such as the x-ray, the microscope, the speculum, sounds (for dilating the urethra and cervix), and forceps further promulgated the role of men in women's care.

The invention of the microscope, in particular, is most likely responsible for gynecologic anatomic and physiologic discoveries, including the follicles of de Graaf and the existence of sperm. Although dissection revealed many anatomic answers, it wasn't until the microscope was invented that researchers were able to confirm the existence of sperm and ova in the 17th century. De Graaf identified the ovarian follicle, and the road was paved for discoveries of tubal pregnancies, the difference between secretions of disease and of normal discharge, and the identification of fibroids and ovarian cysts. Sperm was discovered quite a bit earlier than the ovum, however. It was proposed originally that the father alone gave rise to the fetus, and the uterus was merely the incubator.[1]

The invention of the speculum, used to dilate the vagina and explore the vagina and uterine cervix, dates back to at least the second century A.D., and perhaps earlier than that. It is believed that an early speculum, dating to 1300 B.C. was possibly made from a hollow plant tube, similar to bamboo. Remains from Pompeii revealed evidence of at least two types of specula. The introduction of metal specula came later, in the 1500s.[1] The speculum fell in and out of favor until the 1800s when it started to gain popularity with physicians performing gynecologic surgery.

Sounds for dilating the urethra and cervix became popular in the 1600s, although it is believed primitive types of sounds were used by the ancient Egyptians as far back as 3500 B.C. It is also believed, however, that the early sounds were used strictly for applying medications and for probing wounds rather than as a tool for exploration. Now, with the advent of fiberoptic tools for exploration, application of various treatments through narrow passageways inside the body is again part of the medical regimen.

Perhaps the single most controversial tool introduced into the field was forceps. Not that the forceps themselves were the problem; rather it was the idea of assisted delivery that was questioned. In this area in particular, the practitioner that keeps an eye on historical events will recognize that the idea of nonintervention during delivery may be associated with the earliest uses of forceps. Prior to their introduction, the only assisted deliveries occurred as embryotomies (ie, the extraction of a dead fetus from the womb via dismemberment).

The credit for the first documented delivery of a live child goes to Peter Chamberlen the Elder, but disagreement exists as to whether he invented the forceps, as it was often applied as a secret method. Even the mother was blindfolded when it was used, according to some sources. For the first two centuries or so, obstetricians' use of forceps received little criticism. In the early 1800s, however, public sentiment shifted back in favor of the wisdom of nature, and obstetricians followed suit.

Considerable modification of the forceps has occurred since its appearance in the late 1500s, but the principle of two forces joined to apply traction and leverage continues intact. What has fluctuated over the years is the attitude towards forceps' use. Many believed forceps held the same risk of injury to the mother or fetus as the lever. And in many cases, this fear was justified, as unskilled practitioners did indeed injure mothers and newborns (Figure 1-1). Later, though, forceps were welcomed into the obstetric armamentarium. Many women in danger of losing their own life, or that of their baby during childbirth, believed that any complications potentially imposed by the use of forceps certainly outweighed the risks. Obstetric practice continued with less emphasis on instrumentation until the late 19th century, when technology was viewed as progress. Forceps led the way for technological advancement in obstetrics, an idea that also emphasized the need for delivery in the hospital. "In the early decades of the 20th century, the concept of *prophylactic forceps* fit in well with the idea of delivery as a surgical, scientific procedure best conducted in a hospital setting. Routine instrumentation finally ran aground with the recent backlash against instrumental assistance. What is unclear is whether the pendulum will swing back and whether instrumental delivery will again become popular"[2] (see Figure 1-1).

The only alternative to instrumental delivery was (and is) the Cesarean section. This procedure dates back to 1500 A.D. when a physician, Jacob Nufer, desperately attempted to save his wife. Other Cesarean sections are documented in the 16th century, but these were performed without anesthesia and largely only when the mother's life was in jeopardy. Despite the concerns of modern consumers of obstetric care that Cesarean sections may be

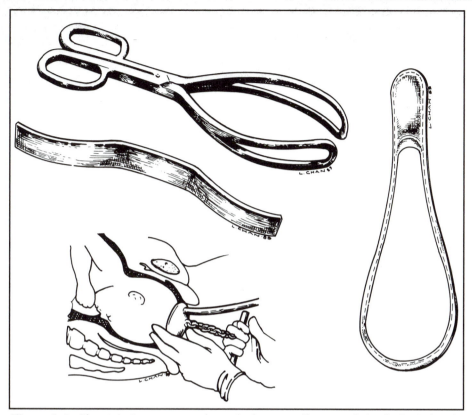

Figure 1-1. Obstetric instruments through the ages: (from top left, clockwise) early forceps, fillet or loop, vacuum extractor, lever. (Reprinted with permission from O'Connor LJ, Gourley Stephenson RJ. *Obstetric and Gynecologic Care in Physical Therapy.* Thorofare, NJ: SLACK Incorporated; 1990.)

performed at the convenience of the caregiver, and not because the mother or fetus needs the procedure, this operation has saved many a life. The advent of anesthesia made this life-saving procedure easier for both physician and patient.

Anesthesia helped not only surgery but forceps application as well. Yet, it was not really popular until notable persons began to demand relief from the pain of labor, once it was known that such relief existed. In fact, Queen Victoria is reported to have asked for chloroform for her eighth delivery in 1853. "Following a discussion with her doctors concerning the proposed and controversial use of this anesthetic, the queen remarked, 'Gentlemen, We are having the baby and We are having the chloroform...' "[2] Even at that time there was objection to the use of anesthesia for spontaneous, uncomplicated deliveries. Some physicians objected to chloroform on the grounds that the mother's pain guided the birth attendant about the progress of the labor. Simpson argued that the contraction of the uterus was the vital element for labor, not the pain. Van Blarcom adds, "Those of us who are accustomed to seeing anesthetics used to relieve patients of the worst of their pain during labor find it hard to realize that until comparatively recent years women went through this suffering without mitigation."[3] Chloroform was often administered only for delivery, not during labor, and strictly as an agent to decrease "the danger of perineal tears, as the accoucheur has better control of the delivery when the patient lies quietly than when she tossed violently about the bed...."[3] There also existed some wariness that too much anesthetic might prolong labor and adversely affect the fetus. Today, this wariness still exists, but more is known about types of anesthesia and analgesia and their effects on the fetus and mother. These effects will be discussed more fully in the chapters on the fetus and on labor.

It seems then that the history of the field has been concerned mostly with advances in technology that allow improved fetal and maternal outcomes. Where in the development of OB/GYN practice does the physical therapist enter, and what services can the physical therapist provide the female patient and the women's health care team?

WOMEN'S HEALTH PHYSICAL THERAPY: DEVELOPMENT OF PRACTICE

Although the practice of physical therapy with women is as old as physical therapy itself, the application of physical therapy skills to the OB/GYN realm is relatively new in the United States. The idea of physical therapists having something to offer the pregnant patient is more firmly entrenched in countries such as England, South Africa, Australia, and Canada. When Elizabeth Noble, an Australian physical therapist, came to the United States, she was disappointed to learn that little (if any) physical therapy practice was conducted in this field. About the closest physical therapists were to treating the obstetric patient was through instructing childbirth education classes; a practice spearheaded by physical therapist Elisabeth Bing in New York in the 1960s. Bing's *Moving Through Pregnancy* was the first American book to apply the concepts of body mechanics training to the pregnant woman. Other foreign books preceded hers: *Relaxation and Exercise for Childbirth*, by Helen Heardman, *Physiotherapy in Obstetrics* by Maria Ebner, and *Preparation for Childbirth*, by Mabel Lum Fitzhugh. In the 1970s came Noble's *Essential Exercises for the Childbearing Year*, a book that meshed nicely with Americans' burgeoning interest in health and exercise. Noble founded the OB/GYN Special Interest Section of the American Physical Therapy Association (APTA) in 1976 and drafted a document of the potential state of practice for physical therapists interested in this field. With much foresight, and based on her experience in her homeland, this document, the Position Paper for the Establishment of the OB/GYN Section, provided a valuable guideline for practitioners and for those therapists wishing to convince department administrations of the need for such a service.[4]

Accounts of the early pioneers in the field in the United States provide us with a feeling of traveling unchartered territory, "Over 30 physical therapists responded to the paragraph in the APTA's August 1976 issue of *Progress Report* concerning a special group in OB/GYN. There must be many more physical therapists involved or interested, probably they are not members of the APTA because in the past this association has had nothing to offer specialists in OB/GYN."

"Unlike other countries, American physical therapists traditionally have not been trained in OB/GYN as undergraduates, employed by women's hospitals, or otherwise involved in this field apart from recent participation in childbirth education.... This leaves glaring deficiencies in early prenatal education, which would stress the role of body mechanics, postural, and other physical adjustments throughout the childbearing year, exercise, and other preventive measures."[5]

"Four out of the six major independent childbirth organizations in the USA were actually founded by physical therapists."[6]

"As physical therapists we have much to offer in the field of childbirth education, and it should not be the sole domain of the RN-CNM (Registered Nurse-Certified Nurse-

Midwife). We've got to get together for the sake of the public's education. The 'man on the street' image of a physical therapist is hazy to begin with. He's confused about what we're doing in respiratory care and burn tanks, and now OB/GYN."

"Unfortunately if the public in unclear about physical therapy, the professional sector is not much better. How does one obtain referrals to childbirth class or post-partum care if the physician thinks of physical therapists as the ladies in the gym."[7]

"Exposure to the OB/GYN area is noticeably sparse in the American physical therapy school curriculum. This seems a logical place to begin to generate interest."[8] "Obstetrical physical therapy... is not a practice in which therapists must train as childbirth educators, but it is a field where therapists practice as therapists."[9]

"I am constantly asked how a physical therapist can get involved with obstetrical patients. For those of you who are hospital-based, Cesarean rehabilitation is an excellent starting place. Our ability to improve the quality of care in this patient population is remarkable. For many of you, the opportunity is there. All it takes is a little initiative to get started!"[10]

And with a little initiative, the role of the physical therapist in treating OB/GYN problems became better understood and welcomed by women who were suffering needlessly. Yet, this role is not totally accepted by the medical profession or even within the field of physical therapy itself.

CURRENT ROLE OF THE PHYSICAL THERAPY PRACTITIONER IN WOMEN'S HEALTH

Today, physical therapists interested in this specialty evaluate, treat, counsel, and monitor OB/GYN patients. Areas of interest within the field now include treatment of gynecologic and urologic dysfunction, breast rehabilitation, and changes associated with pregnancy (physiological, biomechanical, and emotional); instruction in prenatal education, childbirth education, and exercise classes for prenatal, post-partum, and post-Cesarean clients. As recognition grows, so does the need for education. More physical therapy programs offer OB/GYN classes as options for a more indepth view of this specialty. In addition, the Section on Women's Health of the APTA is exploring requirements for clinical competency exams leading to certification as a specialist in this field. With further education, experience, and understanding of the female patient, physical therapists will gain access to clients in need of services.[11,12]

As clinical specialists, physical therapists can treat patients with gynecologic disorders, pre- and post-surgery gynecological and breast; perform musculoskeletal evaluations and treatment of obstetric patients; act as labor support persons; and teach therapeutic exercise for prenatal, post-partum, high-risk, and post-Cesarean clients.

As consultants, physical therapists can expand hospital-based and private practice programs, as well as act as resource persons for the public and medical communities, insurance companies, and the government.

As researchers, physical therapists have their work ahead of them, since the specialty is relatively new and little documentation exists in this field. However, physical therapists have started to explore the effects of exercise, modalities, and current practices; the benefits of cross-cultural approaches to labor and delivery; and the longterm effects of obstetric intervention on both the fetus and the mother.

Lastly, as administrators and educators for physical therapy students, patients, and medical personnel, physical therapists have the opportunity to promote services, knowledge, and experience to increase access to patients. Physical therapists in these roles have the chance to promote not only the OB/GYN specialty, but the profession as a whole as part of the multidisciplinary team approach to patient care.

In the last two decades, the field has progressed somewhat, but we believe that the current status of physical therapists in this specialty has not progressed as it should. Some therapists believe specialists should direct their attention to the care of high-risk OB/GYN patients and market these services to the OB/GYN department. Insurance companies need to know that women may experience fewer complications and may return to work faster after assistance from an OB/GYN specialist. The attitudes of other medical professionals need to shift as well. "Physical therapy is a necessity, not a nicety."[13]

Other therapists have created new positions in their hospitals, such as Coordinator of Obstetrics and Gynecology for Rehabilitation Services, with the emphasis on innovative patient education. "The general public, for example, is not aware that conditions such as pelvic floor dysfunction or high-risk pregnancy can benefit from therapy to alleviate their symptoms."[14] Physical therapists have been instrumental in developing multidisciplinary protocols for high-risk and diabetic patients at major hospitals. For example, a high-risk patient in danger of premature labor due to an incompetent cervix may be on bed rest for 5 days to 5 weeks. Without physical therapy education, such a patient adopts poor body mechanics, like sitting up in jackknife positions or holding her breath when sitting on a bedpan, thereby increasing intra-abdominal pressure and pressure on the cervix. Merely prescribing bed rest is not enough.

Still others have become involved with hospital and clinic prenatal education. As more schools incorporate OB/GYN into their curricula, the greater the exposure for entry-level physical therapists, and perhaps, the greater the interest.[15]

MARKETING PHYSICAL THERAPY SERVICES

With the advent of direct access by the consumer to physical therapists in many states, the physical therapist in private practice and even in some hospital settings has had to rely less on physician referrals and more on creating a market for services. Perhaps that accounts for the success of certain physical therapy practices in some areas and not in others. For instance, orthopedic practice has always had its niche in the rehabilitation of industrially-injured patients. The field of OB/GYN physical therapy, however, has yet to establish such a lucrative niche. Although this specialty has been formally organized since 1977 as a freestanding money-making proposition, it has a way to go before it will be fully accepted by physicians, allied health workers, and pragmatically, by insurance companies.

Some progress has been made through a variety of marketing techniques. In the 1970s the primary marketing techniques were to offer childbirth education classes, early pregnancy workshops, and infant care or infant stimulation sessions. Teaching such classes allowed access to pregnant women and women with problems from previous pregnancies that could be helped with physical therapy. These classes were often taught through hospitals, clinics, for specific physicians, or privately. Many physical therapists, however, found that teaching childbirth education did not allow time to properly treat women with problems, nor was there an opportunity to evaluate or receive financial compensation according to physical therapy protocol.

In the late 1970s and early 1980s, the interest of the general population in exercise boosted a similar interest in the pregnant population. These women sought classes primarily for conditioning, but physical therapists struggled to retain their professional role among minimally trained exercise instructors offering classes through health clubs, adult schools, and city recreation departments. True, a physical therapist could often win the role of exercise instructor, but again, opportunity for thorough evaluation and treatment, plus professional reimbursement by insurance carriers, was lacking. More recently, physical therapists have branched into private practice, from practicing as hospital consultants for women requiring rehabilitation post-Cesarean section, mobility training for high-risk pregnancy patients on bedrest, or for pain relief from the effects of gynecologic cancers. Centers offering a variety of exercise and educational classes, as well as the option of individual evaluation and treatment have appeared throughout the country.

A number of physical therapists have attempted to reach OB/GYN clients by directly working with obstetricians and gynecologic urologists with some success in this field, but it is still young and growing. It will take many more determined physical therapists to guarantee the role of our profession in this specialty area.

To assist beginning practitioners, examples of promotional material successfully used to initiate a private practice in OB/GYN physical therapy are included (Figures 1-2, 1-3, 1-4). It is hoped that, by sharing examples of marketing tools, others may develop their own literature and practices; and in so doing, promote the growth of this field. Brochures with drawings and eye-catching graphics are also helpful in marketing to health care workers and patients alike. The Section on Women's Health of the APTA also offers many brochures that may be personalized for private practice and marketing.

Although direct access now exists in many states, the promotional material directed at obstetric clients urges patients to ask their doctor for a referral to physical therapy. It is the opinion of the authors that the backing of a physician when treating this patient population is wise. However, that does not mean that certain problems cannot be treated within the direct access arena; particularly patients referred by midwives or by other patients. To make a private practice in this field pay, the practitioner will probably need referrals from several sources. Some physical therapists have contracted with women's hospitals or the obstetric units of major general treatment hospitals. Physical therapists can also offer special aches and pains clinics, back classes for pregnant women, and home programs for patients on bed rest, in addition to early pregnancy or labor preparation classes.

CERTIFICATIONS, SPECIALIZATIONS, AND INSTRUCTING EDUCATIONAL CLASSES

Although physical therapists are now able to enter the field through their qualifications as musculoskeletal specialists, teaching classes such as childbirth education, early pregnancy education, refresher for labor and delivery, vaginal birth after Cesarean, preparation for Cesarean, or exercise for prenatal, post-natal, post-Cesarean, or post-gynecologic surgery can bring the physical therapist in contact with women of all ages and provide an atmosphere for relaxed questions and answers. Many physical therapy referrals can be drawn from such sessions. In some areas, however, being a physical therapist is not enough to receive referrals for obstetric clients from other childbirth educators.

There are a few major childbirth education organizations that offer certification as a childbirth educator. This certification is vital to obtain in some cities, because childbirth educators often approach obstetricians via an organization representative to provide a list of

PhysicalTherapy Services for Your Obstetric and Gynecologic Patients with Complaints of:	
Lower or upper back sprain/strain (acute or chronic)	Therapeutic exercise to correct posture; training in safe ways to perform activities of daily living; positioning in sitting, lying, standing, walking, lifting, working; application of local superficial heat, massage, orthoses; TENS for GYN patients; screening for disability referral
Joint dysfunctions or aggravation of previous orthopedic problems (pelvic, wrist, shoulder, elbow, hip, knee, ankle, neck, spine, sacroiliac, symphysis pubis; sprains, strains, tendinitis, bursitis)	Therapeutic exercise to correct dysfunction, training in activities of daily living, gait, positioning for comfort; range of motion; manual muscle testing, heat/cold, massage, orthoses, TENS for GYN, screening for orthopedic referral
Nerve compressions, neuropathy (carpal tunnel, sciatica, paresis, paresthesias)	Neuromuscular reeducation, relaxation, orthosis, TENS for GYN, positioning, functional activities, range of motion, manual muscle testing, exercise, screening for neurologic referral
Muscle weakness (abdominal, pelvic floor causing stress incontinence or mild prolapse, general weakness secondary to bed rest for cervical incompetence or premature labor contractions, diastasis recti abdominis)	Therapeutic exercise to strengthen and promote circulation, manual muscle testing, home visits for gentle exercise, avoidance of Valsalva during movement for bed rest patients, biofeedback, electrical stimulation
Discomforts of pregnancy and reduced mobility (assorted areas of pain weakness)	Relief measures for discomforts, therapeutic exercise, individualized home programs, circulation exercises,
Pain post-Cesarean or post-operative, dysmenorrhea	TENS, positioning, therapeutic exercise, activities of daily living, breathing and coughing

© L. O'Connor, 1987

Figure 1-2. Sample marketing flyer for physicians or health care providers. (Reprinted with permission from O'Connor LJ, Gourley RJ. *Obstetric and Gynecologic Care in Physical Therapy*. Thorofare, NJ: SLACK Incorporated; 1990.)

qualified teachers. Sometimes, being on that list can mean many referrals. The three major childbirth organizations in the United States are the American Society for Psychoprophylaxis in Obstetrics (ASPO/Lamaze), the International Childbirth Education Association (ICEA), and the Academy of Husband-Coached Childbirth (Bradley Method-AAHCC). These certification courses typically involve either home study or a combination of home study and workshops, plus student teaching, observations of labors and deliveries, and perhaps individual design of an entire 6 to 7 week class on preparation for labor and delivery, complete with objectives and teaching materials needed. The entire certification process may take 2 years or more. Other local organizations may offer certification courses

---

Physical Therapy Services for OB/GYN Patients

- Evaluation of muscle strength and range of motion
- Therapeutic exercise for musculoskeletal and minor neurologic dysfunction
- Fitting of orthoses for relief of muscular strain, neuropathies, and varicosities
- Gait training with assistive devices for severe pain on ambulation.
- Preventative instruction for back care and comfort
- Posture evaluation and treatment
- Assessment and treatment of pelvic floor weakness
- Individualized exercise programs for premenstrual syndrome, dysmenorrhea, or osteoporosis
- Post-hysterectomy exercise programs to regain muscle strength in pelvic floor or abdominal muscles
- Individualized prenatal and post-natal exercise
- Application of heat, massage, ice, TENS for pain relief
- TENS for chronic gynecologic pain, including dysmenorrhea
- Breathing control for patients with cervical incompetence during transfers and activities of daily living
- Post-Cesarean TENS and pain relief measures; post-Cesarean exercise
- Relaxation training or breathing control for individual women preparing for labor and delivery

© L. O'Connor, 1988

Figure 1-3. Sample abbreviated list for marketing to health care workers or hospital/clinic administrations. (Reprinted with permission from O'Connor LJ, Gourley RJ. *Obstetric and Gynecologic Care in Physical Therapy.* Thorofare, NJ: SLACK Incorporated; 1990.)

For Obstetric Patients

Some of those aches and pains you have during and after pregnancy may be helped with physical therapy.

Low or upper back ache: hot packs; massage; exercises to correct posture; instruction in proper lifting, carrying, and pushing/pulling/reaching techniques; relaxation; and comfortable positioning for bed or work

Aching muscles, joints, or aggravation of previous orthopedic problems: evaluation of problem and exercise as appropriate for pelvic joints, wrists, neck, hips, knees, ankles, shoulders, elbows, pelvic floor

Tingling or falling asleep of arms or legs: sometimes related to normal swelling of pregnancy and often relieved through positioning and circulation exercises or joint supports

Muscle weakness and discomforts of pregnancy: individualized prenatal/post-natal/post-Cesarean home exercise programs to strengthen and promote circulation, breathing and coughing exercises, pelvic floor exercises

Pain after Cesarean section or after surgery: instruction in how to change positions with minimal pain and without straining muscles, relief from gas distension, posture exercises, strengthening stomach muscles, TENS for pain relief

Ask your doctor for a referral to physical therapy

© L. O'Connor, 1987

Figure 1-4. Sample flyer for marketing to obstetric patients. (Reprinted with permission from O'Connor LJ, Gourley RJ. *Obstetric and Gynecologic Care in Physical Therapy.* Thorofare, NJ: SLACK Incorporated; 1990.)

as well, but these would be specific to an area. Although the training a childbirth educator receives from these organizations is usually valuable, it may not be necessary for the physical therapist wanting to teach the same methods. The physical therapist is trained in the instruction of relaxation methods and the basic understanding of pain mechanisms and relief. It takes only some additional research and reading to understand the actual observations of labor and delivery, the assistance provided by a mentor teacher, and the contacts made by attending such courses. Their potential as referral sources should not be overlooked. Detailed course outlines are provided for teaching educational classes to pregnant women in later chapters.

For those interested in working with gynecologic patients, much of the emphasis today is on muscle reeducation of pelvic floor muscles through exercise, biofeedback, and progressive resistance. There are certification courses in perineometry and numerous product vendors dealing with incontinence products. Physical therapists may also specialize in the treatment of gynecologic cancers and their effects on women and their families, treatment of pelvic pain, and disorders surrounding the menstrual cycle and sexual function. Additionally, physical therapists treat women after breast surgeryso they can regain full use of their arms and trunk.

INTERNSHIPS

Physical therapy interns have had successful experiences in this field. The internship can take many forms—prenatal/post-natal exercise instructor, assisting a private practitioner, designing and implementing an obstetric program for an established clinic or hospital department, or submitting an article to the OB/GYN literature. OB/GYN physical therapy usually takes a lot of conversation: presenting ideas to nursing staff, resident obstetricians, and even anesthesiologists if TENS is part of the proposal. All a student needs to do is to find a practitioner in this field; the best route for that is either through the APTA or through one of the childbirth education associations. At this point in the development of the field, however, the specific criteria for this internship are left to the imagination of the student, academic faculty, and clinical faculty.

RESEARCH NEEDS

Although the physical therapist has much to offer other health team members, as well as the pregnant woman herself, there is a limited amount of literature to provide supportive documentation of physical therapy techniques for inquiring obstetricians, family practitioners, or other referral sources. Therefore, the need for research in all areas of OB/GYN physical therapy is critical. In the last few years, physical therapists have become more interested in performing research in this field. Studies have been published in *Physical Therapy*, journal of the American Physical Therapy Association, and in the *Journal of Obstetric and Gynecologic Physical Therapy*, later known as the *Journal of the Section on Women's Health of the APTA*. There have been clinical studies, literature reviews and critiques of obstetric material published by physical therapists and nonphysical therapists in medical journals, other physical therapy publications, childbirth education material, and lay publications. These studies, though limited in number, help provide a way for physical therapists to convince physical therapy directors, hospital administrative personnel, and insurance copmpanies, that such a service is needed. Research is needed in every aspect of OB/GYN physical therapy, not only in treatment methods, but also in evaluation and incidence of specific disorders.

SELF-ASSESSMENT REVIEW

1. It is useful to know something about history of OB/GYN because:_____.
2. Physical therapists may practice in the field of women's health in a variety of roles. Name three:_____, _____, _____.
3. Name two ways to market physical therapy services in women's health: _____ and _____.

Answers:

1. Changes in the field of OB/GYN are often cyclic and knowledge of history may provide insights for the therapist advising female clients. 2. Clinician, educator, consultant 3. Design practice-specific brochures, inservice other medical personnel

REFERENCES

1. Cianfrani TA. *Short History of Obstetrics and Gynecology.* Springfield, Mass: Charles C Thomas; 1960.

2. O'Grady J. *Modern Instrumental Delivery.* Baltimore, Md: Williams & Wilkins; 1988.

3. Van Blarcom C. *Obstetrical Nursing.* 2nd edition. New York, NY: MacMillan; 1928.

4. Noble E. Position paper. *Bull Sect Obstet Gynecol.* APTA. 1984;8(1):610.

5. Noble E. *Special Interest Group in Obstetrics and Gynecology Newsletter.* 1976;1(1):1.

6. Noble E. *Bull Sect Obstet Gynecol,* APTA. 1977;1(4):1.

7. Frahm J. *Bull Sect Obstet Gynecol,* APTA. 1978;2(3):10.

8. Frahm J. *Bull Sect Obstet Gynecol,* APTA. 1979;3(3+4):1.

9. Iglarsh ZA. *Bull Sect Obstet Gynecol,* APTA. 1982;6(4):18.

10. Kotarinos R. *Bull Sect Obstet Gynecol,* APTA. 1984;8(4):5.

11. Noble E. Reminiscence: Then and now. *Bull Sect Obstet Gynecol,* APTA. 1987;11(2):7-8.

12. O'Connor L. The first 10 years. *Bull Sect Obstet Gynecol,* APTA. 1987;11(2):8-9.

13. Inglarsh ZA. *Telephone interview with R. Gourley.* March 1989.

14. Frahm J. *Telephone interview with R. Gourley.* April 1989.

15. Pipp LM. *Telephone interview with R. Gourley.* April 1989.

Chapter 2

Anatomical Considerations

HISTORICAL INSIGHTS IN FEMALE NOMENCLATURE

Prior to the Renaissance, the only anatomic illustrations of the female depicted her pregnant, nude, and in a squatting position. The uterus was either depicted as bicornuate, multichambered, or shaped like an inverted light bulb. An inner lining encased a fetus, fully formed from conception, and merely growing in size until delivery. During the Renaissance, Leonardo da Vinci's artistic obsession with detail provided both artists and physicians with a new understanding of human development and human anatomy, complete with pictorial observations from various angles, including cross-sectional. But many of da Vinci's illustrations were lost until the twentieth century, and hence, a variety of anatomists' names have been attached to female anatomic structures.[1] Bartholin, Montgomery, Douglas, Cooper, Mackenrodt, Fallopius, and de Graaf are but a few of the anatomists who have been immortalized through their discoveries. This chapter will highlight normal female anatomy with respect to gynecologic and obstetric concerns. Additional anatomical information is provided in the later chapters on obstetric examination, labor and delivery, gynecological treatment, and maternal physiology.

GENERAL FEMALE ANATOMY

The Female Breast

The breast lies superficially to a layer of fascia overlying the pectoralis major, serratus anterior, external abdominal oblique, and the anterior wall of the rectus abdominis sheath, ending in the axillary tail near the axillary lymph nodes. The mammary glands, or breasts, consist of glandular tissue, fibrous tissue, adipose tissue, blood vessels, lymph vessels, and nerves. The fibrous tissue connects 15 to 20 lobes, formed by lobules of alveoli joined by areolar tissue, blood vessels, and lactiferous ducts that drain into lactiferous sinuses.[2] The ducts contain elastic tissue and narrow as they enter the papilla or nipple, encircled by the pigmented areola and areolar glands. The upper fascia is supported by suspensory ligaments (Cooper's) (Figure 2-1).

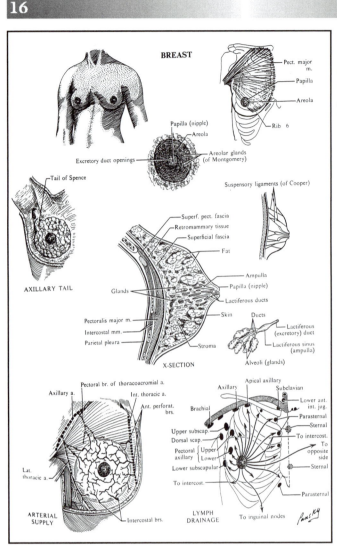

Figure 2-1. The female breast. (Reprinted with permission from Pansky B, House El. *Review of Gross Anatomy.* 2nd ed. New York, NY: McGraw-Hill; 1969.)

The Female Abdomen

The abdominal muscles may be viewed as belonging to two groups, one posterior and one anterolateral. The posterior group is comprised of the quadratus lumborum. The anterior group, which is probably the most stressed during pregnancy, boasts two longitudinal muscles, the rectus and pyramidalis; and three layers of muscles (the external abdominal oblique, internal abdominal oblique, and transversus abdominis) with alternating fiber directions, which extend their aponeuroses to ensheathe the longitudinal muscles. The iliopsoas, although it originates at the lumbar vertebrae and inserts on the lesser trochanter of the femur, serves as a landmark for nerves exiting the lumbar plexus. This muscle group also crosses the sacroiliac joint and runs under the inguinal ligament.[2]

The transversalis fascia covers the quadratus lumborum and psoas muscles and spreads to the lumbar spine and anterior longitudinal ligament. Iliacus fascia extends from the transversalis fascia, attaches to the inguinal ligament, crosses the superior pubic ramus, and blends into the fascia lata.[3]

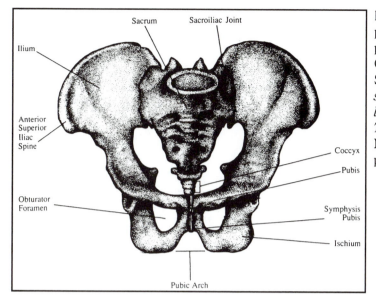

Figure 2-2. The bony pelvis. (Reprinted with permission from O'Connor LJ, Gourley Stephenson RJ. *Obstetric and Gynecologic Care in Physical Therapy*. Thorofare, NJ: SLACK Incorporated; 1990.)

The Female Pelvis

The Bony Pelvis

Forming a continuous cavity with the abdomen, the pelvis serves to support the trunk and provide a site for attachment of the lower extremities. Yet the female pelvis serves another vital function: to protect the reproductive organs and, during the early months of pregnancy, the developing fetus. Bounded by the sacrum and coccyx posteriorly, and by the innominates laterally and anteriorly, the bony structure meets at the symphysis pubis and at two sacroiliac joints (Figure 2-2).

The ilium, ischium, and pubis meet to form the acetabulum and fuse during adolescence to form the coxal or innominate bones. The iliac crest borders the top of the ilium, extending from the anterior superior iliac spine to the posterior superior iliac spine. Muscles attach to a path along the crest between the inner and outer lip of the crest. The anterior and posterior inferior iliac spines are also useful landmarks. The ischium offers a weight-bearing surface in sitting position and forms the greater and lesser sciatic notches.

Joining with the ilium and ischium is the pubis with superior and inferior rami. In the normal, average female the inferior (or descending) rami form a 90 to 100 degree angle for passage of the fetal head (pubic arch is 70 to 75 degrees in males)[4] (Figure 2-3). Ligaments and fibrocartilage join the two pubic portions together at the symphysis pubis. The pubic crest may be palpable as it rises to form the pubic tubercle, which extends laterally to the pectineal line, finally joining the arcuate line and ending at the terminal line. The superior and inferior rami fuse with the ischial ramus and the body of the ischium to form the obturator foramen, through which passes vessels and nerves to the lower extremity.

The sacral promontory projects most deeply into the pelvic cavity, and provides a site for measurement of pelvic size. The normal value for a straight line drawn from the promontory to the sacral apex is 10 cm, and 12 cm along the ventral surface of the sacrum.[5] The anterior of the sacrum hosts four paired foramina, through which pass the anterior divisions of the sacral nerves and tributaries from the lateral sacral vessels. The posterior of the sacrum

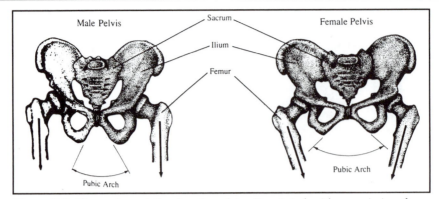

Figure 2-3. The male and the female pelvis. (Reprinted with permission from O'Connor LJ, Gourley Stephenson RJ. *Obstetric and Gynecologic Care in Physical Therapy*. Thorofare, NJ: SLACK Incorporated; 1990.)

also permits passage of the posterior primary divisions of the sacral nerves. Inferior to the median sacral crest at about S4 or S5 is a sacral hiatus that points the way to the sacral canal. The sacral canal is of importance to the obstetric anesthesiologist in that it allows access to the epidural space for caudal conduction anesthesia[6] (Figure 2-4). The lateral portion of the sacrum articulates with the innominate bone. Superiorly it is a facet for articulation with L5 and inferiorly, a facet for coccygeal articulation. The four coccygeal vertebrae are usually fused into one bone, as are the five vertebrae of the sacrum. However, the vertebral canal does not continue into the coccyx.

Those bony landmarks of the pelvis, which are of special significance to the OB/GYN examiner, are summarized in Table 2-1.

The physical therapist treating the adolescent should keep in mind that bony ossification may not be complete until adulthood. The bones of the innominate fuse at different times. At 7 or 8 years of age the inferior rami of the pubis fuses with the ischium, but ossification at the acetabulum occurs later. A Y-shaped cartilage is still present in the acetabulum where the three bones join. The fusion of the ilium and pubis occurs at about 18 years, followed by the joining of the ilium and ischium, and finally the pubis and ischium by 24 to 25 years of age. The sacrum and coccyx, however, may not ossify until 25 to 30 years of age, and the coccyx may totally fuse with the sacrum even later in life.[7]

The two sacroiliac joints and the symphysis pubis are the only articulations of the pelvis. The sacroiliac joints are synovial, with the articular surface of the sacral surface covered by fibrocartilage, and the ilial surface covered by hyaline cartilage. The symphysis pubis is a cartilaginous joint with an interpubic disc of fibrocartilage. Hyaline cartilage on the bony surfaces meets the disc, which varies in shape and thickness. The ligaments, described in Table 2-2, provide support to the pelvis, and may be viewed in five groups. (Figures 2-5, 2-6, 2-7). Although anatomists describe these ligaments from a structural viewpoint, the clinician may find it more helpful to analyze ligamentous support functionally as it relates to presenting symptoms or to the pelvic biomechanics.

Biomechanics of the Female Pelvis

The pelvis has been compared to a ring, appearing as a curved beam in the frontal plane, and as an irregular, angular lever in the sagittal plane.[8] In the frontal plane, the iliolumbar ligament, lumbosacral ligamentous support, posterior back muscles, and lateral abdominal

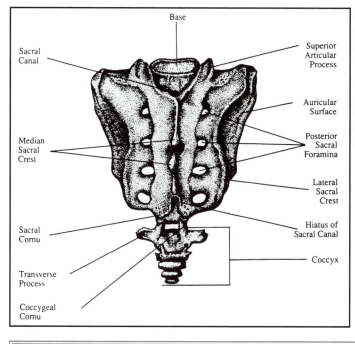

Figure 2-4. Sacrum. (Reprinted with permission from O'Connor LJ, Gourley Stephenson RJ. *Obstetric and Gynecologic Care in Physical Therapy.* Thorofare, NJ: SLACK Incorporated; 1990.)

Base
Sacral Canal
Superior Articular Process
Auricular Surface
Median Sacral Crest
Posterior Sacral Foramina
Lateral Sacral Crest
Sacral Cornu
Hiatus of Sacral Canal
Coccyx
Transverse Process
Coccygeal Cornu

Table 2-1

Bony Landmarks of the Pelvis Palpable During Pelvic Exam

Ischial spine	Determines level of fetal descent into true pelvis and shortest diameter of cavity
Pubic arch	Forms bony framework for vulva and perineum
Pubic tubercle	Provides medial attachment site for the inguinal ligament
Obturator foramen	Allows passage of obturator nerve and vessels
Ischial tuberosity	Marks inferior boundary of pelvis
Sacral promontory	Provides measurement site with sacral tip for dimension of pelvic outlet

---

Table 2-2

Ligaments of the Pelvis

Abdominopelvic Ligaments
Iliolumbar
Inguinal
Lacunar

Sacroiliac Ligaments
Anterior sacroiliac
Posterior sacroiliac
Interosseus

Sacroischial Ligaments
Sacrotuberous
Sacrospinous

Sacrococcygeal Ligaments
Anterior sacrococcygeal
Posterior sacrococcygeal
Lateral sacrococcygeal
Interarticular

Pubic Ligaments
Superior pubic
Arcuate pubic
Pectineal

Figure 2-5. Ligaments of the pelvis. (Reprinted with permission from Warwick R, Williams PL, eds. Gray's Anatomy. 35th British ed. Philadelphia, PA: WB Saunders Co.; 1973.)

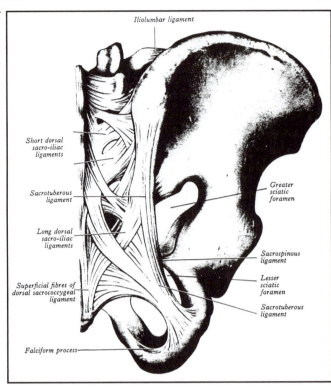

Iliolumbar ligament

Short dorsal sacro-iliac ligaments

Sacrotuberous ligament

Long dorsal sacro-iliac ligaments

Superficial fibres of dorsal sacrococcygeal ligament

Falciform process

Greater sciatic foramen

Sacrospinous ligament

Lesser sciatic foramen

Sacrotuberous ligament

Figure 2-6. Ligaments of the pelvis. (Reprined with permission from Warwick R, Williams PL, eds. Gray's Antomy. 35th British ed. Philadelphia, PA: WB Saunders Co.; 1973.)

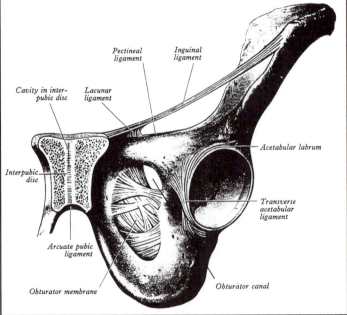

Pectineal ligament

Inguinal ligament

Cavity in inter-pubic disc

Lacunar ligament

Interpubic disc

Acetabular labrum

Transverse acetabular ligament

Arcuate pubic ligament

Obturator membrane

Obturator canal

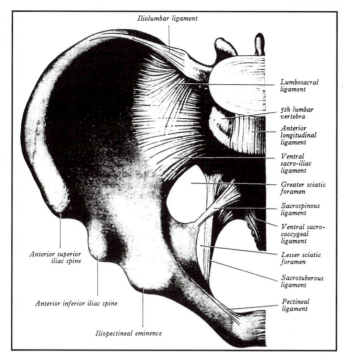

Iliolumbar ligament

Lumbosacral ligament

5th lumbar vertebra

Anterior longitudinal ligament

Ventral sacro-iliac ligament

Greater sciatic foramen

Sacrospinous ligament

Ventral sacro-coccygeal ligament

Lesser sciatic foramen

Sacrotuberous ligament

Pectineal ligament

Anterior superior iliac spine

Anterior inferior iliac spine

Iliopectineal eminence

Figure 2-7. Ligaments of the pelvis. (Reprinted with permission from Warwick R, Williams PL, eds. Gray's Anatomy. 35th British ed. Philadelphia, PA: WB Saunders Co.; 1973.)

muscles maintain stability. When the body is in motion, the ligaments and muscles must control rotatory and translatory movements.

Sacroiliac stress increases on lateral motion. The sacroiliac joint receives weight stress, resulting in both vertical and horizontal components entering the femoral head and neck and entering the symphysis pubis. Shear (horizontal force) is resolved by ligamentous support. Pressure (vertical force) transmits to the femoral head. In the sagittal plane, the line of gravity appears to fall behind the hip joint and anterior to the sacroiliac joint.

Gravity acting upon the pelvis will force the posterior pelvic ring into a downward rotation about the hip axes. If the posterior pelvis is forced downward, the anterior will be forced upward. However, the hip flexors and iliofemoral ligament resist the upward force. The more horizontal the pelvic inclination, the greater the downward force and the lever arm between the lumbosacral junction and the sacroiliac joint. It is believed that, due to the relation of the lumbosacral joint and the sacroiliac joint, rotatory force will first be transmitted to the lumbosacral, and only to the sacroiliac after it passes into the lumbosacral joint and the sacrum.[9]

As the sacrum joins the ilia, the lumbosacral articulation bears the force of the upper body weight. This force is dispersed in two directions. One component attempts to drive the sacrum caudally and dorsally between the ilia, and one attempts to rotate the cephalic sacrum caudally and ventrally into the pelvic cavity.[7] The ligaments then may be identified as preventing the rotational forces imposed upon the sacrum. The interosseus sacroiliac, posterior sacroiliac, and iliolumbar ligaments are positioned to resist the caudal and dorsal drive upon the sacrum, whereas the sacrotuberous, and the sacrospinous ligaments resist ventral rotation of the sacral promontory.[10]

The pubic ligaments assist the disc and maintain the integrity of the joint by the superior pubic ligament and by the arcuate, which supports the pubic arch inferiorly.[5] The natural force of the body weight to push the ilia together may add rotatory and compressive forces to the symphysis. In sitting, the pubic arch resists spreading forces.

OBSTETRIC CONCERNS

Pelvic Axes, Position, Obstetric Diameters, and Shape

When viewed as a whole, the pelvis may be obstetrically divided into a true pelvis and a false pelvis. The linea terminalis separates the true and false pelvis, with the false pelvis lying superiorly to the linea and the true pelvis lying inferiorly. The major, or false pelvis, actually harbors the lower portion of the abdominal cavity. The true, or lesser, pelvis lies below a plane created by the linea terminalis and the sacral promontory; this also identifies the pelvic inlet. The inlet is directed posteriorly and intersects the vertical axis at approximately 30 degrees.[4] The pelvic outlet, however, because of its anatomic structure (the sacrum posteriorly and the pubis anteriorly) lies in an almost horizontal plane.

The cavity of the true pelvis has been compared to a bent cylinder, the top portion directed down and back and the lower portion pointed down and forward.[4] The true pelvis is posteriorly bound by the anterior sacrum, inner ischium, sacrosciatic notch, and sacrosciatic ligaments. Anteriorly, the true pelvis is formed by the pubis, ascending superior ischial ramus, and obturator foramen. It has been estimated that the planes of the walls of the true pelvis converge at the knees.[4]

The irregularity of the pelvis compared to the long bones led anatomists to develop a system of diameters for ease in describing pelvic anomalies. Four planes (pelvic inlet, pelvic outlet, greatest pelvic dimension, and least pelvic dimension) are divided into various diameters and shapes for obstetrical reference (Table 2-3). The inlet diameter of importance is the obstetric conjugate, which is estimated by manually measuring the diagonal conjugate and subtracting a value between 1.5 to 2.0 cm from that distance, depending on the tilt and length of the symphysis pubis. The plane of greatest dimensions, as the name implies, is not of major importance to the obstetric attendant, because this part from S2-S3 to the pubis is the most spacious for the fetal head. However, if any of these other diameters are reduced and cause delay of fetal descent during labor, the pelvis is considered contracted.[11]

Although the pelvic shapes have been carefully delineated, the intermediate type (a combination of shapes) is the usual occurrence. The shapes are based on the line drawn through the transverse diameter to form a posterior and anterior pelvic inlet. The intermediate shapes are described by the posterior division as the pelvic type or hindpelvis; the anterior as the tendency or forepelvis. The gynecoid occurs in over half of all women (see Table 2-3).[11]

Abnormal Bony Pelvis

The abnormal pelvis presents, in some cases, a life-threatening situation for the fetus. Contraction of pelvic diameters may occur at the inlet, outlet, midpelvis (greater and lesser dimensions), or in any combination of the above areas.

A contracted inlet can prevent passage of the fetal head by altering the presentation of the fetus from occiput leading to face or shoulder leading or prolapsed cord or extremities. Cervical dilation may be reduced because of premature membrane rupture and diminished fetal head pressure. Overstretching or rupture of the lower uterine segment may occur, and there may be a predisposition to fistula from impaired circulation. Midpelvis contractions appear more commonly and may result in arrest of fetal descent.

Outlet contraction may contribute to perineal tearing as the fetal head is directed away from the pubic arch. When all or multiple parts of the pelvis are contracted, labor is jeopardized by mechanical resistance and diminished uterine contractions.[11]

Table 2-3

Diameters and Shapes of the Female Pelvis

Pelvic Inlet

Anteroposterior
> Obstetric conjugate- narrowest width-promontory to pubis; 10 cm
> True conjugate- cephalad pubis to promontory
> Diagonal conjugate- caudal pubis to promontory

Transverse–greatest distance between opposite sides of lines terminalis; intersects a/p
    4 cm anterior to promontory

Right Oblique- right sacroiliac synchondrosis to left iliopectineal eminence; about 13 cm

Left Oblique- left sacroiliac synchondrosis to right iliopechneal eminence; about 13 cm

Least Pelvic Dimensions

Interspinous- 10 cm; smallest of pelvis

Anteroposterior- at ischial spines, 11.5 cm

Posterior sagittal- sacrum to intersect with interspinous; 4.5 cm

Greatest Pelvic Dimensions

Anteroposterior- 12.5 cm

Transverse- 12.5 cm

Right and left oblique- unmeasurable

Pelvic Outlet

Anteroposterior- lower pubis to sacral tip; 11.5 cm

Transverse- between ischial tuberosities; 10.0 cm

Posterior sagittal- sacral tip to intersect transverse; 7.5 cm

Shapes

Gynecoid- round and wide

Android- small, narrow, and wedge-like

Anthropoid- oval, narrow, pointed

Platypelloid- shallow and wide

Intermediate- combination of types

Other pelvic abnormalities that may interfere with labor include kyphotic or scoliotic pelvis (lumbosacral kyphosis may obstruct inlet), post-fracture pelvis (malunion or callus formation reduce birth canal), and the coxalgic pelvis (from abnormal development of lower extremity). Tumors arising from the pelvic walls may also obstruct the pelvic cavity.[11]

Mechanical Impact of the Fetus on Anatomic Relations

Influence of Fetal Weight on Blood Supply

The aorta and the vena cava may be occluded by the enlarging uterus, in certain women, when the supine position is assumed for a prolonged period during late pregnancy (supine hypotensive syndrome or aortocaval occlusion). The heart normally becomes slightly rotated, enlarged, elevated, and displaced to the left from the fundal pressure. Other organs with

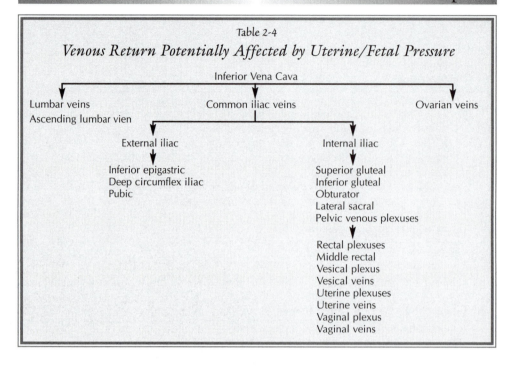

Table 2-4

Venous Return Potentially Affected by Uterine/Fetal Pressure

Inferior Vena Cava

Lumbar veins
Ascending lumbar vien

Common iliac veins

Ovarian veins

External iliac

Internal iliac

Inferior epigastric
Deep circumflex iliac
Pubic

Superior gluteal
Inferior gluteal
Obturator
Lateral sacral
Pelvic venous plexuses

Rectal plexuses
Middle rectal
Vesical plexus
Vesical veins
Uterine plexuses
Uterine veins
Vaginal plexus
Vaginal veins

altered anatomy during pregnancy include a distended gallbladder and enlarged pituitary and thyroid glands.[11]

Of greater interest to researchers has been the partial occlusion of the inferior vena cava and the pelvic veins by the enlarging uterus, not only when the woman lies supine for prolonged periods, but also when she is standing for prolonged periods. This compression not only can reduce venous return, but also may increase venous pressure and contribute to dependent edema in the lower extremities. The inferior vena cava exits the abdomen via the central tendon of the diaphragm at the level of T8. It lies directly anterior to the lower lumbar vertebrae, anterior longitudinal ligament, right-sided psoas muscles, and lumbar sympathetic trunk (among other structures) and its occlusion may directly impact the inferior tributaries. These tributaries include the common iliac veins, the lumbar veins, the ovarian veins, and their tributaries, reviewed in Table 2-4.[6,7,10]

Influence of Fetal Weight and Postural Changes

During pregnancy, laxity around the spine may result in more mobile rib articulations, and the lower ribs flare laterally. The subcostal angle widens, the transverse diameter of the rib cage increases about 2 cm, and its circumference expands approximately 6 cm.[12] With this expansion comes an altered relation to the diaphragm that radiates from the ribs, costal cartilages, sternum, and lumbar vertebrae to the central tendon. In the non-pregnant state, the diaphragm may reach as high as the fifth rib on the right and the fifth interspace on the left during expiration.[2] During pregnancy, the diaphragm rises approximately 4 cm in position, and excursion is thought to be greater than during non-pregnant states. Additional compensatory changes in pulmonary function are not necessarily structurally related.

There appears to be a normal accentuation of the lumbar lordosis during pregnancy, possibly attributable to the stress of added fetal weight anteriorly and to the effects of relaxin, which may cause supporting spinal ligaments, such as the longitudinal ligaments, to allow

Table 2-5

Sensory Innervation of the Lumbar Plexus

Iliohypogasatric (L1)	Symphysis pubis and lateral iliac crest
Ilioinguinal (L1)	Medial thigh, mons pubis, labia majora
Lateral femoral cutaneous (L2, L3)	Anterior thigh
Femoral (L2, L3, L4)	Anterior thigh
Genitofemoral (L1-L2)	Anterior vulva and anterior thigh
Obturator (L2, L3, L4)	Medial thigh

greater spinal joint laxity. Exactly how much accentuation is normal remains unknown. There is little documentation to support observations made by physical therapists that, as the center of gravity shifts upward and anteriorly with increasing fetal weight, the lumbar spine shifts forward. There have also been claims that there are compensatory increases in the dorsal curve and cervical curve as well.[13]

As fetal weight causes an increased lumbar lordosis, the pelvis may tilt anteriorly, and the iliopsoas muscles, with a common insertion, may be stressed. Since part of the lumbar plexus lies within the psoas muscle, strain in this region may cause additional symptoms, particularly irritation of sensory nerves. The ilioinguinal, iliohypogastric, lateral femoral cutaneous, and femoral nerves exit laterally from the psoas, and the genitofemoral nerve travels through the belly. The obturator nerve exits medially and passes through the obturator foramen (see Figure 2-6 and Table 2-5).[2]

The symphysis pubis is able to withstand the force of the fetal head moving beneath it; hence, it appears that most problems of symphyseal separation during pregnancy are related to trauma or faulty pelvic mechanism. If strain of the symphysis pubis occurs, torsion may appear in the sacroiliac joints, and pelvic ring instability may result. Normal separation of the symphysis has been measured at 1 mm to 5 mm, increasing approximately 0.5 mm to 7 mm more during pregnancy, and decreasing by 2 mm on average within the first week post-partum.[14] Labor does not seem to widen this normal separation. There has been no documentation regarding the amount of separation and association with pelvic pain.

The middle segment of the sacrum resists rotational forces as the sacral convexities interlock with the ilial concavities. During delivery, as the fetus descends into the ventral sacrum, this interlocking mechanism of the middle segment, reinforced by the sacrospinous and sacrotuberous ligaments, prevents sacral dislocation.[11] It is believed that during defecation and parturition the coccyx rotates backward at the sacrococcygeal joint.[7] Because of the relaxation of the pelvic articulations and biomechanical forces, pain in the pelvic region may be related to the relaxation of ligamentous attachments to the ischial tuberosity, ischial spine, lateral border of the sacrum and coccyx, posterior iliac spines, pubic bones, or the obturator internus fascia.

As the fetus enlarges, the pressure of the uterus and dependent edema may result in neuropathies or neural compressions, especially of the lateral femoral cutaneous and femoral nerves and its branches as they pass beneath the inguinal ligament (Figure 2-8, Table 2-6, Table 2-7). In addition, the possibility of spinal laxity may create conditions favorable for compressions of spinal or peripheral nerves exiting at the spine, although the incidence of disc herniations is no greater during pregnancy than in the normal population.[15]

Figure 2-8. Relationship of iliopsoas to pelvic nerves. (Reprinted with permission from O'Connor LJ, Gourley Stephenson RJ. *Obstetric and Gynecologic Care in Physical Therapy.* Thorofare, NJ: SLACK Incorporated; 1990.)

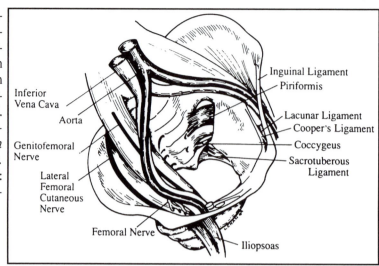

Table 2-6

Muscles of the Trunk and Lower Extremity

Attaching to the Pelvis

Quadratus lumborum	Gemelli
Obturator internus and externus	Piriformis
Glutei	Quadratus femoris
Hamstrings	Adductor group
Tensor fasciae latae	Rectus femoris

Table 2-7

Sensory Innervations of the Nerves

Passing Through the Pelvis

Sacral plexus (L4-S3)

Sciatic:	thigh and leg
Posterior femoral cutaneous:	vulva and perineum

Pudendal plexus (S2-4)

Pudendal:	external sphincter and, urogenital diaphragm, transverse perineal, bulbocavernosus, ischiocavernosus, urethra, skin of vulva, mucosa of vestibule, clitoris and prepuce
Pelvic splanchnics:	bladder, uterus, vagina, distal colon, rectum, external genitalia, erectile tissue, levator and, coccygeus

Coccygeal plexus (S4)

Anococcygeal:	skin over coccyx

Visceral Afferent System
Pathways of abdominal and pelvic pain transmitted through pelvic plexus, superior hypogastric plexus, sympathetic trunks and pelvic splanchnic nerves.

Hormonal Impact of Pregnancy on Anatomic Relations

Although relaxin is a peptide hormone produced by the corpus luteum, and generally associated only with pregnancy and the post-partum, research is contradictory regarding the existence of small amounts of relaxin in non-pregnant and menstruating females and in male seminal fluid.[16-18] Some studies suggest relaxin may only affect cervical and uterine tissues, but other studies offer evidence that relaxin may be responsible for relaxation of the connective tissue, including ligaments, fasciae, and symphyses. It is believed that relaxin softens the ligaments as well as the fibrocartilage of the pelvis; yet this softening does not appear to impair the strength of the joint during childbirth. It is believed that relaxin affects tissues in the pregnant woman immediately after conception, peaks at 3 months, and then either remains at a constant level or drops 20% to 50% to a stable level for the remainder of the pregnancy.[19,20] Some believe there is also an increase prior to delivery,[21] although other studies suggest no rise prior to delivery, but significant rise during labor. Joint laxity associated with relaxin has been recorded in peripheral joints up to 3 to 5 months post-partum,[22] although a recent study showed that serum relaxin levels were not correlated with the increase in joint laxity found in five of seven peripheral joints during pregnancy and post-partum.[23] The cause of the laxity was unexplained. There is also evidence, however, that relaxin levels are higher in some women than in others, and even higher in women with multifetal pregnancies. Studies are mixed regarding relaxin levels and pelvic pain, with some finding an association between higher levels and pain and others finding no association between serum relaxin levels and disabling pain.[24-26] There is also evidence that relaxin may inhibit uterine contractions and maintain the integrity of the cervix during pregnancy.[27]

The influence of relaxin upon ligamentous structures, connective tissue within the breast, and underlying fascia, combined with the increased weight of the breasts during pregnancy and lactation, may cause stress on the chest musculature and upper spine. Thoracic kyphosis associated with lumbar lordosis is a frequent postural change seen in pregnant women. In addition to strain of chest musculature and postural stress, the pull exerted by pendulous breasts and edema of the upper extremities may result in nerve compression, either at the brachial plexus or more distally in the median nerve at the wrist.[3]

As part of relaxin's potential influence on the connective tissue, the fasciae of the trunk and pelvis may be affected as well. As pregnancy advances, the influence of relaxin and the pressure exerted by the growing fetus create new relationships for thoracic and abdominal contents. In some cases, women experience pain or postural discomfort because of normal changes in the abdominal wall during pregnancy. As the fetus enlarges, the abdominal wall must stretch to accommodate,. and as the recti and oblique muscles stretch, some weakening is expected. Yet, this is the time when the abdominal muscles must perhaps work harder than ever before to maintain an upright posture, despite the forces of gravity bearing down on the uterus. On top of this paradoxical situation, relaxin may have an additional influence on the linea alba and a diastasis of the recti may occur.[28] Should diastasis occur, the pregnant woman's ability to provide support without assistance for the enlarging uterus is tenuous at best. Diastasis can occur in varying degrees, and there have been severe cases in which the uterus is partially covered anteriorly only by peritoneum, fascia, and skin.[11]

Anatomically, although undocumented, it is conceivable that the origins of the diaphragm and the influence of relaxin may cause other structures to be influenced by positional changes. The costal origins interdigitate with the transversus abdominis muscle to a slight degree, and the lumbar segments attach to aponeuroses over the psoas and quadratus lumborum muscles. Further, it is possible that the diaphragmatic crura may add stress to the anterior longitudinal ligament in the lumbar area, especially at L1 and L2 into which both

Figure 2-9. Contents of the pelvic cavity. (Reprinted with permission from O'Connor LJ, Gourley Stephenson RJ. *Obstetric and Gynecologic Care in Physical Therapy.* Thorofare, NJ: SLACK Incorporated; 1990.)

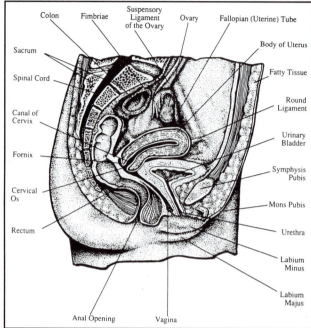

crura attach. The lumbocostal fascial arches also give rise to portions of the diaphragm. Finally, the diaphragm may be responsible for affecting those structures which pass through it, namely the esophagus, the vena cava, hemiazygos vein, lymphatic channels, and splanchnic nerves. The aorta does not pass directly through the diaphragm, although the diaphragm forms a hiatus posteriorly for its passage.[2]

GYNECOLOGIC CONCERNS

Contents of the Pelvic Cavity

Comparing the pelvic cavity to a bowl, Crafts and Kreiger[4] identify the bottom of this bowl as the pelvic floor. Above the floor lies the pelvic cavity proper, and below the floor is the external genitalia. Inside the pelvic cavity is the rectum, which lies anterior to the sacral promontory. The uterus and its peritoneal attachments come between the rectum and the urinary bladder, creating the rectouterine (Douglas) and vesicouterine pouches, respectively. The rectouterine pouch is a continuation of the vagina. The uterine (Fallopian) tubes, ovaries, subserous and parietal fascia, ureters, uterine ligaments, sacral, pudendal and coccygeal plexuses, piriformis muscle, coccygeal muscle, obturator internus muscle, and levator ani muscles also lie within the cavity (Figure 2-9).

The vagina parallels the pelvic inlet, and its superior end encloses the uterine cervix. This relationship causes the vaginal walls to be unequal in length; about 7.5 cm anteriorly and 9.0 cm posteriorly.[4] Anterior, lateral, and posterior fornices surround the cervix. The anterior wall of the vagina relates half to the urinary fundus and half to the urethra. The posterior wall relates in thirds to the rectouterine pouch, rectum, and the perineal body. The rectum lies close to the vagina until the two openings are separated by the perineal body.

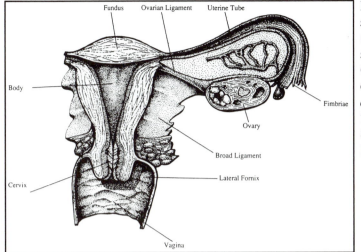

Figure 2-10. Uterine support structures. (Reprinted with permission from O'Connor LJ, Gourley Stephenson RJ. *Obstetric and Gynecologic Care in Physical Therapy.* Thorofare, NJ: SLACK Incorporated; 1990.)

The puborectalis and the external sphincter ani are responsible for fecal continence. The role of the internal sphincter in fecal continence is not clear.[7] The vascularity and position of the anal opening make it subject to both internal and external varicosities. Vaginal plexuses are situated between the vagina and the pelvic diaphragm. The vaginal tissue is mucosal, erectile and muscular.

The uterine tubes are about 10 cm long and are divided into isthmus, ampulla, and infundibulum. The isthmus branches off the uterus, the ampulla extends and caps the ovary, and the infundibulum spreads its fimbriae projections over the ovary.

The ovaries rest against the lateral pelvic walls sheltered by the broad ligament, the ureter, and the external iliac vessels. In standing, the ovary is oriented vertically. The suspensory ligament of the ovary extends past the iliac vessels and the psoas muscles. This is differentiated from the ovarian ligament which connects it to the uterus (Figure 2-10).

The uterus has been compared to an inverted pear the size of a fist. In a non-pregnant state, the uterus is about 7.5 cm long, 5.0 cm wide, and 2.5 cm in thickness. The fundus (top) and body (middle) of the uterus lie over the urinary bladder in an almost horizontal plane, bending (anteflexed) at a 100 to 110 degree angle at the cervix (neck) to meet the vagina. Because of its relation to the urinary bladder, the position and the uterine angle can change with urine volume. The fundus is that portion above the area where the uterine tubes exit the uterus. The body has the greatest amount of broad ligament associated with it, and gives rise to the isthmus, just above the cervix. The cervix is considered the lower 2 cm and it meets the vagina obliquely. The uterus is supported by the pelvic floor and by the surrounding viscera. Anatomists believe that the pelvic floor is essential for support, and that the broad, round, and uterosacral ligaments merely maintain position within the cavity.[4,7,8,11]

The pelvic contents are partially covered by peritoneum and partially embedded in dense connective tissue called the endopelvic fascia. The placement of the uterus creates two peritoneal pouches on either side, but broad ligaments of the uterus reach from the uterus, ensheathing the uterine tubes and the ovaries laterally to the pelvic walls (Figure 2-11). The round ligament of the uterus and the ovarian ligament attach to the side of the uterus below the uterine tube.

The round ligaments keep the fundus forward and spread anterolaterally from the uterine tubes to the labium majora. The uterosacral ligaments maintain a backward and upward position of the cervix and attach to deep fascia and sacral periosteum. These ligaments are augmented by smooth rectouterine muscle. Cardinal ligaments, once thought to be prime

Figure 2-11. Broad ligament. (Reprinted with permission from O'Connor LJ, Gourley Stephenson RJ. *Obstetric and Gynecologic Care in Physical Therapy.* Thorofare, NJ: SLACK Incorporated; 1990.)

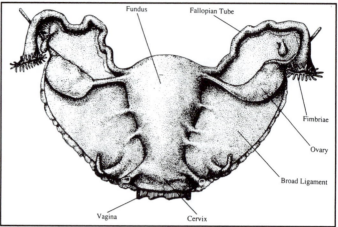

Figure 2-12. Support of the bladder. (Reprinted with permission from O'Connor LJ, Gourley Stephenson RJ. *Obstetric and Gynecologic Care in Physical Therapy.* Thorofare, NJ: SLACK Incorporated; 1990.)

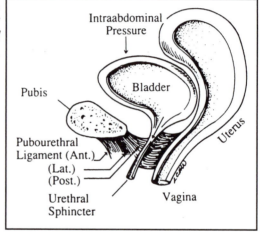

supporters for the uterus, are now believed to be connective tissue covering the uterine blood vessels. The uterosacral ligaments and the cardinal ligaments also carry visceral nerve fibers, sympathetic and parasympathetic efferent fibers, as well as afferent or sensory fibers to thoracic, lumbar, and sacral spinal cord levels.[2]

The urinary bladder lies between the pubis, the vagina, the cervix, and the pelvic diaphragm. The trigone of the bladder rests on the anterior middle third of the vagina. The bladder is attached to and supported by the endopelvic fascia, but remains separate from the vagina. Pubovesical ligaments provide additional support. Nerves reach the bladder through the vesicovaginal ligament, cardinal ligament, and lateral vesical ligaments.[6]

The urinary bladder has an outer longitudinal, middle circular, and inner longitudinal layer that gives rise to the urethral musculature and the trigonal musculature. The trigone is the area in which the muscle tissue changes from the tubular structure of the urethra to the flat, thin sheet of the bladder. The detrusor contraction, or the contraction of muscles that causes a pushing down of the bladder contents, is the sum of many decussating forces. The bladder outlet is surrounded by deep trigonal muscles and middle circular layers. At the outlet there is also a band of muscular tissue called the sling of Heiss that is further supported by the pubourethral ligament. This ligament has three divisions; posterior, lateral, and anterior (Figure 2-12). Through these divisions, the ligament joins with the urethra, the levator

Table 2-8

Divisions of the Female Pelvic Floor

Pelvic Diaphragm:	levator ani and coccygeus
Urogenital Diaphragm:	deep transverse perineal muscle
Urogenital Triangle:	anterior of perineum (pubis to ischium)
Anal Triangle:	posterior of perineum (ischium to rectum)

ani muscles, and the urogenital diaphragm to maintain the relationship of the urethra within the abdomen.

The urethra is supported by the anterior vaginal wall, by the urogenital diaphragm, and by pubourethral ligaments (from endopelvic fascia). The support of the diaphragm assists in providing urethral resistance. Skene's or paraurethral glands and ducts lie within the urethral wall, and empty into the vestibule.

Muscles of the Pelvis and Pelvic Floor/Diaphragm

The terms pelvic floor, pelvic diaphragm, urogenital diaphragm, urogenital triangle, anal triangle, perineum, vulva, and pudendum are frequently used interchangeably and often incorrectly. In addition to confusion about the perineum and the pelvis, there are muscles that technically belong to the lower extremity, but originate in the pelvis, and are therefore part of its anatomy (see Table 2-6). For instance, the iliopsoas tendon inserts on the lesser trochanter, and the iliacus covers the medial surface of the false pelvis. The piriformis, which hosts the sacral and pudendal plexuses, originates from the lateral sacrum, exits the pelvis through the greater sciatic foramen, and inserts into the greater trochanter of the femur. The obturator internus muscle originates from the innominate and obturator membrane, passes through the lesser sciatic foramen, and inserts also into the greater trochanter. Thick fascia covers the obturator inernus and gives rise to the levator ani muscle.[7]

Pelvic floor is probably the most general and abused term, but should probably be used only when referring to the *pelvic diaphragm* (Table 2-8). Arising from the posterior superior pubic rami, the inner ischial spines, and the obturator fascia, the fibers of the pelvic diaphragm insert between the vaginal and rectal openings (perineal body), below the rectal opening, at midline around the vaginal and rectal openings to form sphincters, and into the coccyx. As separate entities, the pelvic diaphragm is composed of the coccygeus and levator ani muscles. The coccygeus muscle arises from the ischial spine and inserts into the lateral coccyx. Anterior to the coccygeus muscle is the levator ani muscle, which is divided by anatomists into three or four parts. A portion (pubovaginalis) blends with the vagina and is sometimes considered separate from the rest of the parts of the levator ani muscle. The puborectalis, pubococcygeus, and the iliococcygeus are the more commonly known divisions of the levator ani muscle. Fibers from the puborectalis merge with the rectum and blend with the opposite corresponding muscle, along with the pubococcygeus and iliococcygeus muscles as they insert into the coccyx. The combination of these muscles creates a sling mechanism to support the internal organs and the openings transsecting the pelvic diaphragm (Figure 2-13).

The *urogenital diaphragm* is a second muscular layer external to the pelvic diaphragm that adds support to the region transsected by the openings of the urethra and vagina. It spans across the ischiopubic rami and is sandwiched between two fascial sheets that fuse near the

Figure 2-13. Urogenital and anal triangles. (Reprinted with permission from O'Connor LJ, Gourley Stephenson RJ. *Obstetric and Gynecologic Care in Physical Therapy.* Thorofare, NJ: SLACK Incorporated; 1990.)

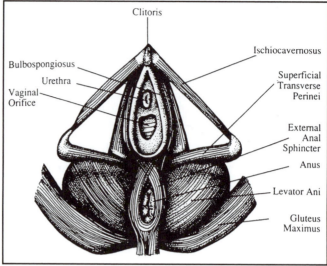

pubis to form the transverse ligament of the pelvis. The muscular portion forms a triangle from the urethral sphincter and the deep transverse perineal muscles; however, this area is different than that called the urogenital triangle of the perineum.[6] The deep transverse perineal muscle arises from the ischial ramus, passes medially and posteriorly to the vagina. It forms a tendinous rapine with contributions from the external sphincter ani and the puborectalis, blending into the vaginal wall. The female sphincter urethrae muscle is an arch of fibers that end in the urethral and vaginal walls.[2]

The *urogenital triangle*, on the other hand, is the anterior portion of the perineum. The urogenital triangle has several layers of its own, primarily fascial. The skin and fatty layer lay superior to the superficial space. The superficial space contains a membranous layer of fascia and a muscular layer. The perineal membrane which stretches across the inferior pubic rami, a muscular layer, and the deep fascia superior to that deep muscular layer make up the deep space. The urogenital triangle may be further divided into the superficial and deep perineal spaces. The deep perineal space hosts the urethra and the lower vagina. The superficial structures of the urogenital triangle of the perineum are also known as the external genitalia, the vulva, or the pudendum. This area includes the mons pubis, labia majora, labia minora, clitoris, vestibular bulb, bulbocavernosus (bulbospongiosus) muscles, greater vestibular glands (Bartholin's), ischiocavernosus muscles, superficial transverse perineum muscles and, in some texts, the urogenital diaphragm.[2]

The posterior portion of the perineum, divided by a line drawn between the ischial tuberosities, is the anal triangle. The anal triangle of the perineum is bordered by the sacrotuberous ligaments, the gluteus maximus, and the urogenital triangle, and contains the anus, external sphincter ani muscle, and the ischiorectal fossae.

The Perineum/External Genitalia

The *perineum*, then, is inferior to the pelvic diaphragm and the urogenital diaphragm (Figure 2-14). The labia majora blend anteriorly to become the mons pubis and taper posteriorly at the anus. The inner skin is smooth, contains sebaceous glands, and borders the areolar and fatty tissue of the labial fold. The labia meet at the anterior and posterior labial

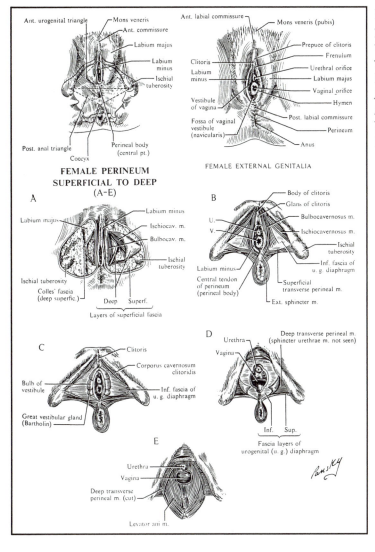

Figure 2-14. Female perineum: superficial to deep. (Reprinted with permission from Pansky B, House El. *Review of Gross Anatomy*. 2nd ed. New York, NY: McGraw-Hill; 1969.)

commissures. Hair and pigment mark the external labia. The labia minora are smooth, cutaneous folds that extend posteriorly from the clitoris for about 4 cm. Between the labia minora is the vestibule of the vagina, which hosts the external urethral orifice, the paraurethral (Skene's) glands, the vagina, and the ducts of the greater vestibular glands. The greater vestibular glands and the vestibular bulbs lie near the vagina. The labium minora form the prepuce and frenulum of the clitoris. Two crura form the clitoris, which angles, by a suspensory ligament to the symphysis pubis, towards the perineum. The clitoris is composed of erectile tissue, assisted by the ischiocavernosus muscles, and covered by epithelium that is sensitive to touch. Arising from the ischial tuberosities passing medially to the central tendinous body of the perineum (perineal body), the superficial transverse perineum muscles stabilize the perineum for other muscle contraction. The external genital area is innervated by the pudendal nerve, vesical plexuses, and vaginal nerves. Lymphatics are rich in this area, which is covered by the superficial perineal fascia (Colles'). This is a space external to the superficial fascia of the urogenital diaphragm.[2]

Three nerves contribute to the cutaneous nerve supply to the vulva and perineum. The iliohypogastric, ilioinguinal, and genital branch of the genitofemoral innervate the anterior vulva. The pudendal nerve and branches innervate the clitoris, vestibule, labia, and perineum; and the perineal branch of the posterior femoral cutaneous nerve innervates the lateral perineum, posterior vulva, and perianal region.

SELF-ASSESSMENT REVIEW

1. Research is inconclusive regarding the action, levels, and effect of _____ on connective tissue in the pregnant woman.

2. Name the five ligamentous groups of the pelvis:_____, _____, _____, _____, and _____.

3. Weight gain and anatomic changes in breast structure may result in the development of _____.

4. During pregnancy, the anterior abdominal wall _____.

5. The enlarged uterus may compress two major blood vessels: _____, _____.

6. Name three important bony landmarks of the pelvis: _____, _____, _____.

7. The pelvic floor can also be referred to as the _____.

8. The ligaments resist _____ forces on the pelvis.

Answers

1. Relaxin. 2. Abdominopelvic Ligaments, Sacroiliac Ligaments, Sacroischial Ligaments, Sacrococcygeal Ligaments, Pubic Ligaments. 3. Thoracic kyphosis. 4. Weakens. 5 .Inferior vena cava, aorta. 6. Pubic arch, sacral promontory, ischial tuberosities. 7. Pelvic diaphragm. 8. Rotatory

REFERENCES

1. Chewning EB. *Anatomy Illustrated.* New York, NY: Simon & Schuster; 1979.

2. Woodburne RT. *Essentials of Human Anatomy.* New York, NY: Oxford University Press; 1973.

3. Massey EW, Cefalo RC. Neuropathies of pregnancy. *Obstet Gynecol Surv.* 34(7):489-492, 1979.

4. Crafts RC, Krieger HP. Gross anatomy of the female reproductive tract, pituitary, and hypothalamus. In: Danforth DN, Scott JR, Eds. *Obstetrics and Gynecology.* Philadelphia, Pa: JB Lippincott; 1986.

5. Warwick R, Williams PL, eds. *Gray's Anatomy.* Philadelphia, Pa: WB Saunders; 1973.

6. Burnett LS. Anatomy. In: Jones HW, Wentz AC, Burnett SL, Eds. *Novak's Textbook of Gynecology.* Baltimore, Md: Williams & Wilkins; 1988.

7. Goss CM, ed. *Gray's Anatomy of the Human Body.* Philadephia, Pa: Lea & Febiger; 1970.

8. Steindler A. *Kinesiology of the Human Body.* Springfield, Mass: Charles C Thomas; 1970.

9. Steindler A. *Mechanics of Normal and Pathological Locomotion in Man.* Springfield, Mass: Charles C Thomas; 1935

10. Basmajian JV. *Grant's Method of Anatomy*. Baltimore, Md: Williams & Wilkins; 1971.

11. Pritchard JA, MacDonald PC, Gant NF. *Williams Obstetrics*. Norwalk, Conn: Appleton-Century-Crofts; 1985.

12. Artal R, Wiswell RA. *Exercise in Pregnancy*. Baltimore, Md: Williams & Wilkins; 1986.

13. Siffert RS, Pruzansky ME, Levy RN. Orthopaedic complications. In: Cherry SH, Berkowitz RL, Kase N, eds. *Rovinsky and Guttmacher's Medical, Surgical, and Gynecologic Complications of Pregnancy*. Baltimore, Md: Williams & Wilkins; 1985.

14. Heyman J, Lundqvist A. The symphysis pubis in pregnancy and parturition. *Acta Obstet Gynecol Scand*. 1932;12:191-225.

15. LaBan MM, Perrin JCS, Latimer FR. Pregnancy and the herniated lumbar disc. *Arch Phys Med Rehabil*. 1983;64:319-21.

16. Quagliarello J, Steinetz BG, Weiss G. Relaxin secretion in early pregnancy. *Obstet Gynecol*. 1979;53(1):62-63.

17. Yki-Jarvinen H, Wahlstrom T, Seppala M. Immunohistochemical localization of relaxin in the genital tract of non-pregnant women. In: Bigazzi M, Greenwood FC, Gasparri F, eds. *Biology of Relaxin and its Role in the Human*. Amsterdam, Holland: Excerpta Medica; 1983.

18. Porter DG. The roles of relaxin in different species. In: Bigazzi M, Greenwood FC, Gasparri F, eds. *Biology of Relaxin and its Role in the Human*. Amsterdam, Holland: Excerpta Medica; 1983.

19. MacLennan AH, Nicolson R, Green RC. Serum relaxin in pregnancy. *Lancet*. 1986;Aug 2:241-243.

20. Kristiansson P, Svardsudd K, von Schoultz B. Serum relaxin, symphyseal pain, and back pain during pregnancy. *Am J Obstet Gynecol*. 1996;175:1342-7.

21. Weiss G. The secretion and role of relaxin in pregnant women. In: Bigazzi M, Greenwood FC, Gasparri F, eds. *Biology of Relaxin and its Role in the Human*. Amsterdam, Holland: Excerpta Medica; 1983.

22. Calguneri M, Bird HA, Wright A. Changes in joint laxity occurring during pregnancy. *Ann Rheum Dis*. 1982;41:126-8.

23. Schauberger CW, Rooney BL, Goldsmith L, et al. Peripheral joint laxity increases in pregnancy but does not correlate with serum relaxin levels. *Am J Obstet Gynecol*. 1996;174:667-71.

24. MacLennan AH, et al. Serum relaxin and pelvic pain of pregnancy. *Lancet*. 1986;Aug 2:243-5.

25. Petersen LK, Hvidman L, Uldbjerg N. Normal serum relaxin in women with disabling pelvic pain during pregnancy. *Gynecol Obstet Invest*. 1994;38:21-3.

26. Albert H, et al. Circulating levels of relaxin are normal in pregnant women with pelvic pain. *Eur J Obstet Gynecol Reprod Biol*. 1997;74:19-22.

27. Norstrom A, et al. Inhibitory action of relaxin on human cervical smooth muscle. *J Clin Endocrinol Metab*. 1984;59(3):379-82.

28. Conant Van Blarcom C. *Obstetrical Nursing*. New York, NY: MacMillan; 1929.

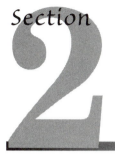

Section

2

Role of Physical Therapy in Gynecologic Care

3

Physical Therapy and the Female Client: Evaluation and Treatment

PRACTICE ISSUES

An area still under debate by physical therapists concerns the application of state practice acts for performing internal evaluation for vaginal and rectal disorders. Some believe the physical therapist is not thoroughly trained to perform an internal pelvic exam. Others believe this is essential to proper management of gynecologic problems with a musculoskeletal basis. The answer probably lies somewhere in the middle. In other words, a complete internal exam should be performed by a gynecologist or urologist prior to a physical therapy referral, to rule out serious pathology and communicable disease.

The physical therapist can assess the strength and tone of the pelvic floor by palpating on the perineum and inserting sterile, gloved, lubricated fingers an inch or two into the patient's vagina. The internal evaluation should be implemented only by physical therapists who are allowed to do so according to their state practice acts. Not only must each physical therapist make their own decision whether this form of assessment is covered by their practice act, but whether it is covered by their malpractice insurance carrier.

If the physical therapist then decides to pursue the treatment of pelvic floor disorders, an extensive resource, beyond what is offered here, is *The Gynecological Manual* developed by the Section on Women's Health of the American Physical Therapy Association.[1] In this manual, specific instructions are provided for a thorough examination of the pelvic floor and influence of related muscles, joints, and ligaments that may contribute to pain and dysfunction. Samples of various evaluations are provided as well as brief discussions of prolapse, musculoskeletal dysfunction, urinary incontinence, bladder dysfunction and hypertonus dysfunction of the pelvic floor. Treatment approaches include: surface electromyographic (sEMG) biofeedback, biofeedback with air pressure (eg, perineometer), electrical stimulation, scar management, vaginal weight training, bladder retraining, and therapeutic exercise for the pelvic floor. Case studies are also included of common problems presented to the physical therapist practicing with patients with gynecological disorders. Psychological factors may also enter into the ultimate diagnosis and treatment.

Restrictions and Cautionary Notes

It is not recommended that physical therapists do internal pelvic exams during pregnancy because of the risk of introducing an infection to the mother and baby. Although an obstetrician does perform them during pregnancy, it is usually infrequent and in the last month of gestation.

Also, some women have been sexually or physically abused in their lives. These women may become clients and their particular history may become an issue in the care that they are receiving from physical therapists. The prevalence of childhood sexual abuse in our society with one in three to five females and one in seven to ten males affected, suggests that physical therapists may unknowingly work with adult survivors on a frequent basis as Candice L. Schachter PhD, PT reports.[2] Physical therapists involved in the treatment of pelvic floor dysfunction should be aware that survivors of childhood sexual abuse may not be comfortable verbalizing their difficulties with treatment. The therapist should be responsive to nonverbal signs such as:

- Body language that demonstrates discomfort such as tension and irregular breathing.
- Difficulty adhering to a treatment plan.
- Difficulty staying focused on treatment.[3]

Women that physical therapists see may be victims of domestic violence. It is important that the practitioner be alert to the indications of abuse. Estimates of domestic violence episodes range from 2 to 4 million per year.[4] Many incidences of abuse go undetected and unreported. The Federal Bureau of Investigation reports that domestic violence is the number one cause of injury to women and occurs more frequently than motor vehicle accidents, muggings and rape combined. The American Medical Association in 1994, reported the 47% of husbands who beat their wives do so three or more times per year and that rape is a prevalent form of abuse in violent marriages.[5] Domestic violence can occur in same-sex relationships or by women against men. However, women are six times more likely to experience violence committed by an intimate partner.[5]

Physical therapists should screen for injuries around the head, face, neck, breasts, abdomen, injuries observed during pregnancy, repeated injuries, gynecological problems, physical symptoms related to stress, self-mutilation and overuse of prescription medication.[4] The American Physical Therapy Association (APTA) has an excellent handbook on "Guidelines for Recognizing and Providing Care for Victims of Domestic Violence" (see resources).[4]

All patients need sensitive health care practitioners who can understand each individual's complexity and decipher patients' behavior that may represent past or present abuse. Patients do consider their past abuse history relevant to the therapeutic relationship and may disclose that information to their practitioner after trust has been established and when given the opportunity in a setting that they feel is safe.[6,7,8] Two types of disclosure are identified here: task-centered disclosure that can be initiated by the physical therapist at the beginning of the treatment and relationship-based disclosure usually initiated by a client after experiencing the physical therapist as trustworthy. Task-centered questions give survivors the opportunity to advise the physical therapist about their sensitivities, such as to touch, disrobing and body positions.

Questions that address abuse directly are not recommended.[8] Physical therapists can ask questions about abuse through open-ended questions: ie, to the client "Is there anything that you consider relevant for a therapeutic relationship here in physical therapy"? Including both types of questions (task-centered and open-ended), provides for different levels of disclosure and addresses the diversity of preferences among survivors. Clients should be given a choice between filling out a patient questionnaire by themselves or with a physical therapist.[8]

By establishing a partnership with the client that conveys an understanding of the survivor's concerns, the physical therapist can maximize the benefits of the physical therapy experience for the client who is a survivor.[6,7] The physical therapist who deals with survivors of abuse must respond carefully to disclosures and be compelled to read more on these topics and have a network of mental health providers on which they can consult and refer to. Furthermore, the women that physical therapists are evaluating may be heterosexual, homosexual, bisexual or transgendered. Ask questions about sexual history in a manner that will get the clinical information necessary to completely treat the client without gender bias. Women with abuse history and gynecological problems often urgently need physical therapy and require a more secure setting in order to reveal their full history.

TAKING AND INTERPRETING A HISTORY

One of the most important aspects of physical therapy evaluation and treatment of the female client is taking the history. Although a careful history is valuable when dealing with any patient, the female patient may tell the physical therapist who takes the time to listen, things about her condition that she has not told her physician. For instance, a busy physician, nurse, or even physical therapist can miss the relationship between symptoms and the menstrual cycle, and therefore miss possible conditions of dysmenorrhea or premenstrual syndrome. Certain types of incontinence can sometimes be determined only through careful history taking. In the latter case, the description of the patient may even determine whether the patient can be helped with physical therapy. However, because limited documentation exists on the benefits of physical therapy treatment of gynecologic problems, and because the next step for many patients is surgery, it's probably worth it to the patient to attempt a trial whether the problem is muscular or neurologic.

Most practitioners find they develop their own system of patient interviewing, similar to developing a standard routine to conduct an evaluation. A sample history questionnaire for incontinence is shown in Figure 3-1. To effectively take a history, evaluate and treat effectively, the practitioner must have a basic understanding of the anatomy (see chapter on Anatomical Considerations) and physiology of the reproductive and urinary system. These systems are extremely complex, and entire books have been written on treatment of gynecological disorders. Therefore, practitioners are advised to use this book as a guide to a basic understanding of the evaluation and treatment of the female client. More important, the methods the physical therapist can employ to treat gynecologic disorders keep expanding; currently the most common include exercise instruction, relaxation training, biofeedback, transcutaneous electrical nerve stimulation (TENS), ultrasound and electrical stimulation.

PELVIC FLOOR EXAMINATION

Frequently the patient with gynecological problems will need a musculoskeletal examination as well as a direct manual exam of the perineum. Included here is a suggested exam so that overlap from pelvic floor dysfunctions and musculoskeletal problems can be treated in harmony. The suggested order of the assessment has the patient supine at the end of the musculoskeletal exam, allowing the clinician to go directly to the manual exam of the perineum with the patient in the lithotomy position. Explain to the patient the order of the exam and what you are going to do. The patient will be more comfortable if she empties her bladder before the start of the exam.

Grading of the pelvic floor can be done with several measurements.[1] This scale presupposes that the examiner has some experience grading pelvic floor muscles and can discrim-

PATIENT INCONTINENCE QUESTIONNAIRE

Name: _____ Home phone: _____ Business phone: _____

Address: _____

Date of birth: _____ Occupation: _____

Responsibilities at home: _____

_____

Level of activity: Sedentary: _____ Light: _____ Active: _____ Very active: ____

Height : _____ Weight: _____ Doctor: _____

Obstetrical History: Number of pregnancies_____ and number of deliveries_____

Date of delivery	Wt of baby	Length of second stage/pushing	Episiotomy/tearing	Difficulty healing

Medications: _____

Problem: _____

1. Is there past or current history of urinary tract disease, infection, injury? _____
2. Is there past or current history of muscular paralysis or disease; diabetes; surgery or trauma to the spine, bladder, pelvis or brain; hysterectomy?_____
3. Was urethral dilatation performed in past?___ Why? _____
4. As a child, was there difficulty holding urine or bed wetting? _____
5. As an adolescent or adult, was or is there difficulty holding urine or bed wetting? ____
6. When urinating, is the amount small, medium, or large? _____
7. Is there difficulty stopping the flow ?_____ Is there dribbling?_____
8. Does urine flow uncontrollably when associated with any of the following: coughing, sneezing, vomiting, standing, sitting, laying down, walking, running, straining, changing position, during intercourse, laughing, lifting, pushing? _____
   Does urine loss occur at the same time or shortly afterward? _____
9. Did the problem start after pregnancy, during pregnancy, after vaginal or abdominal surgery, after Cesarean surgery? _____
10. Is there ever a need for protection?____ When?_____ What is used? _____
    How many a day? _____
11. Are medications used, including over-the-counter or recreational drugs? _____
12. Is the patient aware of urine leaking?___ Does it leak prior to reaching the toilet?   __
13. Is there a strong urge to urinate? Can the urge be controlled? _____
14. Does the patient awaken at night with a strong urge to urinate?_____ Is the bladder full?____ How frequently? _____
15. Is there pain on urination? _____
16. Is there any difficulty passing urine or starting the flow? _____
17. Have other family members had trouble with incontinence or bed wetting in the past or do they now?_____ Age of onset? _____
18. Any pelvic surgery?_____
19. Is there anything else that you consider relevant for me to know in our therapeutic relationship? _____

Figure 3-1. Patient incontinence questionnaire.

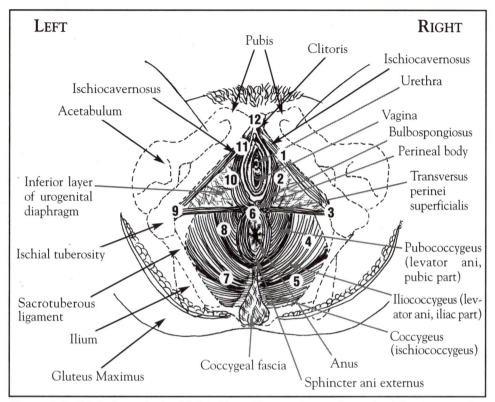

LEFT   RIGHT

Figure 3-2. Pelvic floor clock with locations. The numbers refer to the following muscles and/or groups: 1 and 11 (o'clock) represent the Ischiocavernous muscle; 2 and 10 (o'clock) represent the Bulbospongiosus muscle; 3 and 9 (o'clock) represent the transverse perinei superficialis muscles; 4, 5, 7, and 8 (o'clock) represent the levator ani muscles; 6 (o'clock) represents the perineal body; 1, 2, 3, 9, 10, 11, and 12 (o'clock) represent theurogenital triangle; 4, 5, 7, and 8 (o'clock) represent the anal triangle.

inate between the levels of strength. Lab instruction with an experienced clinician is the only way to learn how to grade pelvic floor muscles. A suggested method for the basic grading is as follows:[1]

0-No contraction
3-Moderate contraction with pelvic floor lift
1-Flicker of contraction
4-Good contraction with pelvic floor lift
2-Weak contraction
5-Strong contraction with pelvic floor lift

A drawing of the pelvic floor with the superimposed bony outlet shows the location of the muscles, ligaments, and urogenital and anal triangles (Figure 3-2). The muscles of the perineum can be assessed in a clockwise direction, starting from the symphysis pubis to the ischial tuberosity (patient's left groin), perineal body and up the patient's right groin to the ischial tuberosity and back to the symphysis pubis. Then the location of any pathology can be done by referring to the position of the pain in relation to the numbers as on a clock, as seen in the evaluation form (Figure 3-3).

Pelvic Floor and Musculoskeletal Examination of the Female Client

Part A. Musculoskeletal Examination

Name: _____

Date: _____

   1. Standing
      A. Posture

Viewed from	Side	Front	Back
1. Head			
2. Shoulders			
3.Mid/upper back			
4. Abdomen			
5. Low back			
6. Pelvis/hips			
7. Knees			
8. Ankles			

      B. Spinal Movements

           FB

   SBL —|— SBR

  RL BB RR

Normal = N
Pain = X
Restricted = 1
Hypermobile = 2

      C. Pelvis
         Level of PSIS and sacral base
         Active movement of Sl joint (Forward bending- landmarks PSISs)

   2. Sitting
      A. Neurologic Strength Lower Extremities

	Right	Left
L1, 2 Psoas		
L3 Quads		
L-4 Tib ant		
L5 Ext. H.L		
S1 Flex H.L		
S2 Hams		

Reflexes	Right	Left
L4 Knee		
S1 Ankle		
UMN Babinski		

Reflexes: 0 = absent
               1 + diminished
               2 + normal
               3 + increased
               4 + clonus

      B. Trunk motions: asymmetries, stability

   3. Prone
      A. Sacroiliac
      B. Spinal palpation (thoracic, low back, sacrum)

    C. Legs- flexibility
        Hip flexors
        Quad length
        TFL length

4. Supine
    A. Sacroiliac joints
        Spring
                Anterior ligaments; Posterior ligaments
            Rotation
                Anterior or Posterior rotation of ilium or sacrum

    B. Hamstring Length
    C. Rectus Diastasis
    D. Hip flexor tightness
    E. Leg lengths

Part B: Pelvic Floor Exam

5. Skin Observation for:
    integrity
    lesions
    scars
    redness
    swelling
    introitus: symmetry, gapping, closed
        excursion-contraction of the pelvic floor

6. Palpation and location:
    A. Sensitivity
    B. Pain and tenderness
    C. Swelling
    D. Tension and scar mobility
    E. Trigger points
        Perineal muscles
        External and Internal palpation

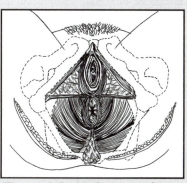

Figure 3-3. Mark areas of pain and tenderness.

7. Pelvic Floor contraction
    Strength (0-5 scale)
    Holding time for one contraction
    Quick repetitions before fatigue
    Overflow to abdominal, gluteal or adductor muscles
    Breath holding

Impression: _____

Goals: _____

Treatment Plan: _____

Frequency: _____

Figure 3-4. Normal menstrual cycle. (Reprinted with permission from O'Connor LJ, Gourley Stephenson RJ. *Obstetrics and Gynecologic Care in Physical Therapy.* Thorofare, NJ: SLACK Incorporated; 1990.)

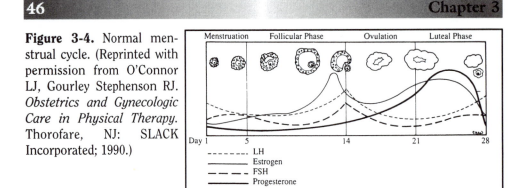

This chart will assist the therapist in organizing a treatment for the pelvic floor patient who may have multiple problems.

Part	Summary of Evaluation Results and Outline for Treatment				
	Signs/Symptoms	Diagnosis	Treatment	Supports	Home Treatment
Head and neck					
Shoulders					
Abdomen					
Pelvis					
Low Back					
Legs					
Feet					
Pelvic Floor					

Additionally, refer to Appendix C for suggestions on use of the *Guide to Physical Therapist Practice* for gynecologic and obstetric practice in physical therapy. With the publication of the *Guide to Physical Therapist Practice*, clinicians may find it necessary to justify techniques, modalities selected, and number of visits when treating patients with gynecologic and obstetric disorders.

FEMALE REPRODUCTIVE SYSTEM

Normal Menstrual Cycle

The menstrual cycle may be divided into the follicular phase, ovulation, and the luteal phase. The follicular phase may be further divided into the primordial, preantral, antral, and preovulatory follicle phases (Figure 3-4). The follicular granulosa cells and the corpus luteum are responsible for producing estradiol, the major estrogen of the human ovary, in response to stimulation from gonadotropins, follicle-stimulating hormone (FSH), and luteinizing hormone (LH). All three classes of sex steroids are produced by the human ovary: estrogens, progestins and androgens. Estrogens, specifically 17 beta-estradiol, produced at a rate of 100 to 300 micrograms/day in the normal, non-pregnant female, exerts a positive feedback effect by stimulating the hypothalamus to release gonadotropin-releasing hormone (GnRH, in the female also known as LHRH). GnRH is secreted from the hypophysis or pituitary gland, and in turn, stimulates the gonadotropins.

It is unclear what governs the number of follicles that grow during a cycle. It has been shown, however, that follicle growth continues during ovulation, pregnancy, anovulatory periods, and at all ages of life.[9] The granulosa-cell covered oocyte selected for ovulation appears to respond to hormonal stimulation, changing in shape and structure to form the pre-antral follicle. At this stage, the follicle develops a membrane, the zone pellucida, surrounded by the theca layer, and estrogen stimulates gonadotropin production in the granulosa cells. FSH directs the dominance of estrogen over the androgens. As the estrogen concentration increases, so does the growth of the follicle, now in its antral stage. Follicular development seems to depend on the conversion of androgen to estrogen via FSH stimulation.[9] It is for this reason that the androgens, as well as prolactin and cortisol, are considered by some to be inhibiting or interfering hormones, as opposed to the releasing hormone, GnRH.[10]

Prior to ovulation, progesterone, a product of the corpus luteum, is released to join with estradiol to influence the endometrial secretion. The entire role of ovarian androgens is yet unexplained, but great progress has been made in recent years in understanding their complex actions within the female reproductive system. It is generally believed, however, that a small amount of androgen enhances follicular development, whereas an excess inhibits this process by causing follicular atresia and granulosa cell death.

The balance of the interfering and releasing hormones is the responsibility of the neuroendocrinologic mechanisms of reproduction. GnRH has been detected in the fetus as early as 10 weeks; FSH and LH by 10 weeks to 13 weeks, peaking at about 20 weeks. However, it seems to be the combined effect of genetics and critical body mass that stimulates puberty, gonadotropin secretion gradually increasing about 3 years to 4 years before the cycle is well established. Both males and females secrete gonadotropins in a pulsating fashion; the male secretion staying at a tonic level, and the female secretion cycling with a surge of both FSH and LH about midcycle. The frequency and amplitude of pulsation is critical, and is apparently regulated by a dual catecholaminergic system that balances norepinephrine and dopamine production from the brain. In fact, the anterior pituitary is now believed to secrete GnRH spontaneously, as well as in response to hypothalamic secretions. Dopamine is thought to inhibit both GnRH and prolactin secretion, although GnRH may also directly stimulate prolactin. Norepinephrine is believed to stimulate GnRH. Previously it was believed that the LH and FSH surge at midcycle was related to GnRH secretion in response to estradiol acting on the hypothalamus. Further research has indicated that the regulation of gonadotropins is directed by stimulation of the anterior pituitary by ovarian steroid feedback.

Estradiol increases as FSH stimulates follicle growth and stimulates the rise of the tropic hormones (hypothalamic releasing hormones and others released from the anterior pituitary). The increase in LH induces ovulation (rupture of the follicle), and the corpus luteum forms. At this stage, the estrogen/androgen balance is particularly important. In the first 12 days of the cycle, the size of the follicle changes from 4 mm to 20 mm, the follicular fluid volume changes from 0.0 ml to 65 ml, and the number of granulosa cells increases from 2 million to 50 million. LH does not appear to any measurable level until day 6 or 7. Prolactin decreases from 60 ng/ml to 5 ng/ml by day 12, and the androgen level theoretically should remain fairly constant.

In addition to this specificity, a variety of growth factors influence cell differentiation, as well as the dominant follicle's own feedback system. This feedback system allows regulation of gonadotropin secretion. The follicular fluid also contains inhibin, synthesized by granulosa cells stimulated by FSH. This peptide is believed to assist in the dominance of one follicle over others. Once inhibin is produced, it acts to stop FSH production at the pituitary, thereby regulating itself. Activin, a releasing substance, does the opposite.

The preovulatory follicle produces estrogen, peaking a day to a day and a half prior to ovulation. The dominant follicle is believed to acquire greater estrogen and FSH concentrations so that the LH surge results in progesterone production in that follicle and an androgen imbalance in less dominant follicles, causing them to yield to atresia. Theca tissue from these lesser follicles produces androgens, causing an increase in androgen levels in peripheral plasma around ovulation. This androgen production theoretically may cause stimulated libido at a time compatible with conception.

In vitro fertilization studies have revealed interesting observations about diurnal ovulation patterns. Ovulation appears to occur in the morning between midnight and 11:00 a.m. in spring, in the evening during fall and winter, and between 4:00 p.m. and 7:00 p.m., from July to February. Ovulation occurs as the follicular wall decomposes in response to the LH surge. This surge also causes the oocyte to resume meiotic activity, the granulosa cells to luteinize, and prostaglandins to synthesize and promote follicle rupture. A combination of prostaglandins, progesterone, histamine, and proteolytic enzymes is thought to assist follicular wall degradation. Following ovulation, there is a rapid decrease in gonadotropin secretion, although the reason for this is unexplained.

In the luteal phase, the granulosa cells grow larger and become yellow from the pigment lutein. The corpus luteum forms, becoming heavily vascularized and able to synthesize the three sex steroids. Progesterone levels rise and peak about 8 days after the LH surge, suppressing new follicle growth This is enhanced by inhibin production. Although it is often believed that the luteal phase is 14 days long, a 1984 study suggests an average of 12 days to 17 days. The corpus luteum degenerates toward the end of this phase, unless pregnancy occurs. Pregnancy stimulates human chorionic gonadotropin (hCG) production to maintain luteal steroidogenesis until the placenta can assume this role around 7 weeks to 10 weeks gestation.

Luteal regression occurs if there is no fertilization. It is believed that PF_2 [9] is synthesized in the endometrium upon stimulation by follicular estrogen. It is locally transported to the corpus luteum through a connection from the ovary to the uterus. This prostaglandin suppresses LH receptor formation in the corpus luteum, contributing to its degeneration and resulting in menstruation.

Abnormal Menstrual Cycles

From the background presented above, it must be clear that regular menstrual cycles are nothing short of a miracle. Things do go wrong sometimes, however, and in a variety of ways. The suffix "rhoea" or rrhea" comes from the Greek "rrhoia," "to flow".[10] Abnormalities of flow are termed amenorrhea (absence of flow), dysmenorrhea (painful flow), or oligomenorrhea (infrequent flow occurring no more than every 40 days and no less than every 6 months). However, the list continues with hypomenorrhea (reduced number of days or amount of flow), and cryptomenorrhea (monthly sign of menstruation without a flow as in an abnormally closed hymen).

Amenorrhea is estimated to occur in less than 5% of women in the normal population, but research suggests that certain groups of women (those imprisoned for great lengths of time, those with nutritional deficiencies, or those who extensively exercise on a regular basis,[12,13] such as long distance runners or ballet dancers), tend to experience menstrual abnormalities at a greater incidence.[9] To further differentiate those cases in which menstruation has not occurred at all versus those in which flow has started but then stops at a later point in the woman's life, the terms primary and secondary amenorrhea have been assigned.

Primary amenorrhea may occur with or without normal sexual development. Sexual features may be limited or abnormal, eg, gonadal dysgenesis, resistant ovary (no follicular development), or damaged ovaries (traumatic or due to administration of anticancer treatments,[14] related to enzyme deficiency, panhypopituitarism (absence of all anterior pituitary hormones), anorexia nervosa, or hypothyroidism. If sexual development occurs normally but no menstruation occurs, it basically rules out abnormality in the hypothalamus, anterior pituitary or ovary. No flow suggests possible obstruction in the uterus or vagina. Secondary amenorrhea is the absence of flow more than 6 months when menstruation was established previously.[15] There is also physiologic amenorrhea (normal state of no flow prior to puberty, during pregnancy, and when lactating). Treatment of flow disorders is generally not within the realm of the physical therapist, but to provide background, the basic causes are summarized in Table 3-1.

Painful Menstrual Cycles

Although treatment for the abnormal cycle disorders is limited, treatment methods for women with painful cycles related to premenstrual syndrome (PMS) and dysmenorrhea are currently being explored by physical therapists.[16,17] Since primary dysmenorrhea is believed to affect between 40% and 95% of menstruating women"[18], this population is one that could potentially benefit greatly from therapeutic assistance. Because many women dislike using medication monthly, (although medication can be highly effective), an offer of a pain relief mechanism such as transcutaneous electrical nerve stimulation (TENS), instruction in relaxation techniques, or designing exercise programs specific to the patient may provide therapists an opportunity to help these women.

Premenstrual Syndrome

Central to an understanding of PMS is the idea that the symptoms occur cyclically, after ovulation. If symptoms occur irregularly or chronically, PMS may not be an accurate diagnosis. Practitioners are becoming increasingly concerned with taking a meticulous history before confirming such a diagnosis.[18]

Premenstrual syndrome has many definitions. Among them: "The symptoms usually begin 10 to 14 days prior to the onset of the menstrual period and become progressively worse until the onset of menstruation or, for some women, several days after the onset."[19] "PMS is the cyclical occurrence of various signs and symptoms beginning near or after ovulation and resolving soon after the onset of menses."[18] It is "the cyclic appearance of a large collection of symptoms, occurring to such a degree that lifestyle or work are affected and followed by a period of time entirely free of symptoms."[4] "PMS is defined as a menstrual related mood disorder that includes the cyclic occurrence of symptoms that are of sufficient severity to interfere with some aspects of life and that appear with a consistent and predictable relationship to menses."[20] The lack of a consistent definition adds to the problems of treatment and identification of this syndrome.

The most common symptoms include abdominal bloating, breast tenderness and swelling, weight gain, fatigue, depression, and irritability. Headache, constipation, acne, rhinitis, and edema may also occur, as well as more uncommon symptoms like paresthesia, sleep disorders, and wide mood swings.[18,20] Other related symptoms may include poor concentration, sensitivity to noise and decreased motor skills.[21] It has been estimated that more than 150 symptoms could possibly be related to PMS. For these reasons, the first step to diagnosis and treatment usually involves the woman keeping a daily menstrual diary

Table 3-1

Overview of Causes of Menstrual Dysfunction

Disorder	Site of Problem	Cause
Primary Amenorrhea	Hypothalamus	Decreased GnRH
		Poor nutrition
		Exercise
		Stress
	Pituitary	Lesions, tumors
	Ovary	Tumors
		Polycystic ovary syndrome
		Turner's syndrome
	Uterus	Defects
		Urinary tract anomalies
Secondary Amenorrhea	Hypothalamus	Lack of LH surge
		Stress
		Dieting
		Exercise
		Post-birth control pill
		Decreased GnRH
	Pituitary	Tumors
	Ovary	Genetic defects
		Autoimmune, thyroid, or adrenal deficiency
		Myasthenia gravis
		Pernicious anemia
		Mumps oophoritis
		Idiopathic early menopause
		Cancer therapies
		Polycystic ovary syndrome
	Uterus	Severe endometriosis
		Chronic granulomatous disease
Excessive Bleeding	Hypothalamus	Failure of LH surge unopposed by estrogen
	Pituitary	Hyperprolactinemia
	Ovary	Menopause
		Polycystic ovary syndrome
		Decreased androgens
		Estrogensecreting tumor
	Uterus	Pregnancy
		Fibroids
		Polyps
		Cancer
		Adenomyosis
		Cystic hyperplasia
		Inflammatory lesions

Symptom (see scale)	Day of Menstrual Cycle																														
	1	2	3	4	5	6	7	8	9	10	11	12	13	14	15	16	17	18	19	20	21	22	23	24	25	26	27	28	29	30	31
Weight gain																															
Bloating																															
Breast tenderness																															
Headache																															
Dizziness																															
Clumsy																															
Forgetful																															
Pain																															
Flow (see scale)																															

Symptom Scale: 0=none, 1=mild,not disabling, 2=moderate, interferes with activities somewhat, 3=severe and disabling
Flow Scale: 0=none, 1=light, 2=medium, 3=heavy, 4=heavy with clots

Figure 3-5. Sample menstrual diary.

(Figure 3-5). It is estimated that between 10% to 90% of women experience some signs of PMS, with only 10% suffering severe debilitating symptoms. It is believed that symptoms increase when the woman is in her 30s and 40s.[21]

Since 1931, the theory of hormonal imbalance has been advocated as the cause of PMS; however, researchers have been unable to confirm the exact nature of that imbalance. "The wide discrepancies among studies are due to: lack of a standard definition for PMS (patients enrolled in studies are not homogeneous populations; many are self-diagnosed); failure to measure hormones at frequent, standardized intervals (estrogen and progesterone levels change during the luteal phase; patients and control samples must be matched to the day past ovulation by basal body temperature charts or the day of LH surge); and failure to recognize that PMS may have multiple etiologies."[18] Another related theory proposes that the ratio of bound to free circulating hormone may be more important than the absolute concentration. Dalton found lower levels of sex-hormone binding globulin (a specific transport protein to which sex-steroids are bound, and by doing so, become inactive at target tissues) in women with PMS than in controls. This, in turn, would cause an increase in free circulating estrogen, thought to be the only active type. Therefore, the total progesterone/estrogen ratio could be unchanged; while in actuality, the estrogenic activity and symptomatology would increase.[22] Other theories of etiology include psychiatric, diet-related hypoglycemic episodes, decrease in luteal-phase endorphins, lower serotonin levels, and possible vitamin deficiencies of A, B, and E.[21]

Whatever the causes of PMS, treatment has traditionally involved medication recently however, innovative physicians and caregivers have experimented with treatments including diet modification, vitamin and mineral supplementation, psychotherapy, and exercise. Diet therapy includes limitation of caffeine and sodium, and an increase of complex carbohydrates and essential fatty acids, despite cravings that might contradict this philosophy. Of the vitamins and minerals, B6 and magnesium are believed to be of some value; but the dosages must be regulated by a physician because of the potential of toxicity. Psychotherapy has been especially valuable for families struggling to understand a family member's mood swings and unpredictable behavior. Finally, but not least important, is exercise.

Physicians and counselors of PMS patients have acknowledged the value of exercise, not only for PMS, but for a variety of health-related ailments. Aside from the physical benefits of exercise, some physicians are encouraging exercise for other reasons as well. One theory supports exercise as an antidepressant, possibly related to the release of endorphins, believed responsible for promoting a feeling of well being. Endorphin levels rise during the early luteal phase of the menstrual cycle; as the corpus luteum function decreases, the endorphins may decrease and a type of withdrawal, similar to narcotic withdrawal, may account for emotional symptoms.[19] Forms of exercise recommended for PMS symptoms include aerobics, particularly bicycling, swimming, and racewalking. Jogging is not the exercise of choice for premenstrual women because of the potential risk of injury, as well as the possible jarring of pelvic organs and breast irritation. Physical therapists can play a role in designing specific exercise programs to fit in with a woman's current lifestyle, coordinate supportive group exercise programs, or even offer TENS, massage or other modalities for symptoms of muscular aching and headache.

Dysmenorrhea

"Primary and secondary dysmenorrhea represent a source of recurrent disability for about 10% to 15% of women in their early reproductive years."[21] In fact, dysmenorrhea is responsible for the most number of missed school and work days by women. Primary dysmenorrhea may begin shortly after menarche and refers to pain related to excess prostaglandins causing painful uterine muscular contractions. Secondary dysmenorrhea may begin years after onset of menses and refers to pain related to factors external to the uterus, inside the uterine cavity or within the walls of the uterus and occurring during menstruation.

For instance, if there is inflammation altering the pressure around the uterus, restricting blood flow or irritating the peritoneum, symptoms may be noticeable during menstruation.[21] If symptoms occur also at other times than during menstruation, chronic pelvic pain may be the correct diagnosis. In other words, the primary form is associated with normal ovulatory menstrual periods, and the secondary form is associated with pathology. Secondary dysmenorrhea encompasses endometriosis (ectopic endometrial tissue), pelvic inflammatory disease, adenomyosis (endometrial tissue within the uterine wall), fibroids, congenital abnormalities, infections, cervical stenosis or painful menstruation associated with wearing an intrauterine device, among other causes. Besides the local symptoms of dysmenorrhea, women may also experience fatigue, nausea, vomiting, low back pain, diarrhea, headache, or dizziness. Differential diagnoses include acute appendicitis, mechanical back pain, ectopic pregnancy, sexual assault, sexually transmitted diseases, urinary tract infection, ovarian cysts, ovarian torsion, and vaginitis or vulvovaginitis.

Contractions of the uterus are believed to be responsible for the local symptoms of dysmenorrhea. Using electrical potentials and direct measurement, electrical activity is highest during menstruation and lowest during the follicular phase. High-frequency waves occurring every 2 to 4 minutes and lasting 30 to 60 seconds have been recorded, producing intrauterine pressures of 100 mm Hg or more. One source cites pressures exceeding 400 mm Hg with increase above baseline of more than 50 mm Hg during menstruation.[21] This type of contraction is comparable to that of some women's labor. In contrast to a normally progressing labor, however, the contractions may be dysrhythmic, sometimes escalating to uterine tetany.

Prostaglandins are synthesized by the endometrium and cause contraction of uterine smooth muscle. In fact, prostaglandins in greater quantities have been identified in the menstrual flow of dysmenorrheic women.[15] This discovery has led to high success rate in some studies with prostaglandinsynthetase inhibitors to relieve menstrual cramping, especially if administered during the first 6 to 12 hours of menstruation when the most severe contractions occur on average.[15] Because prostaglandins affect smooth muscle, contractions elsewhere may be responsible for the nausea, vomiting and diarrhea.[21] Oral contraceptives have also been used in conjunction with nonsteroidal anti-inflammatory medications to inhibit prostaglandin synthesis and prevent ovulation.

Another possible cause of dysmenorrhea is estrogen/progesterone imbalance, but little objective evidence has been collected to support this hypothesis. In addition, placebo administration has relieved certain symptoms in dysmenorrheic patients, suggesting a possible psychogenic component, as well, particularly in women whose mothers had similar menstrual problems. It is more recently the opinion of specialists that psychogenic symptoms may be associated with some dysmenorrheic patients, but that these symptoms are not necessarily the cause of physical complaints. Herbal remedies have sometimes been effective.

Women with dysmenorrhea may also complain of lower abdominal pain, suprapubic pain, pain radiating down the anterior or inner thighs and perineum, or low back pain that is spasmodic in nature. Physical therapists can offer TENS, heat, massage and instruction in exercise. Studies have been published documenting successful treatment of dysmenorrhea with TENS.[16,23,24] Lewers and colleagues attempted to replicate a previous study by Neighbors in which significant differences in relief were found between TENS patients and controls receiving placebo. The Lewers and coworkers study did not replicate this significant difference between groups. However, it was postulated that because their method involved the pre and post-TENS treatment measurement of electrical conductance activity at auricular acupuncture points (for uterus, endocrine, low back, and ovary), any significant differences in pain relief from TENS could have been overshadowed by that obtained via auricular acupressure. As is often true with multiple studies that do not control for exactly the same factors, controversy occurs. These women's symptoms may have merely subsided during the time frame of the study (4 hour no medication period, 30 minute treatment/placebo, and pre and post-treatment auricular measurements, plus 3 hour followup, and following next a.m. wake up). Relief from dysmenorrheic symptoms measured over time may not be valid over an average 12 hour span, if, indeed, symptoms caused by uterine contractions normally subside during this time. However, whether or not this is indeed a placebo/Hawthorne effect, relief via TENS or acupressure can certainly be argued as a less invasive means than prostaglandinsynthetase inhibitors and other medications and should be considered an option for treatment.

Various new products have come on the market and researchers continue to examine different parameters with the TENS device. Two studies by Kaplan, et al examined the efficacy of TENS versus medications and reported over 86% had either marked or moderate pain relief with TENS versus analgesics used for primary dysmenorrhea.[25,266] Effects of high intensity TENS were compared to effects of oral naproxen (500 mg) on the intrauterine pressures and menstrual pain in 12 women. Pain relief was achieved by both modalities, the naproxen relieving pain slightly earlier and lasting longer than the TENS. No change in uterine activity was noted with the TENS, yet pain relief in a segmental fashion was achieved from 30 to 60 minutes after the treatment.[27] TENS and ibuprofen were compared for pain relief of primary dysmenorrhea in 32 women over two cycles. Women received either TENS for two cycles, placebo TENS for one cycle or ibuprofen (400 mg as needed up to 4 times/day) for one cycle. TENS was set at 100 pulses per second with a 100-microsecond pulse width and patient-adjusted amplitude. TENS was found to delay the need for ibuprofen by almost 6 hours. Good to excellent pain relief was recorded in over 40% of the subjects. The best combination was TENS plus a reduced amount of ibuprofen for pain relief in this population.[28] Therefore, practitioners can conclude that the parameters and devices used to help women with primary dysmenorrhea are still under investigation.

Other modalities tried for pain relief of primary dysmenorrhea, though not commonly used, include spinal manipulation, microwave diathermy, and contrast baths. Studies at schools of osteopathy and chiropractic examined the effects of high-velocity, low-amplitude spinal manipulation on electromyographic readings, circulating plasma levels of prostaglandin, women's perceived abdominal pain, back pain and menstrual distress.[29,30] Results based on treatment with 12 women revealed some relief of low back pain associated with reduced EMG activity in the deep lumbar musculature. However, both spinal manipulation and sham manipulation reduced plasma levels of prostaglandin and reduced perceived pain and level of menstrual distress in the spinal manipulation group. Microwave diathermy (45 W for 20 minutes) on the first day of symptoms has been shown to relieve pain. One study reported that a woman with severe primary dysmenorrhea resulting in loss of 1 to 3 work days/month, did not respond to pharmacologic intervention or heat, but with the diathermy she received immediate and lasting relief resulting in no missed days of work for a 7-month period.[31] Contrast baths were believed to be effective for women with primary dysmenorrhea related to neuroendocrine system dysfunction as reflected in psychoemotional and other tests of brain response.[32]

PELVIC PAIN: ACUTE AND CHRONIC

Aside from the disabling effects of dysmenorrhea, gynecologic pathologies such as peritoneal infiltration of endometrial cells, growth of cancerous cells, sexually transmitted diseases and anatomic obstructions may cause severe pain. Indeed, one large study of over 5,000 U.S. women aged 18 to 50 years found that approximately one in seven are affected by chronic pelvic pain. "Estimated direct medical costs for outpatient visits for chronic pelvic pain for the U.S. population of women aged 18 to 50 years are $881.5 million per year."[33] Of about 500 women who were employed, over half reported either time lost from paid work or reduced work productivity.[33] Other causes of pelvic pain include: infection, ovarian cyst, fibroid tumors, ulcerative colitis, irritable bowel syndrome, diverticulitis, mesenteric adenitis, biliary disease, constipation, herniation, parasites, aneurysm, radiculopathy, spondylolisthesis, ankylosing spondylitis, strains, shingles, physical or sexual abuse, stress, and more. Acute pain may be caused by hemorrhage, rupture of a cyst, ischemia, ectopic pregnancy or bowel perforation.[14]

Physical therapists are more likely to be involved with treatment of chronic pelvic pain from musculoskeletal causes, pelvic varicosities, dyspareunia or pelvic relaxation. Today, physicians are more willing to view chronic pelvic pain as having an organic cause rather than solely a psychogenic one,[21] yet referrals do not come automatically. In a study concerned with the frequency of laparoscopic surgery used to diagnose problems in women with chronic pelvic pain, 30% of 500 women had pain related to urologic, myofascial, musculoskeletal, gastrointestinal or psychological causes. Other studies also attribute chronic pelvic pain to non-gynecologic sources.[34-40] In fact, one group of researchers found that hysterectomy did not relieve long-term pelvic pain in up to 40% of the 308 women in their study.[41] Of the other women who had gynecologic sources of pain, endometriosis was the primary finding in almost three-fourths.[42] Yet, several studies suggest that endometriosis still might not be the sole source of that pain.[39,43-51]

Endometriosis is estimated to affect 1% to 2% of all women and 30% to 50% of infertile women. Endometriosis is a pathologic condition of endometrial tissue, which normally lines the uterus, growing in extrauterine locations such as the ovaries, uterine ligaments, cervix, pelvic peritoneum, rectovaginal septum, appendix, umbilicus, laparotomy and episiotomy scars, and even pleural or pericardial cavities.[15] It has been estimated that more than half the teenagers who report chronic pelvic pain will show evidence of endometriosis during laparoscopic exploration.[15] Although the actual cause of endometrial tissue growth in extrauterine sites is unknown, practitioners are becoming more aware of its potential as a cause of infertility, cyclic rectal bleeding, or a number of other clinical signs. In a study of 160 women with endometriosis and no other gynecologic disease, 78% reported dysmenorrhea, 39% reported pelvic pain, and 32% reported deep dyspareunia.

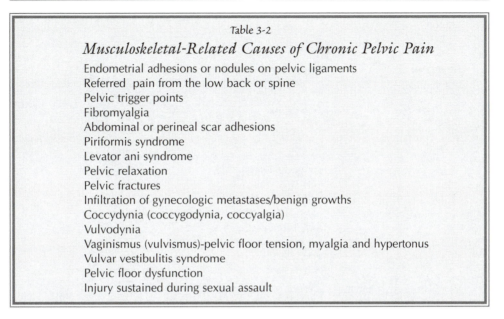

Table 3-2

Musculoskeletal-Related Causes of Chronic Pelvic Pain

Endometrial adhesions or nodules on pelvic ligaments
Referred pain from the low back or spine
Pelvic trigger points
Fibromyalgia
Abdominal or perineal scar adhesions
Piriformis syndrome
Levator ani syndrome
Pelvic relaxation
Pelvic fractures
Infiltration of gynecologic metastases/benign growths
Coccydynia (coccygodynia, coccyalgia)
Vulvodynia
Vaginismus (vulvismus)-pelvic floor tension, myalgia and hypertonus
Vulvar vestibulitis syndrome
Pelvic floor dysfunction
Injury sustained during sexual assault

Each month, when the ovarian hormones signal the uterine lining to duplicate and enlarge to prepare for a fertilized egg, the extrauterine endometrial cells also respond. However, the extrauterine cells are unable to separate from the tissue to slough off, so they may bleed and heal repetitively, causing scarring and adhesions. If adhesions occur in the fallopian tubes or other areas, transport of a fertilized egg may be hindered. Endometrial tissues in the ovaries can cause cysts and adhesions from the large bowel to the pelvic sidewalls are implicated as sources of pain.[52] Symptoms may include increasingly painful periods, moderate to severe lower abdominal pain before or during menstruation, pelvic or low back pain during menstruation, irregular menstrual cycles, premenstrual spotting, pain during or after intercourse, pain on defecation, and infertility. Tender nodules may be found in healed wound scars such as from episiotomy or cesarean section or in uterine ligaments, especially the uterosacral.

In fact, the most common site for endometrial growth is on the uterosacral ligaments, and the patient may present with pelvic pain extending deep between the rectum and vagina. Pain during menstruation, especially with referred pain to the rectum, lower sacrum, or coccyx, can be debilitating. Scarring and adhesions are characteristics of this condition, but the extent of involvement does not necessarily coincide with the severity of symptoms. Pain or infertility are the usual indications for treatment, either with medication or surgery. Oral contraceptives may be prescribed to simulate pregnancy, during which some researchers noted a regression of endometriosis. However, the use of oral contraceptives does not prevent the scarring and adhesions. Other medications have had limited success as well, including antigonadotropins to decrease ovarian estrogen production. No medications so far have proven completely successful. Surgery may attempt to remove all extrauterine endometrial tissue and may involve neurectomy to relieve pain. Laparoscopic surgery resulted in improvement in over 80% of 110 women treated surgically to remove endometrial tissue in uterosacral ligaments with decrease in symptoms related to dysmenorrhea and dyspareunia.[53] Total abdominal hysterectomy is sometimes recommended if pregnancy is no longer desired.

Other causes of pelvic pain are listed in Table 3-2. Physical therapists have a role in helping women seek the proper help for pelvic pain. Most physical therapists are aware of the concepts of referred pain and trigger points. Physicians are increasingly aware that pelvic pain may

Table 3-3

Assessment of Pelvic Pain[1]

Symptoms	Suggested Areas to Assess
Coccygeal pain	pelvic ligaments
Rectal pain	perineum
Episiotomy scar pain	scar tissue pelvic floor/rectal musculature posture abdominal strength coccyx hip/trunk musculature
Abdominal scar pain	posture spinal range of motion lower extremity range of motion strength pelvic floor musculature
Pelvic floor hypertonus/ spasm/tension	posture neurologic biofeedback internal exam/external palpation abdominal strength trigger points lower extremity strength and range of motion pelvic joint integrity emotional status infection/illness

be related to muscular, nerve or soft tissue disorders. The physical therapist and physician can work well together with the physician first ruling out gynecologic concerns and pathology. The woman who is referred for evaluation of pain will require a thorough musculoskeletal examination from head to toe. Referred pelvic pain may originate from the spine or hip, from alignment problems, joint dysfunction or nerve compression. In these situations, orthopedic assessment and treatment is indicated. Several muscular pain syndromes have been identified that affect the pelvic region and are associated with muscle spasm or "hypertonus dysfunctions," including piriformis syndrome, levator ani syndrome, coccydynia, vulvodynia, and vaginismus.[1,54] (Tables 3-3 and 3-4).

Piriformis syndrome has been described in the orthopedic literature since 1928, yet controversy exists as to whether it is indeed an accurate diagnosis and if the treatment for it is appropriate.[55] Piriformis syndrome has been described as a "common cause of buttock and leg pain as a result of injury to the piriformis muscle," with symptoms ranging from buttock tenderness "from the sacrum to the greater trochanter and piriformis tenderness on rectal or pelvic examination."[56] Sciatic paresthesia may occur from nerve entrapment as the sciatic nerve passes under or through the muscle. Dyspareunia has also been reported.[57] Efforts are being made, however, to confirm this syndrome exists through magnetic resonance imaging, computed tomography, and electromyography to detect tension in the piriformis. Stretching is believed to be particularly effective.[57,58] (See Chapter 7 for treatment of piriformis syndrome.)

Levator ani syndrome refers to pain caused by levator ani spasm with irritation of the pudendal nerve. The result may be tenderness in the coccygeal area and chronic rectal pain.

Table 3-4

Treatment of Pelvic Pain[1,54]

Disorder	Selected Modalities
Episiotomy scar pain	ultrasound pelvic floor exercises scar massage
Abdominal scar pain	therapeutic exercise scar massage mobility training postural training myofascial techniques
Pelvic floor hypertonus and pelvic trigger points	therapeutic exercise myofascial techniques deep tissue massage joint mobilization muscle energy stretching exercises friction massage relaxation exercises postural education mobility training biofeedback TENS Interferential/NMES High volt pulsed current Ultrasound Heat/cold agents

Physical therapists have experimented with stretching, massage, heat, electrical stimulation and neuromuscular reeducation.[1,54] Biofeedback has been effective in reducing pain related to levator ani syndrome.[59] A variation of levator ani spasm, also referred to as tension myalgia of the pelvic floor or levator syndrome, may be "intercourse-related vaginal pain syndrome."[60] This syndrome is not to be confused with vulvar vestibulitis, which includes symptoms of severe burning pain on vaginal dilation. Intercourse-related vaginal pain syndrome as described in the literature resolves with term vaginal delivery.[60] (See Chapter 7 for treatment of coccyx dysfunctions.)

In contrast, vulvar vestibulitis is believed to be a form of vulvodynia which may result from vulvovaginal pathogens and is associated with vulvar erythema, tenderness and hypersensitivity of the vestibule, and dyspareunia.[61,62] Vulvodynia may include a variety of symptoms with or without urinary incontinence, but always with vulvar pain. Pudendal nerve block and decompression has been attempted to relieve vulvodynia with some success, but differential diagnosis seems to be the key to the treatment of pain syndromes of the pelvic floor and vulvar area.[63] The chronic pain of vulvar vestibulitis must also be differentiated from actual inflammatory process in response to infection. Medications and surgery have been attempted for chronic pain patients, with recent trials of electromyographic biofeedback of pelvic floor musculature successful in some women.[61,62,64] Criteria to establish the diagnosis more accurately are being developed.[64] Attempts to profile the typical woman with vulvar vestibulitis describe a woman in her 20s, but a strong association between musculoskeletal disorders and gynecological disease was found in women 40 to 42 years old, ie, women with more symptoms and diseases of the genital tract had significantly more musculoskeletal diseases as well.[65] It is unclear whether this finding is simply a factor associated with middle age.

Another cause of pelvic pain is trauma, which may result in fractures, pelvic dislocations or coccydynia. Pelvic fractures were studied in Sweden over a 10-year period. Severe trauma was required to fracture the pelvis in women under 60 years, with more than 80% fracturing the pubic rami.[66] Other injuries may occur at the time of fracture—sciatic nerve injury, soft tissue or symphyseal damage, urethral injuries, vulvar edema, vaginal bleeding, bladder contusions or rupture.[67,68] Treatment for pelvic fractures includes gait training, stabilization exercises, and mobility training. Chronic pain and dyspareunia can result from pelvic fractures and soft tissue damage.

Ligamentous damage may result from delivery trauma or pelvic instability during pregnancy. Terms like pelvic relaxation, pelvic joint syndrome, physiological pelvic girdle relaxation and symptomatic pelvic girdle relaxation can be confusing, but some researchers have assigned the term pelvic relaxation to the loss of the support of internal pelvic organs, physiological pelvic girdle relaxation to the normal softening of ligaments during pregnancy to allow room for the fetus and womb, symptomatic pelvic girdle relaxation to the pelvic instability following pregnancy which resolves spontaneously, and pelvic joint syndrome if pain persists in pelvic joints several months after pregnancy.[69,70] Physical therapists may be involved in the care of all of these conditions.

Pelvic dislocation may rarely occur during a difficult delivery. The symphysis pubis or sacroiliac joints may rupture and pain and neuropathy may result. The authors of related studies recommend conservative treatment with a binder, assistive devices for ambulation, and mobility training, with surgical reduction if symptoms persist.[71,72] The effects of such dislocation or rupture may be long-reaching, however. A Dutch study reported that women may experience increased pelvic pain during subsequent pregnancies or around menstruation. "It is hypothesized that peripartum pelvic pain is caused by strain of ligaments in the pelvis and lower spine resulting from a combination of damage to ligaments (recently or in the past), hormonal effects, muscle weakness, and the weight of the fetus."[73] Another study in the United Kingdom identified 1 in 800 women with symptoms from 2 months to 57 months post-partum. Pubic symphysis separation was confirmed by an abnormal interpubic gap on ultrasonography in all women with symptoms.[74]

Coccydynia may occur not only as a result of trauma from falls or delivery, but from scar adhesions from hysterectomy or episiotomy, sexual abuse or poor sitting posture tilting the pelvis back onto the coccyx. Symptoms arising from coccydynia include: dyspareunia, referred pain to the lower back, sacroiliac area, hip, buttock or groin, difficulty sitting for longer periods, hemorrhoids, and general pelvic relaxation with concomitant muscle imbalance and chronic pain. Coccydynia often responds to gentle internal muscle release techniques (see Chapter 7 on treatment of coccyx dysfunctions for details of techniques and illustration). If perineal or abdominal scarring are sources of pain, techniques for scar management may be appropriate, including massage, ultrasound, and myofascial treatment.[1] If pain results from muscle spasm, weak muscles, tight muscles, muscular imbalance, or nerve compressions or entrapment, other modalities may be effective as well.[54] Contraindications for modalities would include pregnancy, localized infection, malignancies or precancerous lesions, vascular and blood disorders, and insensate areas.

Similarly, various types of body work are indicated for treatment of fibromyalgia, which has been classified by the American College of Rheumatology to occur when a woman has widespread pain in at least 11 or 18 diagnostic points for at least 3 months. These diagnostic points include two each at the neck, throat, shoulder, scapula, rib, elbow, buttocks, hip, and knee. Women with fibromyalgia may also complain of muscular pain, fatigue, insomnia, joint pains, headaches, restless legs, numbness and tingling, impaired memory, leg cramps, impaired concentration, nervousness, and depression. Fibromyalgia may also be associated with irritable bowel syndrome, with symptoms of irregular bowel movements, nausea, diarrhea, constipation, and abdominal gas.[75]

One study of women with chronic pelvic pain and irritable bowel syndrome found an association with lifetime history of depression, panic disorder, somatization disorder, childhood sexual abuse and hysterectomy.[76] Often women who experience pelvic pain have had their symptoms for many years without a confirming diagnosis from a physician. They have frequently seen many doctors in pursuit of information and relief of their pain. Consequently, in frustration, these patients may seem desperate and isolated. They may also experience anger at the medical establishment for not supplying them with answers or assistance. These women often have refrained from sexual relations due to pain and experience strain in their relationships. Generally women with pelvic pain are anxious to try anything that may help them and have often read a great deal about the subject and at times find comfort in support groups (see Appendix).

Following hysterectomy, which may be total (removal of the entire uterus) or partial (removal of the uterine body only) and which may occur through vaginal or abdominal approach, physical therapists can provide the woman with mobility training, gait training, pain reduction methods, scar management, massage to reduce abdominal distention, deep breathing training, and positioning. Neuromuscular re-education is occasionally also necessary as there have been documented cases of sciatic neuropathy and bilateral femoral neuropathy following vaginal hysterectomy.[77,78] Besides cancer, other conditions that may be treated with hysterectomy include: heavy uncontrollable bleeding, fibroids (benign tumors of the uterus), recurrent uncontrolled infection, endometriosis, complications of childbirth where life is threatened, and occasionally for prolapse of the uterus and other internal organs. Various pain reduction methods have been utilized in the management of post-hysterectomy pain. TENS, electroacupuncture, and percutaneous electrical stimulation implants have met with some success in reducing post-hysterectomy.[79-81]

Finally, unremitting pelvic pain may result from gynecologic cancer. According to the Women's Cancer Network, part of the Gynecologic Cancer Foundation, "on average, every 64 minutes a woman in this country will be diagnosed with a cancer of the reproductive organs: ovarian, uterine, cervical, vulvar, vaginal or tubal. Each year approximately 82,000 women will be told they have one of these diseases. Youth doesn't protect you from this disease — it strikes women in their teens as well as post-menopausal women over 50."[82] Ovarian cancer is the fifth leading cause of cancer death among U.S. women, and over half of the women diagnosed with it die within 5 years.[83] The physical therapist dealing with assessment and treatment of chronic pelvic pain must consider the possibility of cancer as a cause. The characteristics of each cancer are listed in Table 3-5.[21] Most cancers are treated with surgical excision if possible, followed by some combination of chemotherapy, radiation or alternative treatments. Physical therapists may be involved in pain reduction, mobility training, gait training, and strength and endurance training for women with musculoskeletal problems associated with cancer. Physical therapists may be called to care for women post-mastectomy, post-hysterectomy, post-abdominal surgery, or post-vaginal surgery.

Table 3-5

Characteristics of Gynecologic Cancers[21]

Type	Risk Factors	Symptoms	5-Year Survival Rate (mets=metastases)
Ovarian	familial never pregnant oral contraceptive use women over 50 women with breast cancer	abdominal swelling/ fullness vaginal bleeding indigestion bowel/ rectal pressure abdominal pressure	92% if local 20% if mets
Uterine	women between 55-70 obesity early menstruation late menopause few or no children estrogen replacement therapy	abnormal bleeding after menopause increasing pelvic pressure	50% (sarcoma)
Cervical	women over 40	abnormal bleeding/ discharge	90% if local
Vulvar	women over 50/under 40	constant burning/ itching/pain change in vulvar appearance abnormal bleeding/ discharge	90% if local 20% if mets
Vaginal	DES in pregnancy women 60-80 (squamous) women 12-30 (adenocarcinoma)	irregular bleeding/ discharge dyspareunia pain on urination pelvic pain	50% squamous 80% adenocarcinoma
Tubal	post-menopausal women	abnormal bleeding/ discharge	70% if local 35-45% if mets
Breast	women over 40	breast mass nipple and skin changes	90% if local 50-70% if mets

URINARY DISORDERS

Pelvic pain syndromes or causes can result in urinary or bowel disorders, which have been alluded to in the prior discussion. However, because the physical therapist has developed a role in the treatment of musculoskeletal and neurologic disorders, practitioners are gaining a stronger position in the treatment of incontinence. The pubourethral ligament, sling of Heiss, deep trigonal musculature, levator ani muscles and the urogenital diaphragm maintain the relative position of the urethra to the urinary bladder (refer to Figure 2-12). Aging, injury, or childbirth are believed to alter the integrity of the pubourethral ligament; when

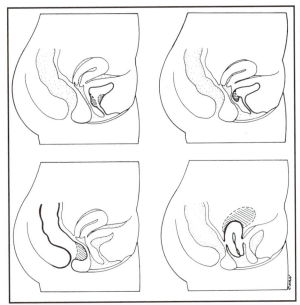

Figure 3-6. Types of pelvic relaxation from top left, clockwise; cystocele, enterocele, prolapse and rectocele (Reprinted with permission from O'Connor LJ, Gourley Stephenson RJ. *Obstetrics and Gynecologic Care in Physical Therapy.* Thorofare, NJ: SLACK Incorporated; 1990.)

combined with pelvic floor weakness, the bladder rotates posteriorly and the urethra falls from its position in the "abdominal pressure zone."[84]

This abdominal pressure zone actually refers to the pressures on the urinary bladder imposed by normal intra-abdominal pressure. Within the bladder (intravesical pressure), the pressure force is the sum of this intra-abdominal pressure plus the detrusor contractions. Intra-abdominal pressure is sometimes estimated by balloon catheter measured via the rectum. This pressure can be increased voluntarily when a woman strains, coughs, or performs the Valsalva maneuver. Urologists have devised ways to measure the detrusor contraction pressure by subtracting intravesical pressure from the intra-abdominal pressure measured rectally. With all these pressures acting on the bladder, how does the bladder hold urine? Fortunately, the bladder connects to a urinary sphincter before leading to the urethra. Maintaining urine in the bladder depends simply on the pressure in the urethra being greater than the pressure in the bladder. To urinate, a woman must relax the urethra to reduce the intraurethral pressure. Detrusor contractions follow to expel urine. Flow, normally at a rate of 20 to 30 ml/sec^2 at midflow (maximal), stops when the bladder is empty. The rate can be enhanced by increasing intra-abdominal pressure.

But what happens when the woman is unable to relax the urethra, detrusor contractions are weak, or the intra-abdominal pressure is reduced because of poor position of the bladder? Frequently, incontinence is the result. In addition to pelvic pain, multiple factors can lead to incontinence including relaxation of pelvic structures (Figure 3-6) (urethrocele, cystocele, enterocele, rectocele, prolapses, and vaginal outlet), fistulas (urethrovaginal, vesicovaginal, uterovaginal, rectovaginal), and neurologic dysfunction. Conditions that contribute to incontinence include pregnancy and childbirth, urinary tract or vaginal infections, sphincter weakness, pelvic relaxation, radiation therapy, pelvic injury or surgery, hormonal deficiency and neurologic diseases, eg, stroke, parkinsonism, or multiple sclerosis. Relaxed ligamentous and fascial structures, similar to those mentioned with the sling of Heiss, contribute to "celes" from the Greek word for hernia. The urethra, bladder, rectum, or posterior vagina may herniate into the vaginal canal. These herniations are described as first degree, second degree, or third degree, third degree being the most severe. The symptoms of

Table 3-6
Spinal Cord Reflexes Associated with Micturition[84]

Storage of Urine

Sympathetic detrusor inhibiting reflex
Sympathetic sphincter constrictor reflex
Perineodetrusor inhibitory reflex
Urethrosphincteric guarding reflex

Initiation of Flow

Perineobulbar detrusor facilitative reflex
Detrusodetrusor facilitative reflex

Control the Flow

Detrusourethral inhibitory reflex
Detrusosphincteric inhibitory reflex
Urethrodetrusor facilitative reflex
Urethrodetrusor facilitative reflex II
Urethrosphincteric inhibitory reflex

Stop the Flow

Perineobulbar detrusor inhibitory reflex

each, however, can be quite different. A cystocele may cause no incontinence, in fact, no symptoms at all, until the posterior urethrovesical angle becomes so acute that the patient has difficulty initiating voiding, or retains urine, leading to a urinary tract infection. In the patient with an urethrocele, on the other hand, the posterior urethrovesical angle decreases to the point that incontinence results. Enteroceles produce few symptoms until severe; they may herniate through the vagina. Often accompanying an enterocele is a rectocele, which may block bowel movement. Although there are other causes, fistulas (unnatural openings) usually result from carcinoma or trauma, sometimes as a result of other gynecologic surgery. In the United States, this surgery is commonly abdominal hysterectomy. In a severe vesicovaginal fistula, the urinary stream may be continuous through the vagina. Less severe fistulas of this type may cause intermittent watery vaginal discharge. The treatment for large fistulas is almost always surgery.

Four neurologic pathways have been identified in the control of micturition: cerebral cortexbrain stem detrusor nucleus (loop I), brain stem spinal detrusor muscle nucleus/sacral (loop II), bladder sacralurethral sphincter (loop III), and sacral-cerebral (loop IV).[15] Voluntary control is mediated by loops I and IV, the former over the micturition reflex, and the latter over the striated external urethral sphincter. The fourth mediates voluntary control. The second and third loops regulate detrusor contractions to empty the bladder and coordinate the efforts between the detrusor and the urethra. In addition to these links to the cerebrum and brain stem, there are four reflexes that assist in continence and storage of urine, two that assist in initiation of flow, five that coordinate the actual flow, and one that stops the flow and reestablishes storage mode. With 12 reflexes (Table 3-6), it is a wonder that this system works so well in so many people for as long as it does.[84] Three basic reflex mechanisms are involved: a vesicosympathetic reflex to relax the bladder and tighten the urethra, a vesicoparasympathetic reflex to contract the detrusor and relax the urethra, and

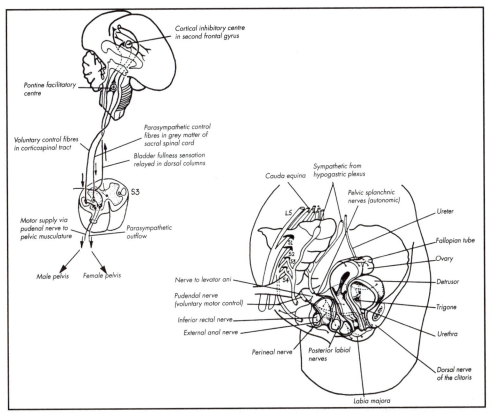

Figure 3-7. Micturition pathways in the female.

a vesicopudendal reflex at S3 which controls the striated pelvic floor musculature and the external sphincter which is inhibited upon micturition. "Micturition involves complete relaxation of volitional control. The external sphincter and pelvic floor relax and the local reflex is allowed to take over. As the detrusor contracts, the bladder neck is pulled open and this combined with inhibition of the weak internal sphincter, allows urine to flow by combination of rising intravesical pressure and gravity."[85] (Figure 3-7).

Physical examination by a urologist or gynecologic urologist includes checks for hernias, prolapse, pelvic relaxation, fistulae, or diverticula. Tests that may easily be performed by the physical therapist include neuromotor evaluation of sensory and motor function of the lower extremities and of the voluntary sphincters. Standard tests for lower extremity sensation via dermal distribution should be performed, as well as tests of motor strength for lumbar and sacral nerves. Deep tendon reflexes should also be evaluated at the knee and ankle, as well femoral, popliteal, and pedal pulses. It is believed that control over the external voluntary anal sphincter links to control of the pelvic floor musculature, so anal sphincter integrity is assessed as well. Should expected responses not occur, the problem may be related to central or peripheral nerve dysfunction and referral to a neurologist is warranted.[84]

Urinary incontinence is classified by international standards.[86] (See summary Table 3-7, and Table 3-8) Although stress incontinence is a term bandied about, it can result from many disorders. "The term stress incontinence, on its own, only designates the symptom and the sign, but is not the diagnosis."[84] Types of urinary incontinence include genuine stress, urge, mixed, reflex, and overflow. Genuine stress incontinence is pressure-related. One

Table 3-7
Urinary Incontinence Classification by the International Continence Society

Problem	Types	Symptoms
Failure to Store	1. Overactive bladder	Urge incontinence, elevated bladder pressure
	2. Underactive outlet	Stress incontinence, decreased outlet resistance
Failure to Empty	1. Underactive bladder	Decreased bladder pressure
	2. Overactive outlet	Increased outlet resistance

Table 3-8
Anatomic and physiologic explanations for types of incontinence[1]

Problem	Types	Symptoms
Reflex Incontinence	1. Detrusor hyperreflexia (suprasacral lesion)	Any amount of urine leakage without warning
	2. Detrusor areflexia (Infrasacral lesion)	Any amount of urine leakage without warning
	3. Involuntary sphincter relaxation	Any amount of urine leakage without warning
Stress Urinary Incontinence		Involuntary loss of urine during physical exertion
Urge Incontinence	1a. Motor-detrusor instability	Loss of urine occurring with a strong desire to urinate with little warning
	b. Detrusor hyperreflexia	Reflex incontinence
	2. Sensory urge	Frequency and urgency
	3. Detrusor hyperactivity with impaired contractility	Seen in the elderly, obstructive or stress symptoms
	4. Urethral instability	
Mixed Stress and Urge Incontinence		Leakage with both movement and urge. She urinates and goes just in case
Overflow Incontinence	1. Outlet obstruction from prolapse, tumor, stricture, tight sling repair or constipation	Urine leaks and dribbles when bladder overfills. Can have urge or stress symptoms. Reduced urine stream, tenderness of the suprapubic region, enlargement of the bladder.
	2. Underactive detrusor: neurologic or systemic illness, sacral neuropathy	
	3. Functional incontinence	Leakage when mobility, dexterity or cognition is impaired. No urinary tract dysfunction.
	4.Iatrogenic incontinence- caused by health care provider	Change in bladder symptoms post-operatively, or after starting a new or changing medication.

exceeds the other. As a symptom, stress incontinence occurs when exercising, coughing, sneezing or laughing; as a sign, it occurs as intra-abdominal pressure increases. Genuine stress incontinence should be differentiated from an unstable bladder, in which physical stress results in a delayed loss of urine as detrusor contractions occur that the patient cannot control. A patient may have both types of incontinence problems, however. Two studies suggest that almost half of all pregnant women experience genuine stress incontinence, and about 10% to 20% may have episodes of urge incontinence by the third trimester.[87] Urge incontinence is loss of urine with a strong urge to urinate. It may have a motor component (uninhibited detrusor activity) or sensory component. Although treatment of this type usually focuses on the bladder, recent studies suggest unstable urethra may be a factor with or without unstable bladder.[88] Mixed incontinence is a combination of stress and urge. Reflex incontinence, again, may occur without a sensation to urinate and is related to neurologic dysfunction. Overflow incontinence is caused by a bladder that does not respond to stretch feedback. (Enuresis, a subset of incontinence, is any involuntary loss, particularly bothersome as nocturnal enuresis or bedwetting, during sleep.)

Other noninvasive tests for types of incontinence, excluding flow studies (urodynamics), include stress tests, voiding diaries, and pad tests. The stress, or cough, test requires the patient to cough while standing. Small amounts of urinary leakage when coughing suggest genuine stress incontinence. If leakage is considerable, or occurs after the cough, an unstable bladder (patient cannot control detrusor contractions) may be responsible. The patient who keeps a voiding diary records times during the day when incontinence occurs, amount of fluid intake and urinary output, as well as whether an urge is associated with leakage. One-hour and 12-hour pad tests may be conducted to assess the effect of normal activities on continence. The pads are weighed to determine volume of urine output over time.[84]

Methods of physical therapy management for genuine stress incontinence include pelvic floor (Kegel) exercise instruction, resistive pelvic floor exercise (vaginal weights), dietary counseling to avoid diuretic and bladder-irritating substances (such as caffeine), biofeedback via perineometer and or sEMG, and electrical stimulation. Instruction in pelvic floor exercise should be offered to any woman who comes in for physical therapy. Dr. Arnold Kegel conducted several studies to assess the efficacy of strengthening pelvic floor musculature to control continence. He and others reported improvement in three-fourths of women included in study samples.[89] In the "Kegel" or pelvic floor exercise, loop IV is activated to use cortical impulses to contract fast twitch and slow twitch, striated periurethral sphincter muscles via the pudendal nerve It is believed that these muscle fibers can hypertrophy with prolonged training, but physicians and patients may become impatient with this method. No optimal number of repetitions has been standardized, but several protocols have been proposed[54] for strengthening, endurance, and functional retraining. Exercise training for the pelvic floor is as specific as for any other muscle group, and may depend on the tissue integrity of each woman, often a factor of age[90] and race.[91] Although early studies suggested isolation of the pubococcygeus muscle was the optimal way to strengthen it, more recently practitioners believe that overflow contractions through lower extremity and abdominal muscle contractions may enhance pelvic floor muscle training.[54,92] Evaluation, therefore, may include external and internal assessment. Additionally see the section on Teaching About Pelvic Floor Toning in Chapter 4 and Table 4-20, Handout for Pelvic Floor Exercises and Table 3-9, Exercise Prescription for Pelvic Floor Strengthening for a variety of ways to teach pelvic floor exercises.

Table 3-9

Exercise Prescription for Pelvic Floor Strengthening

Adapted from Lynne Assad, PT, from seminar notes from "Evaluation and Treatment for Urinary Incontinence for Physical Therapist". August 1999.[93]

Goal is to perform maximal isometric contraction. The duration of one maximal contraction is more important than the duration of any contraction(DiNubile)

• Long Holds: Overload the muscle by 2+ seconds of what was determined by subjective report, internal exam or sEMG of when the muscle fades in contraction. Prescribe 8-10 maximal repetitions of this hold time.(DiNibule) Rest twice as long as the length of time that the contraction was held.

• Quick Flicks: "Squeeze and let go". Use rapid, maximal squeezes with good techniques. Overload 2 repetitions determined by subjective report, internal exam or sEMG of when the muscle fades in contraction. Stress the importance of completely letting go between each contraction. Amount of repetitions is not as important as the speed of initiation of contraction.

• Complete 3-5 sessions per day

Incorporate functional use of the pelvic floor by contracting prior to and during activities which normally create leakage: coughing, laughing, sneezing, lifting and jumping.

• Self Progression-
  • First 3-5 days do exercise as prescribed. Monitor muscle soreness. Watch for signs of overuse which include suprapubic soreness, rectal pain, constipation, and worsening of leakage.
  • During first set each day, retest and hold time and number of quick flicks. Add two seconds to hold time and two repetitions to quick flicks and work up to 8-10 repetitions of long holds. Good proprioception and body awareness are necessary for true increase of muscle bulk and tone. (Bo)

• Duration of exercise period
  • Three to six months (Tschou, Adams, Bo 1990)
  • Initially there is more effective recruitment of motor units and increased frequency of excitation (Di Nubile)
  • Increase in cross sectional area takes at least 5 months (Bo)

• Encourage general fitness

References

DiNubile NA. Strength training. *Clin Sports Med.* 10(1):33-62,1991.

Bo K, Hagen RH, Kvarstein B, Jorgensen J, Larsen S. Pelvic floor muscle exercise for the treatment of female stress urinary incontinence: III. Effects of two different degrees of pelvic floor muscle exercises. *Neurourol and Urodyn.* 9:489-502. 1990.

Tschou D, Adams C Varner RE, Denton B. Pelvic floor musculature exercises in treatment of anatomical urinary stress incontinence. *Phys Ther.* 68:652-655. 1988.

PELVIC FLOOR TRAINING

The goals for pelvic floor training are to:
• Increase the muscular shelf which supports the bladder, vagina/uterus and rectum which will improve the urethrovesical angle so the bladder neck remains sealed.
• Improve strength and response time of fast fibers of the external urethral sphincter during sudden increases intra-abdominal pressure(ie, during coughing, sneezing, lifting and jumping).
• Dampen any hyperactivity of the autonomic pelvic nerve to the bladder which causes urge incontinence. Clinically named detrusor instability.[93]

Initial Training

• Describe a proper contraction of the pelvic floor muscles and instruct in a quick flick with no holding, and a long hold which is a contraction holding for 10 seconds.
• Give verbal cues: "pull up and in, close the vagina and rectum, squeeze as if holding in a tampon while pulling on the string."
• Check for a Valsalva: abdomen rise with red face and breath holding.
• Can the client isolate the pelvic floor? The client should not use the abdominals, gluteals, hip adductors to do a bridge or a pelvic tilt.
• Client should appear to be concentrating and demonstrate a subtle pulling in of the abdominal muscles.
• Have her hold until she feels the muscle melt or fade in contraction.
• Instruct her to repeat the quick flick until she feels that she is no longer feeling the contraction.[93]

Position

• Subjective reports of the client of the position for best proprioception
• Position of best technique for visual inspection
• Need for isolation: For patients who have difficulty isolating, try abducting and externally rotating the hips in supine or quadraped as this will decrease other muscle groups and isolate the contraction.
• Need for facilitation by:
   Supine or sitting with use of a proper abdominal/pulling in contraction, gluetal set, adductor squeeze
   Supine with PNF resistance
   Quick stretch manually by the therapist
   Supine or sitting with use of internal sensor for proprioception
• sEMG results-(surface electromyographic biofeedback)
• MMT strength grade
   1/5 to 2/5 place client in the supine position with the knees up and the feet flat or knees supported on pillows
   3/5 to 5/5 place client in any position including quadraped with buttocks up (except in pregnancy and the post-partum period)

To assess the quality of contraction of the pubococcygeal muscle, physical therapists can be trained in internal examination, depending on their state practice acts. Physical therapists do not perform full pelvic examinations; they assess the strength and integrity of pelvic floor muscles by inserting the distal phalanx of the finger of a gloved hand, inside the vagina to assess the introitus, then, if needed, continue insertion to the level of the proximal interphalangeal joint of the finger to assess the levator ani muscles. Muscle condition, sensation, muscle tone, and strength can be assessed this way, but practitioners are strongly encouraged to take a training course if expecting to work with this population. Several references detail procedures for examination and additional strength grading than what is included in this chapter.[1,47] Other vital considerations are infection control and having a third person in the room with the examiner to act as a witness of proper procedure since this is a delicate area.

A side note to physical therapists who will be doing internal assessments. Allergic reactions to latex found in gloves and some theraband is on the rise according to *The PT Bulletin*, September 18, 1998. All health care practitioners are cautioned to use powder-free, low-protein gloves or non-latex gloves to reduce exposure to airborne latex particles. Frequent users of latex product, client or professional, may develop sensitivities to the latex proteins with resulting allergic reactions which vary from mild to life-threatening.

Sometimes treatment may require several months of persistent exercise to achieve continence. This is where perineometers have value — not only as a biofeedback device for the woman to become aware of the correct muscle contraction, but also as a resistance and assessment device.[94] The perineometer is a pneumatic resistance device, measuring contraction in millimeters of mercury (mm Hg), or cm of water, or inches of water pressure when inserted into the vagina. As the patient contracts the pubococcygeal muscle, located one to two inches inside the vagina, the meter reflects pressure change and can provide objective information regarding the contraction. Several perineometers are available, including computerized units with a printout. If a biofeedback device is used, the patient must be trained in proper use and will insert it herself with instruction. Single use or personal pressure probes are recommended.

Additionally, surface electromyographic (sEMG) biofeedback can be used for assessment and treatment. Unlike air pressure biofeedback, sEMG measures the electrical activity generated leading to an action potential. This electrical activity is correlated to recruitment of muscle fibers therefore indirectly is a measurement of strength.

Yet another form of therapeutic intervention for incontinence is through electrical stimulation of the pelvic floor. Neuromuscular electrical stimulation, interferential, TENS, and high-volt pulsed current have been used with varying success.[1,54] Although electric current was first applied to the pelvic floor and bladder via surgical implants, external units were found to have fewer complications and a higher success rate. Inflatable vaginal cuffs with electrodes, intra-vaginal electrodes, and intra-anal electrodes are available. There are even some that the patient can wear during the day. In either case, stimulation should be intermittent to avoid muscle fatigue. Electrical stimulation has been used successfully in cases of sphincter weakness, as well as to promote bladder inhibition (Table 3-10). Recommended frequencies also vary, and no one protocol has proven effective in all cases.

Another intervention is resistive exercise training, using specially designed weighted cones placed inside a condom and inserted into the vagina. These weights also provide proprioceptive feedback for better awareness for urinary control. Exercise with the cones may start in a gravity-assisted position and progress to antigravity positions. Studies have been initiated to explore the value of conditioning using vaginal cones. One sample of 38 women with either genuine stress incontinence, mixed stress/urge incontinence or no incontinence found that 80% of the women with incontinence were either cured or improved after 4 weeks.[95] However, another group of researchers treated 30 women with genuine stress incontinence with pelvic floor exercise training once a week over 12 weeks. Thirty women used the cones and were seen every 2 weeks over the 12-week period. Almost half of the women in the cone group withdrew

Table 3-10

Electrical Stimulation Treatment for Gynecological Conditions[1]

Types	Conditions	Parameters	Duration
Neuromuscular Electrical Stimulation	Weak pelvic floor ms (MMT 0-3)	(Overall Paramenters) Amplitude 0-100mA	Muscle weakness: 8-12 weeks
	Urinary stress incontinence genuine or mixed	Lower amplitude <35mA for afferent stimulation	
	Urge incontinence		
	Fecal incontinence	Higher amplitude >65mA for efferent stimulation	Urge incontinence need 2-4 months BID
	Incoordination of pelvic floor ms		
	Decreased urethral closure pressures	Voltage units are 7.9V or higher	
	Short urethra	Frequency 5-100 Hz	
	Pelvic pain	5-20 Hz for bladder inhibition	
		5-50 Hz for strengthening	
		80-100 Hz for pain	
		Wave form- symmetrical or asymmetrical biphasic pulsed	
		Duty cycle adjustable 25% for weak ms 50% for moderate weakness	
Interferential	Weak pelvic floor muscles- MMT 0-3		30 minutes daily
	Urinary stress incontinence (Weakness/laxity) (genuine or mixed)	Genuine stress incontinence (weakness) Sweep of 10-50 Hz so 10-20 Hz slow twitch and 30-50Hz for fast twitch will be fully stimulated	30 minutes 3x week to start with 15 minute treatments initially
	Urge incontinence Incoordination of pelvic floor ms Decreased urethral closure pressures	Urge incontinence-5-10 Hz.) Sweep 10 usec to 500 usec	30 minutes 3x week
	Pelvic pain	Sweep of 10-50 Hz so 10-20 Hz slow twitch and 30-50Hz for fast twitch will be fully stimulated	30 minutes 3x week to start with 15 minute treatments initially
TENS	Pelvic pain Endometriosis Dysmenorrhea Pelvic inflammatory disease Coccydynia Vulvodynia	Electrode placement for dysmenorrhea, endometriosis, PID Vulvodynia, dyspareunia, coccyxdynia two electrodes placed under the	Treatment time and mode to be determined by the physical therapist depending on the client's condition,

Table 3-10 Continued

Electrical Stimulation Treatment for Gynecological Conditions[1]

Types	Conditions	Parameters	Duration
	Perineal Pain	ischial tuberosities and two placed over the obturator foramina or four electrodes crossed over the S2-4	age and severity of pain. Start with 20-30 minutes as tolerated. (Brief intense mode should only be used for 10-12 minutes. For dysmenorrhea may use continuously for first 2-3 days of flow
High volt pulsed current	Weak pelvic floor muscles Urinary stress incontinence Sexual dysfunction related to pelvic floor weakness	Urinary incontinence and weak pelvic floor muscles use vaginal or rectal electrode at a comfortable setting	2x day for 15-20 minutes
	Rectal pain Levator Ani Syndrome	Levator Ani Syndrome vaginal or rectal probe at pulse frequency 80 Hz voltage starting at 0 and gradually increase until patient has mild discomfort then reduce voltage until client is comfortable (usually 250-400 volts)	60 minute treatment time

from the study, and the researchers concluded that the cones were no different in effectiveness than weekly pelvic floor training.[96] Another research group found the use of cones helps women with mild stress incontinence, but not with severe stress incontinence.[97] Finally, in a single-blind, randomized controlled trial of pelvic floor exercises compared to electrical stimulation, vaginal cones, or no treatment with 107 women with genuine stress incontinence, researchers concluded that pelvic floor muscle training was superior to the other modalities. One factor that may influence these results is the pelvic floor training occurred with the physical therapist in weekly sessions, in addition to self-directed exercise at home.[98]

BREAST REHABILITATION

Physical therapy management of breast cancer has become focused on treatment of lymphedema, decreased shoulder and upper extremity function, scar management and pain reduction. Depending on the type of reconstruction, whether submuscular implants and muscle flaps are involved, physical therapists may also need to address problems in the shoulder joints, scapular muscles, trunk muscles, abdominal muscles, cervical musculature, fascial tissues, and in the brachial plexus. Submuscular implants include: silicone, saline, temporary tissue expanders, and permanent tissue expanders. Muscle flaps use the ipsilateral muscle resected with it's blood supply and fat to form a breast mound. These include transverse rectus abdominus muscle flap or TRAM, and latissimus dorsi muscle flap LAT.[99]

It is generally believed that post-mastectomy rehabilitation by the patient should continue at least through the first year after surgery, as women may tend to lose range of motion, function, and edema may become chronic, especially if they had shoulder problems prior to the surgery. Studies show that although the woman with local excision and axillary dissection with radiation may have more chest wall tenderness at 1 and 2 years after surgery and were slower to regain preoperative range of motion compared to women who had modified radical mastectomy,[100] both groups can regain preoperative range within 3 months post-operatively.[101]

Maintaining that motion and function can be a problem, however.[102,103] Immediately after surgery, positioning of the arm is important. Resting and elevating the arm on a pillow, and completing gentle active elbow and hand exercises will help reduce edema. Controversy exists whether to start immediate range of motion at the shoulder or wait a week for wound healing. One study showed no significant difference in wound drainage whether range was started immediately or was delayed, and no differences were found regarding wound complications or shoulder function after 6 months.[104] However, another study found that women who received immediate physical therapy and shoulder motion instruction had less volume of lymph drainage, more shoulder motion, and less pain at day 7 compared to women who had neither or who performed shoulder motion only.[105] These differences in rehabilitation practice can be reflected nationally and internationally. The physical therapists working with breast surgery clients need to have a relationship with the referring surgeon to best understand their particular guidelines for recovery.

Lymphedema management has become a specialty area of treatment, both related and unrelated to breast surgery. Management usually involves some combination of range of motion exercises, compression (either by intermittent pneumatic pump, compression garments or by wrapping the extremity with bandages), and various systems of manual lymphatic drainage massage. This approach may also be referred to as complex or complete decongestive physical therapy.[106] Ultrasound and myofascial release of chest wall adhesions have also been applied, with varying success. Regardless of the approach, it is generally agreed that the practitioner should address "the functional, cosmetic and emotional sequelae of this potentially disabling condition."[107]

Manual lymphatic drainage techniques developed by various practitioners basically focus on the same things in different ways. Components that may vary: are the rate of movement, depth of pressure, the areas of the body treated, the desired direction of lymph flow, and how scar tissue is addressed.[106, 108-111] Courses in specific nontraditional methods are available and are recommended for physical therapists working with this population, as currently, most physical therapy programs in the United States are teaching only traditional methods.[112]

Treatment of the breast surgical patient begins with an assessment of: posture, neck arm and trunk range of motion, strength, arm girth measurements, skin palpation, pain level, ADL's and functional abilities (Table 3-11).

THE AGING FEMALE

Anatomical and Physiological Changes

The aging female offers the physical therapist a different challenge. In addition to any of the problems mentioned in this chapter, the unstoppable effects of time bring other consid-

Table 3-11

Physical Therapy Goals and Treatment After Breast Surgery. *
Adapted from Mauria Vallas "Exercise after Breast Surgery".[99]

Treatment Goals	Physical Therapy Treatment	Client Self Treatment
Elimination of pain and swelling	• Myofascial release techniques • Muscle energy techniques • Deep tissue massage techniques • Electrical stimulation • Manual lymph drainage • Heat/ice applications	• Self massage • Therapeutic exercises • Heat/ice • Positioning • Adapt functional activities
Stretching	• PNF Diagonals • Shoulder ROM • Trunk ROM • Cervical ROM • Swiss ball exercises	• ROM with cane • Overhead pulleys • Neck ROM • Trunk ROM
Strengthening	• Resisted PNF • Weight training • Lumbar stabilization • Aerobic conditioning • Neuromuscular reeducation-abdominal or latissimus muscle • Swiss ball exercises	• Resume functional activities • Therapeutic exercises • Aerobic conditioning
Education	• Caution on swelling • Prevent infection • Functional mobility for safety • Check for scar integrity	• Follow through with wound care • Adapt home for safety • Adapt home for ADL's and functional activities

erations when treating the woman who is coming to the end of her childbearing years or who has lived past them. Anatomical changes are the most obvious. The breast changes considerably at puberty and during lactation. Consisting primarily of ducts in childhood, after puberty the ducts, stimulated by estrogen, develop potential alveoli. Premenstrually, the glandular tissue increases, vascular engorgement occurs, and the lumen of the ducts enlarges. During pregnancy, stimulation from estrogen and progesterone from the placenta causes the alveoli to open and secrete milk, the adipose tissue increases, circulating blood increases, and the areola darkens and enlarges. Lactation lasts on an average about 5 or 6 months, but can last longer if estrogen and progesterone continue to interact with hypophysial hormones, prolactin, and growth hormone. There are many variations in lactation function. After lactation, milk is absorbed, alveoli shrink, and the glandular tissue rests. The glandular tissue atrophies after menopause and the ducts degenerate, as does the connective tissue support.

The sacroiliac joint cavities acquire fibrous or fibrocartilaginous adhesions, and synostosis may occur.

The uterus enlarges, swells, and changes color during menstruation. During pregnancy, the uterine fibers hypertrophy and new fibers develop. The uterine walls grow thinner as pregnancy advances. After childbirth, the uterus involutes, but the cavity remains larger than prior to pregnancy, and it is believed that the muscular layers are thicker. The aged uterus is atrophied and portions are more defined.[113-115]

The external genitalia generally atrophy as well and secretions diminish often requiring lubrication during intercourse.

Menopause

The ultimate cause of less frequent menses and abnormal cycles is menopause. The tricky part of this diagnosis is that menopause may occur any time within a 20 year span for the female population. "About one-fourth of women experience spontaneous menopause before age 45 years, about one half experience it between 45 and 50 years, and the remaining one fourth experience it after age 50. Many gynecologists, however, are impressed with the frequency with which apparently regular menstruation may persist well into the sixth decade."[15] The gradual extension of the lifespan of the human female, now averaging about 77 years in Western countries, virtually places the woman in a post-menopausal state for about one third of her life.[15] With this increasing longevity, new problems for female clients have developed. As a woman ages, the number of follicles with oocytes decreases, and the ovary begins to decrease in size and weight. Follicles tend to degenerate and, in combination with fewer oocytes, the amount of estrogen and inhibin decreases as well. As the inhibin decreases, FSH increases, follicles are stimulated, and short menstrual cycles occur. As the number of follicles decreases and estrogen production level falls, it becomes impossible to induce an LH surge, and ovulation tends to occur irregularly. As steroidogenesis by the follicles decreases, ovarian stroma increases. When combined with adrenal cell production of steroid hormones, a certain amount of steroidogenesis continues, although the level of estrogen and progesterone production is markedly decreased. However, the post-menopausal ovary produces mostly androgens, which are converted peripherally to estrogens. Yet this peripheral conversion cannot compensate for the direct secretion by the ovaries premenopausally of over 90% of the estradiol. As long as the ovaries respond to produce moderate amounts of estrogen, there will be episodic bleeding. Levels of gonadotropin increase as ovarian function diminishes. Menopause can be correctly diagnosed after 1 year of amenorrhea. Although there is variation, the average age for menopause is 51. Usually the bleeding decreases over 1 to 3 years, the interval between menstrual periods increases (amenorrhea), and the amount of bleeding decreases. In some women, however, the periods stop abruptly and permanently.

Occurring at the time of menopause is a variety of physical and psychological symptoms including some strictly associated with menopause and others related to aging. Researchers may view the symptoms of menopause as four associated endocrine syndromes (anovulatory cycles, hot flashes, vaginal atrophy, and osteoporosis), as problems related to estrogen withdrawal (disturbed menstrual pattern, vasomotor instability, psychological symptoms, atrophic conditions, headache, insomnia, myalgia, altered libido), or as health problems secondary to long-term hormone deprivation (osteoporosis and cardiovascular disease). Hot flashes (flushes), hirsutism, voice changes, vaginal dryness and itching, dry mouth, and loss of skin integrity are among the symptoms related to hormonal changes. Other symptoms include stress incontinence, with or without frequency or urgency, uterovaginal prolapse, backache, and fractures associated with bony changes. After menopause, the vagina actually becomes smaller, the mucosa atrophies, and cervical secretions decrease. Cystoceles and rectoceles may be encouraged to develop by waning hormones.[15]

Treatment of specific menopausal symptoms is primarily centered around estrogen replacement therapy, but additional problems sometimes result from this form of assistance. Spontaneous excessive estrogen can cause irregular uterine bleeding, endometrial hyperplasia, and has been linked to endometrial cancer. Estrogen-progestin therapy has been associated with thromboembolism, metabolic disorders, hypertension, and breast tumors, but only at dosages used in oral contraceptives. The amounts of hormone used post-menopausally are believed to be low enough that risk for these complications does not increase.[9]

Psychological Changes

With the onset of the climacteric (menopause), women are faced with many changes. Anatomical changes, loss of function and physical limitations may cause psychological reflection and introspection. Childbearing is over. Children are often grown and on their own, and women are facing, in full force, the slowing down and aging process of their bodies. Unlike pregnancy, when the changes are dramatic and last only 9 months; in menopause, the changes are permanent. It is not unusual for women to experience feelings of loss, hopelessness, self-condemnation, depression, anxiety, and tension. She will often reflect on her own life goals and accomplishments, and possibly experience decreased sexual appetite due to libido changes and discomfort from atrophic vaginitis. A woman, during menopause, may have many fears: death, loneliness, a partner's death, dependency upon her children, helplessness, and physical limitations. Understanding this period in life, its biologic basis, and the time needed for readjustment, can be reassuring for the menopausal women. In a recent survey of 750 women over half the women believed that "menopause is the beginning of a new and fulfilling stage of life."[116]

Cardiovascular and Other Systemic Changes

"Heart disease is the leading cause of death in women, accounting for about 28% of all deaths."[117] The multiple risk factors associated with coronary heart disease, such as heredity, hypertension, diabetes mellitus, hyperlipidemia, obesity, smoking, decreased activity, and stress make it difficult to fully understand the specific influence of menopause on heart disease. Studies show that the incidence of cardiovascular disease, hypertension, and stroke is lower in premenopausal women than in men of the same age. For men, there is a marked increase in coronary vascular disease after age 40; whereas for women, the risk factors do not increase until after menopause. After this time, the rate of cardiovascular disease in women increases, rapidly approaching the rate of men 10 years younger.[117] The most common cardiovascular disorders in women are hypertension, coronary artery disease, congestive heart failure, and chronic atrial fibrillation. Angina pectoris, myocardial infarction and sudden cardiac death occur most commonly. Differential diagnoses for chest pain in women are arthritis pain, gastroesophageal reflux and other chest conditions. Although it has been theorized that ovarian function appears to have a protective effect against cardiovascular disease in young women, there is not an abrupt rise after cessation of ovarian function. Cardiac output at rest decreases and the ability of the cardiovascular system to respond to stress declines. Systolic blood pressure increases, vascular resistance increases, and maximum-exercise heart rate decreases.[109] Other effects of aging can be seen in every system (Table 3-12).

Osteoporosis, Falls, and Fractures

Women experience an abrupt increase in bone loss after menopause, either naturally from decreased estrogen production or as a result of gynecologic surgeries. Bone sensitivity to parathyroid hormone increases, along with bone resorption and calcium absorption from the intestines.[119] Osteoporosis occurs more in white than in black, Asian or Hispanic women,

Table 3-12

Systemic Changes with Aging in Women[117]

System	Changes
Cardiovascular	Cardiac output decreased
	Systolic blood pressure increased
	Vascular resistance increased
	Maximum-exercise heart rate decreased
Pulmonary	A/P chest diameter increases
	Respiratory muscle strength decreased
	Costal cartilages calcify
	Vital capacity decreases
Gastrointestinal	Gut mucosa atrophies
	Vitamin absorption decreased
	Hiatal hernia in 70% of women over 70
Renal	Renal blood flow decreased
	Glomerular filtration rate decreased
	Sodium conservation impaired
Musculoskeletal	Arthritis
	Bone mass decreased /osteoporosis
	Muscle mass decreased

more in thin than fat, more in smokers than nonsmokers, and finally, more in physically inactive females than in active ones. Post-menopausal women lose bone on the average of 1% to 2% a year. Consequently, by their 80s, they may have lost half of their total bone mass. One quarter of women and half of women over 65 years are affected by osteoporosis. Twenty percent of women will have a femoral neck fracture by age 90 years, 80% because of osteoporotic bone. Twenty-five percent of those over 50 years develop compression fractures of the vertebrae, resulting in pain, height loss, deformity, impaired mobility and pain.[120] When falls result in fractures, more than two-thirds are women about 75 years old.[121] The most common fracture sites in women are hip, distal radius, pelvis, vertebrae, and rib. Women fall more than four times as frequently as men,[122] and older women have 50% greater lower extremity stiffness when stepping down off a platform.[123] Current pharmacologic intervention includes 1200 to 1500 mg elemental calcium/day, vitamin D (400 to 800 IU/day), antiresorptive agents (eg, alendronate), hormone replacement therapy, and nasal calcitonin.[122] It has been shown that estrogen may stop or slow the process of osteoporosis; however, there are risks involved with estrogen therapy. In women with low bone mineral density without vertebral fractures, alendronate increased density and reduced the risk of clinical fractures in women with osteoporosis.[124] Physical therapy for women with osteoporosis includes stretching, strengthening, balance exercises, fall prevention instruction, and impact exercise.[125-126] The effects of increased activity have been shown to slow bone loss and demineralization levels. "Resistance training has a positive effect on multiple risk factors for osteoporotic fracture in previously sedentary post-menopausal women."[127] Similarly, a 10-week ambulatory program for osteoporotic women with at least one vertebral fracture and pain within the 3 years prior found that physical therapy with balance training, muscle strengthening, and lumbar stabilization exercises resulted in significant decrease in analgesic use and pain level and improved quality of life, quadriceps muscle strength and back extensor muscle strength.[128] Home exercise programs alone do not seem to be as successful group classes which work on more than static exercises.[129]

CASE STUDIES

Client with Genuine Stress Incontinence

Subjective: Client is 35-year-old female with stress incontinence that started after her third child was delivered.(Her first was 5 years ago, second was 3 years ago and she is now 6 months post-partum with her third.) She had an episiotomy with the first child and had a one degree tear in her second and third deliveries. She complains that now she must wear a small pad and change it 3 to 5 times a day. She notices that she uses more pads when she is menstruating (up to 7 pads). She has given up running for recreation as she will leak and now walks for exercise. When she has a cold and repeatedly coughs, she is unable to control leaking.

Objective: Initial evaluation
- External exam shows a healed tear on the perineum
- Minimal excursion of the pelvic floor on contraction
- Internal exam MMT 1/5
- Inability to hold a contraction for more than 2 seconds
- Abdominal strength –3/5 and protruding

Assessment:
- Stress incontinence
- Weak pelvic floor muscles
- Weak abdominals

Plan:
  Goals-Short term:
  - Complete bladder diary for base line
  - Hold pelvic floor contraction for 5 seconds
  - Independent home program for quick and long contractions and functional exercising of the pelvic floor muscle
  - Train client to use home electrical stimulation unit

  Long term
  - Muscle strength 3+ to 4/5
  - No leakage, no need for pads
  - Return to all recreation activities without accidents

  Treatment in Physical therapy- Client will be instructed in proper contraction of the pelvic floor muscles and set up with a home exercise program with progression. At her second treatment she will be fit with a home electrical stimulation unit and retested. Her subsequent treatments will include biofeedback training in the clinic and instruction in abdominal strengthening and use of pelvic floor contractions while completing functional and recreational activities

Client with Vulvar Vestibulitis

Subjective: A 55-year-old female who suddenly developed vestibulitis after she had a yeast infection. Her symptoms have increased over the last year and she is unable to wear underwear, tight jeans or pants, preferring skirts and dresses. Pain was 8 out of 10 on a 0 to 10

scale, 10 being the worst She has had intercourse only once in the last year with her husband and found the pain unbearable. She recently saw a vulvar specialist who placed her on neurotin and a low oxalate diet. She has noticed that she had some relief with pain at a 6.

Objective: Initial examination
- On external examination she had little excursion of the pelvic floor.
- On palpation the area in the six o'clock position of the perineum was red and painful.
- MMT was 2/5 and she was unable to hold the contraction for more than 4 seconds.

Assessment:
- Severe vulvar pain
- Pelvic floor weakness
- Dyspareunia

Plan:

Goals: Short Term
- Decrease pain to level 4 on 0 to 10 scale
- Hold contraction for 8 seconds
- Start physical therapy treatments for pain reduction

Long Term
- Resolve of vulvar pain
- Pelvic floor strength 4/5
- Intercourse without pain

Treatment: Client will be instructed in proper contraction of the pelvic floor muscles and set up with a home exercise program with progression. She will be instructed in perineal massage techniques to decrease sensitivity. Her therapy will include perineal ultrasound and myofascial techniques and ice. After her pain has decreased she will be instructed in the use of vaginal dilators to stretch the perineum and vagina. The size of these will be increased as she is able to tolerate.

Client with Osteoporosis

Subjective: An 88-year-old female is referred to physical therapy 8 weeks after she developed severe discomfort in the upper to mid dorsal spine area after bending over to pick something off the floor. On x-ray, a T7 osteoporotic compression fracture was found with thoracic kyphosis accentuated focally at the T7 level. The bone scan reported that the bones were demineralized and the compression of T7 was 30% of its normal height. She has pain on rolling in bed and coming to standing and ADL activities.

Objective: Initial examination
- Poor balance in static and dynamic activities with mininal resistance
- Pain on range of motion
- MMT throughout trunk muscles is -3/5
- Difficulty in activities of daily living, ie, coming to standing, rolling in bed

Assessment:
- Poor balance
- Weak trunk muscles
- Pain on movement
- Inability to complete all ADL's

Plan:

Goals- Short Term

- Able to stand on one leg with eyes open for 45 seconds
- No pain on rolling
- Initiate strengthening home exercise program
- Fit for TENS unit at home with the assistance of her partner

Long Term

- Good balance in static and dynamic activities with maximal resistance
- Trunk strength 4/5 throughout
- No complaints of pain
- Independent in all ADL's
- Independent in home and group exercise programs

Treatment: The client will be started with a home exercise program that strengthens all her back muscles (cervical to sacrum areas). She will be tested for balance at each visit and given progressive balance training in the clinic and at home. Training will be given on how to move on all levels without trunk rotation so as to decrease pain and move without compromise to her osteoporotic spine. All safety precautions will be taught so she can protect herself from future injury. With assistance she will use a TENS machine at home to decrease her pain as she becomes stronger. In addition to her home program she will enroll in a group exercise program for weight bearing conditioning and weight training for muscle strengthening.

SELF-ASSESSMENT REVIEW

1. Of utmost importance for the physical therapist conducting a gynecologic patient evaluation is _____.

2. Physical therapists wishing to conduct an _____ exam on patients referred for pelvic floor dysfunction or incontinence problems should review their state practice act and contact their insurance carrier .

3. Even in states with direct access, it's a good idea to recommend patients be examined by a gynecologist or urologist before physical therapy to rule out _____ or _____.

4. Genuine stress urinary incontinence is largely a symptom related to a difference in _____.

5. _____ pelvic support may result in rectocele, cystocele, urethrocele, or enterocele.

6. The physical therapist who examines a patient referred because of genuine stress incontinence should perform a neurologic screening to include:

7. Name and define at least three types of incontinence.

8. Name at least one way in which to treat women with the following: premenstrual syndrome, dysmenorrhea, genuine stress incontinence, post-hysterectomy, post-gynecologic surgery.

Answers

1. Taking a careful history. 2. Internal. 3. Pathology or communicable disease. 4. Pressures. 5. Relaxed. 6. Sensory and motor tests of lower extremities and sacral nerves, deep

tendon reflexes. 7. Genuine stress, urge, reflex (see text for definitions). 8. Exercise, relaxation, TENS (see text).

REFERENCES

1. Wilder E, ed. *The Gynecological Manual*. Section on Women's Health. Alexandria, Va: American Physical Therapy Association; 1997.

2. Schachter CL. Working sensitively with adult survivors of childhood sexual abuse. *American Physical Therapy Association Annual Conference Compendium*. June 1999: 181-183.

3. Schachter CL. *An interview with CL Schacter, PhD, PT*. October 1999.

4. Guidelines for Recognizing and Providing Care for Victims of Domestic Violence. *American Physical Therapy Association*. Alexandria, Va; 1997. No. P-138.

5. Diagnostic and Treatment Guidelines on Domestic Violence. *Washington American Medical Association*. Washington, D. C.: 1992.

6. Schachter CL, Stalker CA, Teram E. Toward sensitive practice: issues for physical therapists working with survivors of childhood sexual abuse. *Phys Ther*. 79:248-261.

7. Teram E, Schachter Cl, Stalker CA. Opening the doors to disclosure. *Physiotherapy*. 85(2)88-97.

8. Rothstein JM. The sensitive practitioner, editor's note. *Phys Ther*. 79.

9. Speroff L, Glass RH, Kase NG. *Clinical Gynecologic Endocrinology and Infertility*. 4th ed. Baltimore, Md: Williams & Wilkins; 1989.

10. Federman DD. Ovary. In: Scientific American. Endocrinology. *Scientific American*. 1986.

11. Dox I, Melloni BJ, Eisner GM, eds. *Dorland's Illustrated Medical Dictionary*. 24th ed. Philadelphia, Pa: WB Saunders; 1965.

12. Russell JB, Mitchell D, Musey PI, Collins, DC. The relationship of exercise to anovulatory cycles in female athletes: hormonal and physical characteristics. *Obstet Gynecol*. 1984;63(4):4525.

13. Bachmann GA, Kemmann E. Prevalence of oligomenorrhea and amenorrhea in a college population. *Am J Obstet Gynecol*. 1982;144(1): 98-102.

14. Gomel V, Munro MG, Rowe TC. *Gynecology: A Practical Approach*. Baltimore, Md: Williams & Wilkins; 1990.

15. Jones HW, Wentz AC, Burnett LS, eds. *Novak's Textbook of Gynecology*. 11th ed. Baltimore, Md: Williams & Wilkins; 1988.

16. Mannheimer JS, Whalen EC. The efficacy of transcutaneous electrical nerve stimulation in dysmenorrhea. *Clin J Pain*. 1985;1:75-83.

17. Pomerantz E. Premenstrual syndrome. Concerns for the OB/GYN physical therapist. *Bull Sect Obstet Gynecol*. 1987;11(3):89.

18. Chihal HJ. *Premenstrual Syndrome: A Clinic Manual*. Durant, Okla: Creative Infomatics; 1985.

19. Lark S. *Premenstrual Syndrome Self-Help Book*. Los Angeles, Calif: Forman Publishing; 1984.

20. Glass RH. *Office Gynecology*. 3rd ed. Baltimore, Md: Williams & Wilkins; 1988.

21. Beckman CR, Ling FW, Barzansky BM, et al. *Obstetrics and Gynecology*. 2nd ed. Baltimore, Md: Williams & Wilkins; 1994.

22. Dalton K. *The Premenstrual Syndrome and Progesterone Therapy*. Chicago, Ill: Year Book Medical Publishers; 1983.

23. Lewers D, Clelland JA, Jackson JR, Varner RE, Bergman J. Transcutaneous electrical nerve stimulation in the relief of primary dysmenorrhea. *Phys Ther*. 1989;69(1):3-9.

24. Neighbors LE, Clelland JA, Jackson JR. Transcutaneous electrical nerve stimulation for pain relief in primary dysmenorrhea. *Cliff J Pain*. 1987;3:1722.

25. Kaplan B, Peled Y, Pardo J, et al. Transcutaneous electrical nerve stimulation (TENS) as a relief for dysmenorrhea. *Clin Exp Obstet Gynecol*. 1994;21:87-90.

26. Kaplan B, Rabinerson D, Lurie S, Peled Y, Royburt M, Neri A. *Clinical Evaluation of a New Model of a Transcutaneous Electrical Nerve Stimulation Device for the Management of Primary Dysmenorrhea*. 1997;44:255-259.

27. Milsom I, Hedner M, Mannheimer C. A comparative study of the effect of high-intensity transcutaneous nerve stimulation and oral naproxen on intrauterine pressure and menstrual pain in patients with primary dysmenorrhea. *Am J Obstet Gynecol*. 1994;170:123-129.

28. Dawood MY, Ramos J. Transcutaneous electrical nerve stimulation (TENS) for the treatment of primary dysmenorrhea: a randomized crossover comparison with placebo TENS and ibuprofen. *Obstet Gynecol*. 1990;75:656-660.

29. Kokjohn K, Schmid DM, Triano JJ, Brennan PC. The effect of spinal manipulation on pain and prostaglandin levels in women with primary dysmenorrhea. *J Manipulative Physiol Ther*. 1992;15:279-285.

30. Boesler D, Warner M, Alpers A, Finnerty EP, Kilmore MA. Efficacy of high-velocity low-amplitude manipulative technique in subjects with low-back pain during menstrual cramping. *J Am Osteopath Assoc*. 1993;93:203-8, 213-4.

31. Vance AR, Hayes SH, Spielholz NI. Microwave diathermy treatment for primary dysmenorrhea. *Phys Ther*. 1996;76:1003-8.

32. Ushakova OE, Davydova OB, Iarustovskaia OV, Filina LF, Lebedeva OD, Iazykova TA. The effect of contrast baths on central nervous system function in patients with a disordered menstrual function. *Vopr Kurotol Fizioter Lech Fiz Kult*. 1997;Jul-Aug:25-7.

33. Mathias SD, Kuppermann M, Liberman RF, Lipschutz RC, Steege JF. Chronic pelvic pain: prevalence, health-related quality of life and economic correlates. *Obstet Gynecol*. 1996;87:321-7.

34. Ryder RM. Chronic pelvic pain. *Am Fam Physician*. 1996;54:2225-32,2237.

35. Banerjee R, Lauger MR. Reproductive disorders associated with pelvic pain. *Semin Pediatr Surg*. 1998;7:52-61.

36. Savidge CJ, Slade P. Psychological aspects of chronic pelvic pain. *J Psychosom Res*. 1997;42:433-44.

37. Duleba AJ, Keltz MD, Olive DI. Evaluation and management of chronic pelvic pain. *J Am Assoc Gynecol Laparosc*. 1996;3(2):205-27.

38. Rapkin AJ, Kames LD. The pain management approach to chronic pelvic pain. *J Reprod Med*. 1987;32:323-7.

39. Baraldi R, Ghirardini G. Partial detachment of round ligament found at laparoscopy for chronic pelvic pain in a female adolescent. *J Pediatr Adolesc Gynecol*. 1998;1:189-90.

40. Browning JE. Mechanically induced pelvic pain and organic dysfunction in a patient without low back pain. *J Manipulative Physiol Ther*. 1990;13:406-11.

41. Hillis SD, Marchbanks PA, Peterson HB. The effectiveness of hysterectomy for chronic pelvic pain. *Obstet Gynecol*. 1995;86:941-5.

42. Carter JE. Diagnosis and treatment of the causes of chronic pelvic pain. *J Am Assoc Gynecol Laparosc*. 1996;3:S5-6.

43. Hurd WW. Criteria that indicate endometriosis is the cause of chronic pelvic pain. *Obstet Gynecol*. 1998 Dec;92(6):1029-32.

44. Dmowski WP, Lesniewicz R, Rana N, Pepping P, Noursalehi M. Changing trends in the diagnosis of endometriosis: a comparative study of women with pelvic endometriosis presenting with chronic pelvic pain or infertility. *Fertil Steril*. 1997;67:238-43.

45. Laufer MR, Goitein L, Bush M, Cramer DW, Emans SJ. Prevalence of endometriosis in adolescent girls with chronic pelvic pain not responding to conventional therapy. *J Pediatr Adolesc Gynecol*. 1997;10:199-202.

46. Lopes P, Mensier A, Laurent FX, Besse O. Pelvic pain and endometriosis. *Rev Fr Gynecol Obstet*. 1995;90:77-83.

47. Barlow DH, Glynn CJ. Endometriosis and pelvic pain. *Ballieres Clin Obstet Gynaecol.* 1993;7:775-89.

48. Stovall DW, Bowser LM, Archer DF, Guzick DS. Endometriosis-associated pelvic pain: evidence for an association between the stage of disease and a history of chronic pelvic pain. *Fertil Steril.* 1997;68:13-8.

49. Peveler R, Edwards J, Daddow J, Thomas E. Psychosocial factors and chronic pelvic pain: a comparison of women with endometriosis and with unexplained pain. *J Psychosom Res.* 1996;40:305-15.

50. Wechsler RJ, Maurer PM, Halpern EJ, Frank ED. Superior hypogastric plexus block for chronic pelvic pain in the presence of endometriosis: CT techniques and results. *Radiology.* 1995;196:103-6.

51. Weather L Jr. The frequency of endometriosis in women with pelvic pain and large leiomyomata uteri. *J Am Assoc Gynecol Laparosc.* 1996;3:S55.

52. Keltz MD, Kim A, Arici A, Olive DL. Large bowel to pelvic sidewall adhesions associated with chronic pelvic pain. *J Am Assoc Gynecol Laparosc.* 1996;3:S21-2.

53. Chapron C, Dubuisson JB, Fritel X, et al. Operative management of deep endometriosis infiltrating the uterosacral ligaments. *J Am Assoc Gynecol Laparosc.* 1999;6:31-7.

54. Sapsford R, Bullock-Saxton J, Markwell S. *Women's Health: A Textbook for Physiotherapists.* London England: WB Saunders Co., Ltd.; 1998.

55. Silver JK, Leadbetter WB. Piriformis syndrome: assessment of current practice and literature review. *Orthopedics.* 1998;21:1133-5.

56. Barton PM. Piriformis syndrome: a rational approach to management. *Pain.* 1991;47:345-52.

57. Kouvalchouk JF, Bonnet JM, de Mondenard JP. Pyramidal syndrome: apropos of 4 cases treated by surgery and review of the literature. *Rev Chir Orthop Reparatrice Appar Mot.* 1996;82:647-57.

58. Fishman LM, Zybert PA. Electrophysiologic evidence of piriformis syndrome. *Arch Phys Med Rehabil.* 1992;73:359-64.

59. Heah SM, Ho YH, Tan M, Leong AF. Biofeedback is effective treatment for levator ani syndrome. *Dis Colon Rectum.* 1997;40:187-9.

60. Monif GRG, Belatti RG Jr. Intercourse-related vaginal pain syndrome: a variant of vulvar vestibulitis syndrome? *Am J Obstet Gynecol.* 1993; 169:194-6.

61. Glazer HI, Rodke G, Swencionis C, Hertz R, Young AW. Treatment of vulvar vestibulitis syndrome with electromyographic biofeedback of pelvic floor musculature. *J Reprod Med.* 1995;40:283-90.

62. Glazer H, Jantos M, Hartmann EH, Swencionis C. Electromyographic comparisons of the pelvic floor in women with dysesthetic vulvodynia and asymptomatic women. *J Reprod Med.* 1998;43:959-962.

63. Shafik A. Pudendal canal syndrome as a cause of vulvodynia and its treatment by pudendal nerve decompression. *Eur J Obstet Gynecol Reprod Biol.* 1998;80:215-20.

64. White G, Jantos M, Glazer H. Establishing the diagnosis of vulvar vestibulitis. *J Reprod Med.* 1997;42:157-60.

65. Ostensen M, Schei B. Sociodemographic characteristics and gynecological disease in 40-42 year old women reporting musculoskeletal disease. *Scan J Rheumatol.* 1997;26:426-34.

66. Ragnarsson B, Jacobsson B: Epidemiology of pelvic fractures in a Swedish county. *Acta Orthop Scand.* 1992; 63:297-300.

67. Pohlemann T, Bosch U, Gansslen A, et al. The Hannover experience in management of pelvic fractures. *Clin Orthop.* 1994;305:69-80.

68. Chan L, Nade S, Brooks A, et al. Experience with lower urinary tract disruptions associated with pelvic fractures: implication for emergency room management. *Aust NZ J Surg.* 1994;64:395-9.

69. Dietrichs E, Kogstad O. Pelvic girdle relaxation—suggested new nomenclature. *Scand J Rheumatol Suppl.* 1991;88:3

70. Moen MH, Kogstad O, Biornstad N, Hansen JH, Sudmann E. Symptomatic pelvic girdle relaxation. Clinical aspects. *Tidsskr Nor Laegeforen.* 1990;110:2211-2.

71. Kharazzi FD, Rodgers WB, Kennedy JG, Lhowe DW. Parturition-induced pelvic dislocation: a report of four cases. *J Orthop Trauma.* 1997;11:277-81, 281-2.

72. Snow RE, Neubert AG. Peripartum pubic symphysis separation: a case series and review of the literature. *Obstet Gynecol Surv.* 1997;52:438-43.

73. Mens JM, Vleeming A, Stoeckart R, Stam HJ, Snijders CJ. Understanding peripartum pelvic pain: implications of a patient survey. *Spine.* 1996;21:1363-9.

74. Seriven MW, Jones DA, McKnight L. The importance of pubic pain following childbirth: a clinical and ultrasonographic study of diastasis of the pubic symphysis. *J R Soc Med.* 1995;88:28-30.

75. Triadafilopoulos G, Simms RW, Goldenberg DL. Bowel dysfunction in fibromyalgia syndrome. *Dig Dis Sci.* 1991;36:59-64.

76. Walker EA, Glefand AN, Gelfand MD, Green C, Katon WJ. Chronic pelvic pain and gynecological symptoms in women with irritable bowel syndrome. *J Psychosom Obstet Gynaecol.* 1996;17:39-46.

77. McQuarrie HG, Harris JW, Ellsworth HS, Stone RA, Anderson AE. Sciatic neuropathy complicating vaginal hysterectomy. *Am J Obstet Gynecol.* 1972;113:223-32.

78. Hsieh LF, Liaw ES, Cheng HY, Hong CZ. Bilateral femoral neuropathy after vaginal hysterectomy. *Arch Phys Med Rehabil.* 1998;79:1018-21.

79. Fassoulaki A, Papilas K, Sarantopoulos C, Zotou M. Transcutaneous electrical nerve stimulation reduces the incidence of vomiting after hysterectomy. *Anesth Analg.* 1993;76:1012-4.

80. Fassoulaki A, Sarantopoulos C, Papilas K, Zotou M. Nerve stimulation in patients undergoing hysterectomy under general anesthesia. *Anaesthesiol Reanim.* 1994;19:49-51.

81. Christensen PA, Rotne M, Vedelsdal R, Jensen RH, Jacobsen K, Husted C. Electroacupuncture in anaesthesia for hysterectomy. *Br J Anaesth.* 1993;71:835-9.

82. *Women's Cancer Network Web Page.* http://www.wcn.org/ 4/13/99.

83. *Facts about Ovarian Cancer.* Ovarian Cancer National Alliance. http://www.ovariancancer.org/cancer/ fact_sheet.shtml 4/13/99.

84. Ostergard DR, ed. *Gynecologic Urology and Urodynamics: Theory and Practice.* 2nd ed. Baltimore, Md: Williams & Wilkins; 1985.

85. Patten J. *Neurological Differential Diagnosis.* 2nd ed. London, England: Springer-Verlag; 1996.

86. Pauls JA. *Therapeutic Approaches to Women's Health: A Program of Exercise and Education.* Gaithersburg, Md: Aspen; 1995.

87. Francis WJA. Disturbance of bladder function in relation to pregnancy. *J Obstet Gynaecol Br Emp.* 1960;67:35366.

88. Ulmsten U, Henriksson L, Iosif S. The unstable female urethra. *Am J Obstet Gynecol.* 144:9397, 1982.

89. Jones KG, Kegel AH. Treatment of urinary stress incontinence. *Surg Gynecol Obstet.* 1952;94:17988.

90. Faber P, Heidenreich J. Treatment of stress incontinence with estrogen in post-menopausal women. *Urol Int.* 1977;32:2213.

91. Zacharin R. A Chinese anatomy: the pelvic supporting tissues in the Chinese and occidental female compared and contrasted. *Aust NZ J Obstet Gynaecol.* 1977;17:111.

92. Glazer H, MacConkey D. Functional rehabilitation of pelvic floor muscles: a challenge to tradition. *Urol Nurs.* 1996;16:68-9.

93. Assad L. *"Evaluation and Treatment of Urinary Incontinence for the Physical Therapist" class notes from seminar.* Aug 1999.

94. Burgio KL, Robinson JC, Engel BT. The role of biofeedback in Kegel exercise training for stress urinary incontinence. *Am J Obstet Gynecol.* 1986;154:5864.

95. Fischer W, Linde A. Pelvic floor findings in urinary incontinence—results of conditioning using vaginal cones. *Acta Obstet Gynecol Scand.* 1997;76:455-60.

96. Cammu H, Van Nylen M. Pelvic floor exercises versus vaginal weight cones in genuine stress incontinence. *Eur J Obstet Gynecol Reprod Biol.* 1998;77:89-93.

97. Kato K, Kondo A. Clinical value of vaginal cones for the management of female stress incontinence. *Int Urogynecol J Pelvic Floor Dysfunc.* 1997;8:314-7.

98. Bo K, Talseth T, Holme I. Single blind, randomized controlled trial of pelvic floor exercises, electrical stimulation, vaginal cones, and no treatment in management of genuine stress incontinence in women. *BMJ.* 1999;318:487-93.

99. Vallas M. Exercise after breast surgery. Lecture notes for Combined Sections Meeting. APTA; Feb. 1997.

100. Gerber L, Lampert M, Wood C, Duncan M, D'Angelo T, Schain W, et al. Comparison of pain, motion, and edema after modified radical mastectomy vs. local excision with axillary dissection and radiation. *Breast Cancer Res Treat.* 1992;21:139-45.

101. Gutman H, Kersz T, Barzilai T, Haddad M, Reiss R. Achievements of physical therapy in patients after modified radical mastectomy compared with quadrantectomy, axillary dissection, and radiation for carcinoma of the breast. *Arch Surg.* 1990;125:389-91.

102. Sugden EM, Rezvani M, Harrison JM, Hughes LK. Shoulder movement after the treatment of early stage breast cancer. *Clin Oncol.* 1998;10:173-81.

103. Hladiuk M, Huchcroft S, Temple W, Schnurr BE. Arm function after axillary dissection for breast cancer: a pilot study to provide parameter estimates. *J Surg Oncol.* 1992;50:47-52.

104. Jansen RF, van Geel AN, de Groot HG, Rottier AB, Olthuis GA, van Putten WL. Immediate versus delayed shoulder exercises after axillary lymph node dissection. *Am J Surg.* 1990;160:481-4.

105. LeVu B, Dumortier A, Guillaume MV, Mouriesse H, Barreau-Pouhaer L. Efficacy of massage and mobilization of the upper limb after surgical treatment of breast cancer. *Bull Cancer.* 1997;84:957-61.

106. Rinehart-Ayres ME. Conservative approaches to lymphedema treatment. *Cancer.* 1998;83(suppl 12):2828-32.

107. Brennan MJ, Miller LT. Overview of treatment options and review of the current role and use of compression garments, intermittent pumps, and exercise in the management of lymphedema. *Cancer.* 1998;83(suppl 12):2821-7.

108. Leduc O, Leduc A, Bourgeois P, Belgrado JP. The physical treatment of upper limb edema. *Cancer* 1998;83(suppl 12):2835-9.

109. Kasseroller RG. The Vodder school: the Vodder method. *Cancer.* 1998;(suppl 12):2840-2.

110. Casley-Smith JR, Boris M, Weindorf S, Lasinski B. Treatment for lymphedema for the arm—the Casley-Smith method: a noninvasive method produces continued reduction. *Cancer.* 1998;83(suppl 12):2843-60.

111. Lerner R. Complete decongestive physiotherapy and the Lerner Lymphedema Services Academy of Lymphatic Studies (the Lerner school). *Cancer.* 1998;(suppl 12):2861-3

112. Augustine E, Corn M, Danoff J. Lymphedema management training for physical therapy students in the United States. *Cancer.* 1998;83(suppl 12):2869-73.

113. Goss CM, ed. *Gray's Anatomy of the Human Body.* Philadelphia, Pa: Lea & Febiger; 1970.

114. Danforth DN, Scott JR, eds. *Obstetrics and Gynecology.* Philadelphia, Pa: JB Lippincott; 1986.

115. Warwick R, Williams PL, eds. *Gray's Anatomy.* Philadelphia, Pa: WB Saunders; 1973.

116. Kaufert P, Boggs PP, Ettinger B, Woods NF, Utian WH. Women and menopause: beliefs, attitudes, and behaviors. *The North American Menopause Society 1997 Menopause Survey.* 1998;5:197-202.

117. Byyny RL, Speroff L. *A Clinical Guide for the Care of Older Women.* Baltimore, Md: Williams & Wilkins; 1990.

118. Lewis CB, Bottomley JM. *Geriatric Physical Therapy: A Clinical Approach.* Norwalk, Conn: Appleton & Lange; 1994.

119. MacKinnon JL. Osteoporosis—a review. *J Am Phys Ther Assoc.* 1988;68:1533-9.

120. Lyles KW. Management of patients with vertebral compression fractures. *Pharmacotherapy*. 1999;19:21S-24S.

121. Mayo NE, Korner-Bitensky N, Levy AR. Risk factors for fractures due to falls. *Arch Phys Med Rehabil*. 1993;74:917-21.

122. Pavol MJ, Owings TM, Foley KT, Gabiner MD. The sex and age of older adults influence the outcome of induced trips. *J Gerontol A Biol Sci Med Sci*. 1999;54:M103-8.

123. Hortobagyi T, DeVita P. Altered movement strategy increases lower extremity stiffness during stepping down in the aged. *J Gerontol A Biol Sci Med Sci*. 1999;54:B63-70.

124. Cummings SR, Black DM, Thompson DE, et al. Effect of alendronate on risk of fracture in women with low bone density but without vertebral fractures: results from the Fracture Intervention Trial. *JAMA*. 1998;280:2077-82.

125. Lane JM, Nydick M. Osteoporosis: current modes of prevention and treatment. *J Am Acad Orthop Surg*. 1999;7:19-31.

126. Heinonen A, Kannus P, Sievannen H, Pasanen M, Oja P, Vuori I. Good maintenance of high-impact activity-induced bone gain by voluntary, unsupervised exercises: an 8-month follow-up of a randomized controlled trial. *J Bone Miner Res*. 1999;14:125-8.

127. Evans WJ. Exercise training guidelines for the elderly. *Med Sci Sports Exerc*. 1999;31:12-7.

128. Malmros B, Mortensen L, Jensen MB, Charles P. Positive effects of physiotherapy on chronic pain and performance in osteoporosis. *Osteoporos Int*. 1998;8:215-21.

129. Kerschen K, Alacamlioglu Y, Kollmitzer J, et al. Functional impact of unvarying exercise program in women after menopause. *Am J Phys Med Rehabil*. 1998;77:326-32.

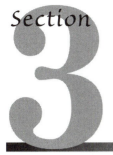

Role of Physical Therapy in Obstetric Care

4

Maternal Physiology

Physiologic changes during the life of the human female are numerous, occurring in every system of the body. The most frequent changes, however, occur during and immediately following pregnancy. Remarkable altered functions in the reproductive, renal, neurologic, cardiovascular, gastrointestinal, respiratory, endocrine, and dermatological systems, and exercise responses will be discussed. Most information is in chart form, for easy reference. Understanding the physiological basis of these changes will assist the physical therapist in making clinical decisions for treatment, prescribing exercise and finding supportive positions.

REPRODUCTIVE CHANGES

Table 4-1 lists the changes and effects on the reproductive system during pregnancy

RENAL CHANGES

This hydroureter usually occurs more frequently on the right side. Although blood flow in the non-pregnant woman is maximal when she is supine, the assumption of this position by a pregnant woman may compromise vena cava renal blood flow because the uterus compresses the great vessels. For this reason, left-side lying is recommended in pregnancy[4,5] (Table 4-2, Figures 4-1 and 4-2).

CARDIOVASCULAR CHANGES

Table 4-3 summarizes the changes to the cardiovascular system during pregnancy. Through increased blood volume and alterations in cardiac output, stoke volume and heart rate the mother and fetus are well supplied during pregnancy (Figures 4-3, 4-4, and 4-5).

Table 4-1

Reproductive Changes in Pregnancy

Structure/Function	Change	Outcome
Uterus – 1st half of pregnancy	Growth due to hypertrophy of muscle cells, increase in total amount of elastic tissue, and increase in size and number of blood vessels.	Most uterine weight is gained by 20th week of pregnancy
	Myometrial walls become thicker	
Uterus – 2nd half of pregnancy	Myometrial walls become thinner.	To allow for growth of fetus.
	Myometrial contractions cause thickening of upper uterine segment as lower segment expands	Expansion of lower segment allows for dilation of cervix and easier passage of infant
Uterine Blood Flow	Averages 500 ml/min at term as opposed to 50 ml/min in nonpregnant state.	
Braxton-Hicks Contractions	Irregular, usually painless contractions	Sometimes felt during second trimester; increase after 30 weeks
Cervix	Hypertrophied glands and softening of cervical tip (Goodell's sign) evident soon after conception. Increased vascularization.	Evident by 6th week.
	Mucus secretion is increased and thickened, forming large plug at cervical opening.	Serves as a barrier to protect fetus from bacterial or mechanical disruption.
Round Ligaments	Become elongated and hypertrophied	Helps to stabilize uterus.
Fallapian Tubes	Become elongated, edematous and hyperemic	
Ovaries	Become enlarged and elongated due to an increase in vascularity	
	Ovary containing corpus luteum is markedly longer and reaches maximum development during third month.	Corpus luteum is the endocrine body that produces progesterone at site of ruptured follicle. Ovulation discontinued due to pituitary inhibition
Vagina	Becomes congested and cyanotic (Chadwick's sign).	Evident by 8th week and is an objective sign of pregnancy.
	Secretions are highly acidic (3.3 to 5.5) due to increased glycogen content of the epithelium.	To prepare vagina for delivery.
	Connective tissue decreases, mucosa thickens, and muscular wall hypertrophies	
Vulva	Increases due to edema and increases vascularity	In multiparous women, this increased edema reaction feels as if they are "sitting on something" [1,2,3]

Table 4-2

Renal Changes in Pregnancy

Structure	Change	Outcome
Urine	Increase related to increased renal function	Early complaint is present in 80% of all women at some stage
Renal (Kidney)	Increased function	
Renal Blood Flow	Increases 60 – 80% by end of first trimester; assisted by increases in cardiac output	Maintained to term
Glomerular Filtration Rate (GFR)	Increases by 50%[4]	Increased extretion of many therapeutic drugs so doses may need to be increased
Ureter	May be obstructed by expanding uterus at level of pelvic brim	Causes ureteral bladder distension with urine (hydroureter)
Renal Plasma Flow	Increases 20 – 30%	Causes increased GFR
Extracellular Fluid (ECF)	Increases due to increase in plasma volume	Affected by salt intake and retension occurs after 13th week[4]
Volume Regulation	Intravascular fluid and extracellular fluid are normal	Levels are reset; protects from dramatic shrinking and expanded volumes

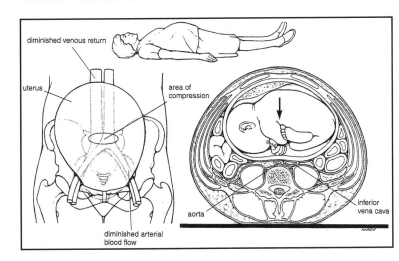

diminished venous return

uterus

area of compression

aorta

inferior vena cava

diminished arterial blood flow

Figure 4-1. After the 20th week, the woman may experience a sense of dizziness in the supine position due to the pressure of the baby interfering with the blood flow in the inferior vena cava and aorta. (Effects of Supine Position on the Pregnant Woman. American Journal of Nursing. May 1982, 810.)

Figure 4-2. Effects of shift in position by the pregnant woman. By shifting the woman's position to side-lying or semiside-lying, the supine hypotension syndrome can be avoided. (Effects of Supine Position on the Pregnant Woman. American Journal of Nursing. May 1982, 811.)

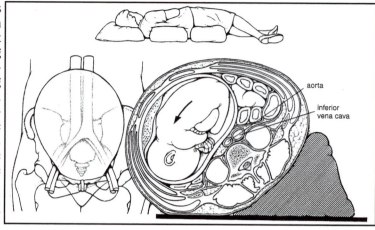

aorta

inferior vena cava

Table 4-3

Cardiovascular Changes in Pregnancy

Structure/Function	Change	Outcome
Blood Volume	Increases by 40–50% above non-pregnancy values. Increases more with twins than singleton gestation.	Largest increase during first 20–30 weeks of pregnancy.
Blood Plasma	Increases unequally with red cell mass. Leads to hemodilation and physiologic anemia; supplemental iron alleviates this outcome.	See Figure 4-1.
Cardiac Output	Increase at 12th week and peaks at 28–32 weeks to 30–50% above non-pregnancy values (see Figure 4-2).	"Vena Cava Syndrome", see Figure 4-1, 4-2.
Stroke Volume	Increases 20 – 40% in mid-pregnancy. Decreases after 28–32 weeks of pregnancy until term.	Increased cardiac output is related to tachycardia.
Heart Rate	Increases throughout pregnancy.	At term, heart rate reaches peak of 10–15 beats/min above non-pregnancy values (when measured in lateral position).
Arterial Blood Pressure	Decreases end of first trimester and throughout pregnancy.	Substantial fall in systemic vascular resistance (2-3 mm Hg systolic and 5–10 mm Hg diastolic).

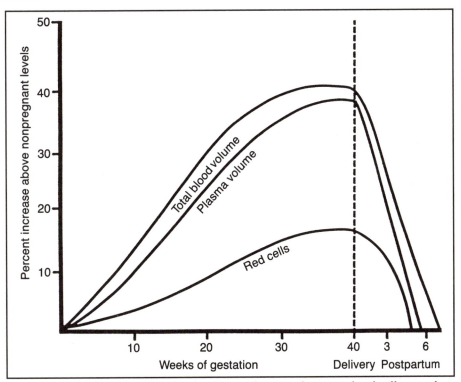

Figure 4-3. Changes in total blood volume, plasma volume, and red cell mass during pregnancy and puerperium (From Wilson JR, Carrington ER, Ledger WJ. *Obstetrics and Gynecology.* 7th ed. St. Louis, Mo: CV Mosby Co; 1983, 235).

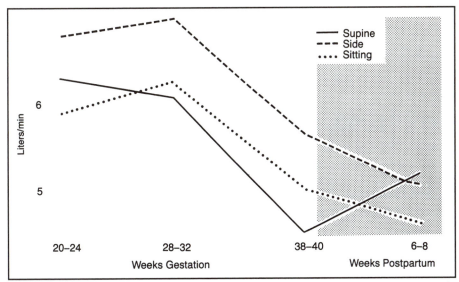

Figure 4-4. Cardiac output at different stages of pregnancy and puerperium according to patient's position. (From Veland K, et al. *American Journal of Obstetrics and Gynecology.* 104: 856,1969).

Parameter	Patient Position	1st Trimester	2nd Trimester	3rd Trimester	Post-Partum
Heart Rate	L	77 ± 2	85 ± 2	88 ± 2	69 ± 2
(beats/min)	S	76 ± 2	84 ± 2	92 ± 2	70 ± 2
Stroke Volume	L	75 ± 2	86 ± 4	97 ± 5	79 ± 3
(ml/min)	S	82 ± 5	85 ± 4	87 ± 5	79 ± 3
Cardiac Output	L	3.53 ± 0.21	4.32 ± 0.22	4.85 ± 0.27	3.30 ± 0.17
l/min/m^2	S	3.76 ± 0.24	4.19 ± 0.21	4.54 ± 0.28	3.33 ± 0.21
Left ventricular	L	302 ± 2	290 ± 5	281 ± 4	310 ± 5
Ejection Time	S	301 ± 3	286 ± 4	260 ± 4	307 ± 5
(msec)					
Systolic Blood	L	98 ± 2	91 ± 2	95 ± 2	97 ± 2
Pressure	S	106 ± 2	102 ± 2	106 ± 2	110 ± 2
(mm Hg)					
Diastolic Blood	L	53 ± 2	49 ± 2	50 ± 2	57 ± 2
Pressure	S	57 ± 2	60 ± 1	65 ± 2	65 ± 1
(mm Hg)					
L, lateral; S, supine					

Figure 4-5. Hemodynamic parameters throughout pregnancy (Key TC, Resnik R; Danforth DN, Scott JR, eds. *Maternal Changes in Pregnancy in Obstetrics and Gynecology.* 5th edition. Philadelphia, Pa: J.B. Lippincott; 1986.)

NEUROLOGIC CHANGES

There is no neurologic disorder that occurs solely during pregnancy. There are diseases of the peripheral and central nervous systems that occur more frequently in pregnancy or in the puerperium, and pregnancy may cause a recurrence of a preexisting neurologic disorder. These diseases and disorders will be discussed at length in Chapter 5.

GASTROINTESTINAL CHANGES

Alterations in gastrointestinal function arise from hormonal changes, as well as from structural adaptations to the fetus. Nausea, vomiting, appetite preference, constipation, heartburn, hemorrhoids, and minor abdominal pains are common in pregnancy. Various degrees of nausea and vomiting, called "morning sickness", are experienced by 50 to 90% of women during the first trimester. However, 20% of women experience nausea on and off during the entire pregnancy. Gastric disturbances can range from a mild, transient form, to a continual, severe type, hyperemesis gravidarum, that threatens the life of the mother.

Nausea is more likely to occur first thing in the morning or before meals when the stomach is empty. There are several theories, both biological and psychological, as to why nausea and vomiting occur. Human chorionic gonadotropin (hCG) is secreted in large quantities by the placenta, and may be a contributing cause. Additionally, the byproducts of rapid development of the trophoblastic cells that form the placenta give off degenerative products that may produce nausea and vomiting.[7] There are also metabolic and endocrine factors that predispose women to nausea and vomiting. Increased progesterone prolongs esoplageal, gastric, small bowel motility, and stomach emptying due to smooth muscle relaxation. In addition, studies have also shown that possibly a psychological overlay of an unwanted preg-

Table 4-4
Gastrointestinal Changes in Pregnancy

Location	Change	Etiology and outcome
Mouth	Gum hypertrophy, increased caries, ptyalism	Unknown
Esophagus	Decreased lower esophageal sphincter tone, increase of nonperistaltic contraction in distal esophagus; heartburn	Possibly progesterone; pressure reduced in lower esophageal sphincter
Appetite	Increased food cravings and aversions, occasionally pica (craving unnatural foods or substances)	Unknown
Digestion	Nausea and vomiting, improvement in lactose digestion	Possibly estrogens, hCG*, possibly progesterone, decreased intestinal motility
Stomach	Decreased motility, tone, and acid secretion; increased incidence of hiatal hernia	Possibly progesterone; mechanical effects of expanding uterus
Small, large intestine	Possibly decreased motility	Possibly progesterone
Liver	Cholestasis, pruritus gravidarum (generalized itching)	Liver cell response to estrogen
Appendix	Displaced upward as pregnancy develops	Mechanical effects of expanding uterus
Gallbladder	Decreased emptying time, possible buildup of cholesterol; gallstones	Possibly progesterone
Colon/anus	Constipation, hemorrhoids	Decreased tone in rectal sphincter; pressure of expanding uterus; possibly progesterone; slower passage of food results in hard, dry feces difficult to expel

*hCG-human chorionic gonadotropin
Adapted from Manual of Obstetrics, Niswander, 1987.[3]

nancy and women's negative assessment of their relationship with their own mothers, causes more nausea and vomiting.[8]

It has been shown that many women have improved physiological adaptation to lactose digestion during pregnancy. Women who were previously lactose-intolerant in early pregnancy, improve enough to digest milk during the third trimester, therefore increasing their supply of calcium.[9] This change may be the result of a progesterone-induced decrease in intestinal motility. Slower peristalsis allows for increased contact time with the layers of the intestine for lactose digestion. The influences of pregnancy on the gastrointestinal system are listed in Table 4-4 by location, changes, and etiology.

BREAST CHANGES

Breast changes are often one of the earliest signs of pregnancy. Typically, a tingly feeling with increased sensitivity develops. Breast enlargement is usually noted by the eighth week

Table 4-5 *Maternal Weight Gain with a Singleton Pregnancy*	
Fetus	7.5 lb.
Placenta	1.5 lb.
Amniotic fluid	2.0 lb.
Increased uterine muscle mass	2.5 lb.
Increased blood volume	3.5 lb.
Increased breast tissue	2.0 lb.
Increased interstitial fluid	2.0-3.0 lbs.
Additional fat storage	4.0 lb.

as venous supply to the breasts increases. The areola deepens in color and forms small, palpable papules. These hypertrophied sebaceous glands are called glands of Montgomery. After the 10th week, colostrum (a clear substance) can be expressed, and is the forerunner of the milk that comes 2 to 3 days after delivery to prepare the infant's intestinal system for mother's milk. (Full lactation is inhibited by high estrogen-progesterone levels prior to delivery). Estrogen stimulates production by the ducts, and progesterone increases the proliferation of the lobule-alveolar tissue. This is completed by mid-pregnancy. After delivery, the suckling of the infant stimulates the secretion of prolactin by the anterior pituitary gland, which then stimulates the production and secretion of milk.[1,2,10]

WEIGHT GAIN

Historically, physicians' opinions fluctuate about weight gain in pregnancy. In the mid-1950s, women were often restricted to a 15-pound gain, and some physicians even advised diet pills. Now it is known that weight gain not only affects fetal well-being but also alters the infant's ability to thrive after birth. Currently physicians believe the average woman with a singleton pregnancy should gain an average of 25 to 26 lbs., distributed as shown in Table 4-5.

Therefore, the uterus and its contents account for approximately 13.5 pounds, and maternal gains are about 11.5 to 12.5 pounds on the average. Fetal maternal weight gain ranges from 20 to 40 pounds for a single birth. The general recommendation for weight gain during the first trimester is 2 to 4 lbs.; and in the second and third, an average of slightly less than 1 pound per week. Extra fluid, protein, and fat are deposited as emergency stores in case the nursing mother is unable to get proper nutrition. The recommended daily allowance for women between the ages of 23 and 53 is about 2000 calories/day. During pregnancy, a mother should add 300 calories slightly more for a teen mother, and during lactation an extra 500 calories (above the 2000 calories/day base).

In singleton pregnancies, women of normal weight who have high gestational weight gains have babies with increased birth weight compared with women who have moderate weight gains. After delivery these women (with normal weight prior to pregnancy) returned to their normal weight despite large weight gains.[11]

Maternal weight gain for a multiple births can range from 40 to 80 lbs. depending on the number of fetuses. Luke reported in 1998 weight gains of 45 to 50 lbs. in triplet gestations and 45 to 80 lbs. gains in quadruplet pregnancies. A low early weight gain before 24 weeks of gestation is associated with poor intrauterine growth and higher morbidity among twins.[12] The Food and Nutrition Board of the Institute of Medicine (IOM) recommends a weight

Table 4-6
Summary of Weight Gain and Birth Weight in Multiple Gestations
MATERNAL GAIN

Plurality	No. of Infants*	% LBW (<2500 g)	% VLBW (<1500 g)	To 24-wks (lb)	Total (lb)	Range of Gestation (weeks)	Average Birth Weight (g)
Singletons	3,851,109	6	1	12	25-35	38-41	3,700-4,000
Twins	97,064	50	10	24	40-45	36-38	2,500-2,800
Triplets	4,233	90	32	36	50-60	34-35	1,900-2,200
Quads+	361	98	75	50	65-80	31-33	1,500-1,800

LBW = low birth weight; VLBW = very low birth weight.
*1994 U.S. live births.

Adapted from Luke B. What is the influence of maternal weight gain on fetal growth of twins? Clinical Obstetrics and Gynecology. 4(1)63,1998.

gain of 35.2 to 45 lbs. weight gain overall in twin gestations and a rate gain of 1.65 lbs./week during the second and third trimesters (Table 4-6).[12]

METABOLIC CHANGES

Profound metabolic changes occur during pregnancy. Metabolism of proteins, carbohydrates, fats, minerals, oxygen, and fluids is altered (Table 4-7).

RESPIRATORY CHANGES

Dyspnea is some times a first sign of pregnancy indicating how quickly the pregnant women adapts to the multiple respiratory changes in pregnancy (Table 4-8).

Pulmonary function is not impaired, because the respiratory system accommodates the changes of pregnancy (Figures 4-6 and 4-7).

ENDOCRINE CHANGES

During pregnancy, the major sources of hormone production are the adrenal, thyroid, parathyroid, anterior pituitary glands, and the placenta. After delivery, hormone secretions return to preexisting levels.

It is through the constant interaction of the fetus, placenta, and maternal system that steroid hormone levels increase (Tables 4-9 and 4-10).

DERMATOLOGIC CHANGES

There are many skin changes that occur during pregnancy, including increased pigmentation, abdominal wall tissue modification, cutaneous vascular markings, skin tags, sweating, itching, hair growth or loss, and nail alteration (Table 4-11).

Table 4-7

Metabolic Changes in Pregnancy

Structure/Function	Metabolic Change	Outcome
Protein	Increase due to demands of increase in tissue growth (eg, uterus and breasts).	Protein stored causing positive nitrogen balance.
		Nitrogen balance occurs early in gestation and increases through third trimester.
Carbohydrate	Insulin is elevated due to plasma expansion and blood glucose is reduced for a given insulin load.	Islet cells are stressed and may unmask a latent deficiency in islet cell secretion.
	Renal threshold for glucose is 100–150 mg/dl (drop from prepregnancy value 150 – 200 mg/dl) due to increase in glomerular filtration rate	May account for glycosuria and low blood sugar fasting levels in pregnancy; first evidence of diabetes.
Minerals	Sodium, potassium and calcium are stored for maternal use.	
	Sodium–Stored in amniotic fluid, placenta, tissues, and 33% in fetus.	At delivery, newborn's magnesium, phosphorous, and total ionized calcium levels are increased over mother's normal levels.
	Potassium–48% stored in fetus, additionally in breasts, uterus, and placenta.	
	Calcium–90% stored in fetus.	Maternal serum calcium diminishes during pregnancy, ionized calcium is increased until delivery.
	Iron–NOT stored in pregnancy. 1000 mg daily iron must be supplied to meet demands of mother and fetus.	500 mg daily requirement utilized by fetus, placenta and maternal red cell mass. 450 mg remain in the maternal store. 150 mg lost during delivery.
Fats	Increase in maternal fat stored and related increase in insulin resistance.	Elevated level of free fatty acids gives an anti-insulin effect by interfering with peripheral use of.
	Progesterone may reset fat thermostat in hypothalamus.[10]	Stores energy for mother and fetus during periods of starvation or extreme physical exertions.
Fluids	Increase in sodium and water retension.	Maternal edema – 50% may develop eyelid edema; 70% may develop edema of lower extremities (not associated with preclampsia or eclampsia).
	Increased capillary permeability from additional circulating placental ovarian and adrenocortical hormones.[10]	Edema present in morning and decreases with activity.

Table 4-8

Respiratory Changes in Pregnancy

Change	Cause	Outcome
Oxygen consumption increases by 14% (half to fetus and placanta, half to uterine muscle and breast tissue).	Half each to supply needs of fetus, placenta, and uterine muscle and breast tissue.	Respirations and cardiac function increase.
Increased levels of progesterone.	Hyperventilation	Decreased concentration of carbon dioxide in the alveoli which favors diffusion of carbon dioxide from fetal to maternal circulation.
Increased elevation of diaphragm.	Enlarged uterus.	Excursion decreases; breathing is more costal than abdominal.
Central part of diaphragm flattens.		Constant pulmonary function remains.
Dyspnea in first and second trimester ("hyperventilation of pregnancy").	Increased respiratory tidal volume.	Increase in respiratory minute volume by 26%.
Maternal plasma bicarbonate and total base values decreased.	Respiratory alkalosis caused by lowering the PCO2 of the blood.	Increase of sodium to compensate for alkalosis with little change in blood pH.

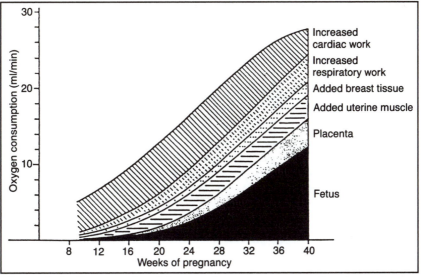

Figure 4-6. Components of increased oxygen consumption in pregnancy (From Hytten FE, Leitch I. *The Physiology of Human Pregnancy.* Blackwell, Oxford, 1964).

Figure 4-7. Components of lung volume in late pregnancy and in non-pregnant state (from Hytten FE, Leitch I. *The Physiology of Human Pregnancy*. Blackwell, Oxford, 1964).

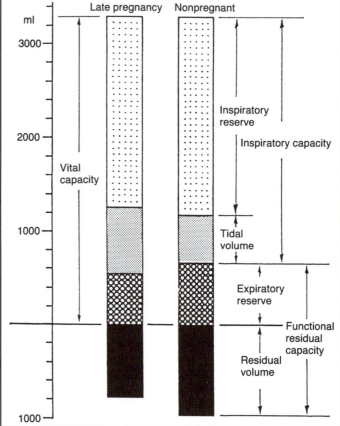

Table 4-9

Endocrine Changes in Pregnancy

Change	Cause	Outcome
Adrenal glands increase through pregnancy	Hyperplasia at the adrenal cortex	
Thyroid is increased by more than 50%[1]	New follicale formation, Increased vascularity, cell foration	Basal Metabolic Rate increased 10 – 30% by 16th week
Hypertrophy of *parathyroid glands*	Increase in fetal calcium demands	Maternal extracellular fluids for the fetus maintain normal calcium ion concentration. Calcium is absorbed from maternal bones.
Maternal *pituitary gland* enlarges. *Anterior lobe* increases 20–40% *Posterior lobe* does not hypertrophy. Secretion of oxytocin and ADH (antidiuretic hormone) increases in pregnancy	Due to prolactin-containing "pregnancy cells". Increase in estrogen. Increase requirement for antidiuretic hormone because of increased glomerular filtration rate and possible antagonistic effect of progesterone on antidiuretic hormones[1]	Marked prolactin production until gestation and allows for start of milk production ADH changes the osmolarity of blood oxytocin, helps contact uterus, and causes ejection of milk from milk ducts

Table 4-9 continued

Endocrine Changes in Pregnancy

Change	Cause	Outcome
Ovaries secrete relaxin at site of ruptured ovarian follicle (*corpus luteum*).[15]	Increased ligamentous length through body.	Larger pelvic outlet; easier delivery.
Placenta acts as am endocrine gland. After delivery there is a sudden loss of estrogen and progesterone secretion by the placenta.	Acts in respiration, nutrition, and excretion for the fetus. Allows for marked prolactin production by the pituitary gland.	Maintain the pregnancy and support of fetus until gestation. This process stimulates production of fat and lactose by the mammary glands which secrete colostrum.

*It is through constant interaction of the fetus, placenta, and maternal system that steroid hormone levels increase.

Table 4-10

Hormones and their Functions in Pregnancy

Hormone	A. Where Produced B. When Occurs	Function
hCG Human chorionic gonadotropin	A. Placenta, by the trophoblastic tissues of the early fertilized ovum into the fluids of the mother B. Soon after fertilization	Augments, maintains endometrial bed; causes persistence of corpus luteum to secrete larger quantities of progesterone and estrogen, prevents menses
HPL Human placental lactogen, also known as human chorionic somato-mammotropin (hCS)	A. By trophoblastic tissue, placenta, third week after ovulation in the trophoblast B. 5th week, progressing with pregnancy	Plays a major role in development of mother's breast prior to birth of baby; inhibits action of insulin to cause glucose transport through cell membranes; promotes cell growth and provides increased circulation of free fatty acids for energy for maternal metabolism and fetal nutrition; inhibition of glucose uptake and gluconeogenesis in mother; anti-insulin action raises levels of insulin, which favors protein synthesis and ensures mobilizable source of amino acids for transport to the fetus
Human chorionicthyrotropin (HCT)	A. Produced by the placenta B. Evident in early pregnancy and rises until term	Increases secretion of thyroid hormones to stimulate incorporation of inorganic phosphates into thyroid to be neutralized by antipituitary TSH (pituitary thyrotropin)
Human chorionic adrenocorticotropin HCACTH (HCCG)	A. Pituitary-like hormone produced by placenta B. Evident by 10th week of gestation	Placental steroidogenesis

Table 4-10 continued
Hormones and their Functions in Pregnancy

Hormone	A. Where Produced B. When Occurs	Function
Estrogen	A. Produced by ovarian follicle, placenta and adrenal cortex. B. Appears mid-pregnancy	Levels used to assess fetal and placental functions; necessary for a viable placenta, healthy fetus; intact fetal circulation
Progesterone	A. Formed by maternal adrenals, corpus luteum, placental syncytial cells, and fetal adrenals. B. Corpus luteum in early gestation; placenta in late pregnancy; polypeptide protein secreted by corpus luteum, evident by missed period	Development, maintaince of endrometrial bed; relaxation of pelvic ligaments and connective tissue, softening of the cervix, inhibition of uterine motility
Prolactin	A. Produced by anterior lobe of pituitary gland. B. Produced immediately after birth of baby[7,15,16]	Stimulates milk production

Table 4-11
Dermatologic Changes in Pregnancy

Change	Cause	Outcome
Chloasma (Mask of Pregnancy)	Increase in pigmentation around eyes, over cheekbones and around breast areola.	Disappears at end of pregnancy, but may last for several weeks.
Linea Alba	Increased pigmentation resulting in brownish-black streak down middle of abdomen.	Usually regresses after delivery
Breast Areola	Increased pigmentation.	Usually regresses after delivery.
Striae Gravidarum (stretch marks) along breasts, abdomen and thighs.	Changes in the collagen elastic fibers of the deep layers of the skin resulting in purplish irregular lines. Elevated levels of adrenal steroids may cause thinning of fibers.	Color of lines fades to white after delivery but the lines do not disappear.[1,2]
Spider Nevi appear in two-thirds of Caucasians and one-tenth of African American women.	Cutaneous vascular changes marked by small red elevations with radiating branches from a central body on face, upper chest and arms due to an increase in estrogen production.	Usually disappear at end of pregnancy.
Telangiectasia around ankles and thighs.	Capillary dilations due to an increase in estrogen production.	Related to varices but not painful. Subside to an extent but not completely after delivery.
Palmer Erythema appears in two-thirds of Caucasian and one-third of African American women.	Reddening of the palms due to an increase in estrogen production.	Usually disappear at end of pregnancy.[17]
Skin Tags (molluscum fibrosum gravidarum)	Skin colored, fleshy growths 1–5 mm in length on sides of	Usually form in second half of pregnancy and may progress or disappear

Table 4-11 continued

Dermatologic Changes in Pregnancy

Change	Cause	Outcome
	face and neck, anterior portions of chest, axilla and feet. May result from endocrine changes.	after delivery.[17]
Increase in Sweating	Increased weight and thyroid activity causing the increased glandular activity. Palmer sweating may result from adrenocortical secretion	Effect of pregnancy on acne is unpredictable; may lead to some types of eczema. Axillary sweat glands may actually decrease during pregnancy possible causing a rebound effect post-partum
Pruritus (itching) – generalized or localized.	May be from hepatic disorder. May be related to mild form of intrahepatic cholestases.	Affects approx. 20% of pregnant women. Begin in third month and continue to last; usually does not continue post-partum.
Hirsutism seen in most women in early pregnancy.	Related to increased adrenocortocotrophic hormone and adrenocorticosteroid secretion. Hair may increase on face, arms, legs and sometimes back. Women with darker or more body hair experience greater growth.	After delivery, new fine hair is replaced with coarse hair.
Hair Loss	May be due to changes in endocrine balance and/or stress.	By 4–12 weeks post-partum, hair loss is noticeable and may continue for several months. Regrowth usually occurs within 6 to 15 months but hair may never be abundant as before pregnancy.
Nail Changes – transverse grooving, softening, increased brittleness, loosening, overgrowth of skin beneath nail (subungual keratosis).	Not fully understood.	Occur as early as sixth week.
Autoimmune progesterone dermatitis of pregnancy–severe acniform eruption in first trimester. Increase in eosinophilic hyperglobulinemia and hanstent arthritis.	Related to hormone-dependent mechanisms because of cell-mediated immunity against endogenous progesterone produced in pregnancy.	Associated with spontaneous abortion.
Herpes Gestationis-generalized itching followed by red papules, plaques and lesions around umbilicus which spread over entire body.	Autoimmune dermatitis unique to pregnancy.	Areas of pigmentation may reoccur in subsequent pregnancies.
Marked by severe local burning, fever and large number of eosinophils in the blood.		Symptoms clear within a few days of delivery.
Impetigo Herpetiforms – very rare serious inflammatory dermatitis of pregnancy. Occurs at any stage of pregnancy or puerperium. Primary pustule surrounded by red oozing crushed lesions usually in genitoanal area.	Systemic reaction including fever, leukocytes, tachycardia, vomiting and electrolyte imbalance. Cause unknown.	Delivery of fetus as soon as there is lung maturity. Disease reoccurs with subsequent pregnancies.

Table 4-11 continued
Dermatologic Changes in Pregnancy

Change	Cause	Outcome
Papular Dermatitis – generalized eruption of intensely pruritic papules covered with bloody crusts over generalized distribution.	Extremely high levels of urinary hCG.	High stillbirth rate. Eruptions clear after delivery but reoccurs in subsequent pregnancies.
Prurigo Gestationis – small highly pruitic papules covered by bloody cysts from scratchng on extensor surfaces of extremities, abdomen and rib cage.	Specific to pregnancy.	Clears spontaneously after pregnancy leaving small hyperpigmentation areas. No fetal affect.
Pruritic Urticarial Papules (PUPPP) – appear in last trimester. Eruption of red papules that change to a urticarial (wheal) followed by a papule on abdomen, thighs, buttocks and arms.	Specific to pregnancy.	Clears after pregnancy. No fetal or maternal mortality.

MULTIPLE PREGNANCIES

Multiple pregnancies occur in 1% of all gestations carried beyond 20 weeks, and account for 10% of all perinatal mortality.[1] The frequency of twins increases with both maternal age and parity and is more likely to occur after the use of drugs for induction of ovulation, after discontinuing oral contraceptives, and as a result of in vitro fertilization. Over the last 20 years women have chosen to delay motherhood. With the increased age, there has been an increased chance of multiples. The incidence of twin, triplet, and quadruple plus births has been rising at rates faster than for singletons. Between 1974 and 1994, there has been a 21% increase in singleton births, a 68% increase in twin births and a 357% rise in triplet and higher order births.[12] Fertility treatments have a 25% to 50% greater chance of resulting in twins and a 5 to 7% chance of triplets and higher order of multiples. The rates for monozygotic twinning (occurs as a result of division of one fertilized ovum early in gestation) is constant in all races and throughout the world at the rate of 3 to 4 per 1,000 births. Dizygotic twins (when two separate ova are fertilized by two different sperm) vary from country to country and is likely a reflection of maternal nutrition. Women who conceive dizygotic twins tend to be older, overweight, obese, taller, have had more children and a family history of dizygotic twins. These mothers of spontaneous multiples have an earlier onset of menses, a shorter menstrual cycle, and an earlier onset of menopause.[1,12] Women with multiples after fertility treatments tend to be more educated, white, and older.[12]

Multiple gestations are suspected when uterine size is greater than expected for gestational age, but ultrasound and auscultation of the heartbeat can identify twins as early as 6 or 7 weeks. Human placental lactogen levels are higher in twin pregnancies than they are in normal single ones. Monozygotic twins occur as a result of division of one fertilized ovum early in gestation. These identical twins may have four different configurations of chorions (the outermost layer of the amniotic sac and placenta). The most common arrangement is one shared placenta, two amniotic sacs, and one chorion. Next common is two chorions, two amniotic sacs, and two fused placentas; followed by two chorions, two amniotic sacs, and two distinct placentas. The rarest arrangement is one chorion, one amniotic sac, and one placenta.

Pre-term birth (before 32 weeks of gestation) occurs in less than 2% of singleton births, 11% of twins and 31% of triplet births. Birth before 37 weeks of gestation occurs in 11% of singleton births, 48% of twin births and 88% of triplet births. Twenty-five percent to 40% of all twin pregnancies result in premature labor and delivery due to the volume of intrauterine expansion that exceeds what the myometrium can accommodate.[12] Congenital anomalies, abnormal placentation, and the effect of the uterine contents on cervical integrity may also initiate premature labor and delivery.[1] Perinatal mortality among twins is three to four times that of singleton births because of low birth weight, prematurity complications, intracerebral hemorrhage, respiratory distress syndrome, traumatic delivery, or sepsis. During pregnancy, a mother carrying twins will easily gain 60 pounds, and blood volume increases 50% or more (30% to 40% with singletons).[1] This leads to a disproportionate increase in plasma volume over red cell volume, resulting in hemodilution or "pregnancy anemia".[1] The risk of iron deficiency is two to three times that of a singleton pregnancy because of the increased fetal and maternal demands. Other maternal complications include a greater risk of hemorrhage antepartum, intrapartum, and post-partum because of increased risk of abruptio placenta, placenta previa, and uterine atony, related to complications from surgical deliveries.

EXERCISE

Exercise in pregnancy is of concern to the physical therapist because of the possibility of exceeding safe metabolic, respiratory, and cardiac thresholds of the mother and fetus. The types of exercises advocated have changed dramatically since the 1930s, when physicians in Great Britain simply encouraged "activity" for expectant mothers, based on an observation that working-class women had easier births.

Recommendations for treatment from research on exercise in pregnancy must be applied cautiously. There are many legal and ethical standards that limit not only the scope of research studies but the relation of results from animal studies to humans. Physiologic parameters that differ between animals and humans, such as heat elimination from sweating versus panting and venous pooling from standing, are but two variables that make it impossible to directly apply results to humans. Therefore, this discussion will focus only on exercise in human pregnancy.

The adjustment to exercise depends upon age, sex, body size; type of exercise, body position, light, moderate, or heavy work; frequency; the environment, temperature, water, altitude, pollution, as well as; the health and nutritional status of the subject. It should also be understood that there are no consistent methods of training nor consistent test protocols. This makes extrapolations from research difficult to apply to activities of daily living. Of importance, however, are maternal physiologic responses to work and exercise, including oxygen consumption, circulation, cardiovascular response, respiration, hormonal changes, body temperature, energy expenditure, and physical work capacity, as well as fetal and placental responses.

Maternal Responses to Exercise

Artal has summarized the literature for cardiovascular responses to exercise during pregnancy as follows: there is a slight increase in cardiac output during mild and moderate exercise with a significant drop in maximal cardiac output; there is an increase in stroke volume on any given work load; there may be an increased heart rate at low intensity exercises, a normal heart rate at normal intensity exercise, and a reduced maximal heart rate; there is no difference in arteriovenous oxygen difference between work and pregnancy; and then there

Cardiovascular Changes That Influence Exercise Capacity during Normal Pregnancy			
Function	**Non-Pregnant**	**Pregnant**	**Percentage Change**
Blood volume (ml)	2500	3900	55
Heart volume (ml)			12
Heart rate (bpm)			
Rest	70	85	20
Exercise	190	170	15
Cardiac output (ml/min)	4500	6000	30[a]
Stroke volume (ml/beat)	60-70	85-90	30[b]
A-V oxygen difference (ml)	45	40	12
Arterial pressure			
Systolic	120	112	5
Diastolic	75	70	5
Systemic vascular resistance (dynes/sec/cm^5)	1700	1250	30

[a]*Greatest during mid-pregnancy.*
[b]*Greatest by the end of the second trimester.*

Figure 4-8. Cardiovascular changes that influence exercise capacity during normal pregnancy (From deSwiet M, Hytten F, Chamberlain G, eds. *Clinical Physiology in Obstetrics,* Oxford, England: Blackwell Scientific Publications; 1980).

may be an error associated with the prediction of maximal work capacity from a submaximal heart rate (Figure 4-8).

The oxygen consumption per unit time (VO_2) at rest in pregnancy increases with advancing gestation to a maximum value near term.[18] This increase may be due to a higher metabolic rate, increased tissue mass, or extra work needed to perform vital functions. Increased VO_2 during exercise results from increased muscle work involved in changing body position, respiration, and cardiac function.[18] The highest measurements of VO_2 have been recorded at term during maximal exercise.[18] Lotgering reported a logical increase in VO_2 during a treadmill test in a pregnant woman, as compared to her non-pregnant value. It is believed that there is a training effect evident in pregnancy (unless a sedentary lifestyle is adopted), because every activity requires a higher absolute VO_2 In addition to maternal demands, uterine oxygen consumption also increases during pregnancy due to the expanding demands of the fetus and placenta. During exercise, uterine blood flow may reduce markedly, but the uterine VO_2 is maintained secondary to hemoconcentration and increased oxygen extraction by the myoendometrium.

Exercising women may experience increasing difficulty as their pregnancy advances because of the inability to transfer oxygen and carbon dioxide from the air to the cells. Along with a significant increase in hemoglobin and cardiac output, there is an excess demand that leads to a decrease in arteriovenous oxygen difference. Non-pregnant women compensate by increasing pulmonary diffusion capacity and increasing alveolar ventilation. The pregnant woman compensates for these physiologic and associated anatomic changes by breathing more deeply. As weight increases during pregnancy, exercise produces a greater oxygen debt, and results in a longer recovery rate.

Artal compared pulmonary responses to exercise at mild, moderate, and VO_2 max (maximum oxygen consumption) levels (Figures 4-9 and 4-10). He found that in mild exercise,

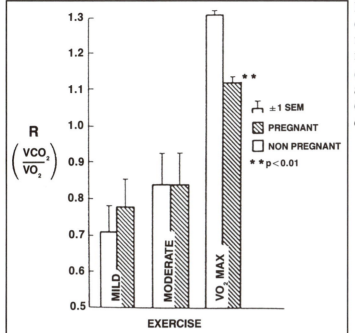

Figure 4-9. Comparison of respiratory exchange ratio (R) during mild, moderate, and VO_2 max exercise (from Artal R, et al. *American Journal of Obstetrics and Gynecology*)

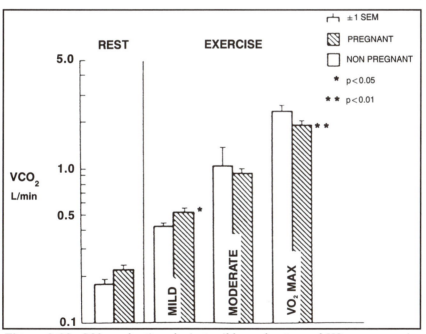

Figure 4-10. CO^2 production during mild, moderate, and VO_2 max exercise (from Artal R, et al. *American Journal of Obstetrics and Gynecology*).

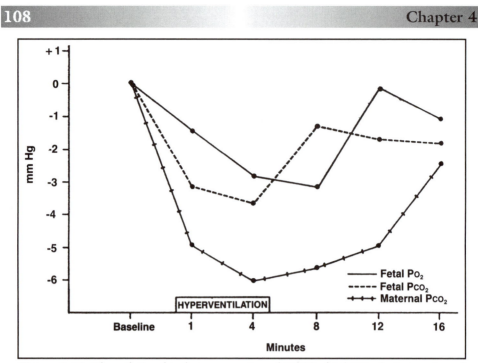

Figure 4-11. The relationship between maternal PCO2, fetal PO$_2$ during maternal hyperventilation (from Miller FC, et al. *American Journal of Obstetrics and Gynecology* 120: 489,1974.)

respiratory frequency was significantly higher than in controls. Overall, pregnant women responded to exercise with increased ventilation at mild and maximal exercise levels. At moderate exercise, they responded with a more efficient ventilation. This may be the result of primary respiratory alkalosis of pregnancy. Pregnant subjects were found to have lower respiratory frequencies and tidal volumes equal to controls.

Hyperventilation, during rest in pregnancy, increases with exercise (Figure 4-11) and results in a lower carbon dioxide tension, lower bicarbonate concentration and buffering capacity, and a moderate increase in pH with a negligible change in oxygen tension.[18,19] In addition to the findings of Artal, research has shown that respiratory frequency during and after bicycling or weightbearing exercises slightly increases, but not significantly. Gas exchange during exercise increases to the same levels in pregnant women and controls as an effect of increased pulmonary diffusion capacity and increased alveolar ventilation.[20] In a study of pregnant women during moderately strenuous bicycle exercise, lower carbon dioxide tensions were found at rest and during exercise, with hyperventilation displayed during exercise. No change in arterial carbon dioxide content was found during mild exercise in pregnant and non-pregnant women (see Figure 4-10). Mean arterial blood pressure may increase up to 20% in response to exercise in human pregnancies, mainly because of systolic pressure increases proportionate to the level of exercise at moderate work loads. Increased weight from pregnancy may be a factor in this alteration in pressure (Figure 4-12). Diastolic pressure decreases about 10% below non-pregnant values in early and midgestation, although systolic pressure decreases only slightly.

During pregnancy, the whole blood volume increases slowly by 50% near term because of a 30 to 60% increase in plasma volume and a 20 to 30% increase in erythrocyte mass.[18,20] Because of this hypervolemia, there may be an increase in mean systemic pressure that, combined with a decreased peripheral resistance, mediates the increase in stroke volume and

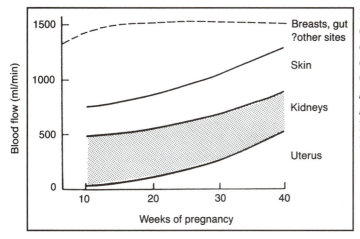

Figure 4-12. Distrubution of increased cardiac output during pregnancy (From de-Sweten M, Hytten F, Chamberlain G, eds. *Clinical Physiology in Obstetrics.* Oxford, England: Blackwell Scientific Publications; 1980).

resting cardiac output. Plasma volume, however, decreases during exercise (depending on intensity) to a maximal low of 15% at about 60% VO_2 max. This occurs within the first 10 minutes and does not change with further exercise. In studies of pregnant cardiac patients, it has been demonstrated that heart disease does not affect blood volume or plasma but does reduce cardiac reserve. As a consequence, these patients respond with increased stroke volume and tachycardia.

By using indicator dilution and electromagnetic flow probes with the patient under anesthesia or in a compromising supine position, a dramatic increase in uterine blood flow can be demonstrated (see Figure 4-11). Because the woman is anesthetized, the actual changes in uterine blood flow may be further increased under physiologic conditions.[18,20] Urine tests measuring 5-hydroxyindolacetic acid suggest that there is a decrease in visceral blood flow in pregnant women during exercise compared to controls.[20]

Cardiac output, peripheral resistance, arterial blood pressure, left ventricular work, and arteriovenous oxygen difference adjust to within normal limits during exercise,[18] as long as there is no pre existing cardiac problem. Cardiovascular function is impaired in cases of patients with heart disease and pregnancy-induced hypertension. The increased blood pressure at rest noted in patients with pregnancy-induced hypertension appears to be the result of increased systemic vascular resistance. Vigorous exercise for these patients is contraindicated and needs further study.

Cardiovascular responses to isometric exercises in patients with pregnancy-induced hypertension was studied by Nisell and colleagues.[21] Although the isometric hand-grip test increased blood pressure, heart rate, stroke volume, cardiac output, epinephrine, and norepinephrine concentrations in arterial plasma in both the pregnancy-controlled group and the pregnancy-hypertensive group, these factors did not differ significantly. Nisell and colleagues concluded that pregnancy-induced hypertension does not seem to be associated with exaggerated cardiovascular or sympathoadrenal reactivity to isometric exercise compared with normal pregnancy.[21] The increase in blood pressure appeared to be a response to an increase in cardiac output for both groups.

Cardiovascular conditioning during pregnancy has been of interest as a possible means to shorten or decrease the intensity of labor. Many studies have tried to relate physical fitness to pregnancy outcome,[18,22] and there is some evidence to suggest that physical fitness may shorten labor in multiparas.[22] Results of studies of labor in primiparas are mixed; some show a shorter labor, and others do not.[18] More control is necessary to accurately assess the question of labor duration and level of previous exercise. Lactate levels studied by Erkkola and

Rauramol[18] revealed that fit women worked harder during labor and delivery than the non-fit. The study also showed that fit women had higher oxygen-carrying capacities to compensate for metabolic acidosis.

The mother's basal body temperature rises by about 0.5° C immediately following ovulation, increases to a maximal level at midgestation, and then decreases to normal.[18] This rise in temperature is due to progesterone, which increases through term. The decline in basal body temperature after midpregnancy reflects the opposing effect of increasing estrogen concentrations. Body core temperature may also be affected by prolonged maternal exercise, which may cause an increase high enough to produce teratogenic effects on the fetus. Animal studies show that core temperatures above 39°C may be teratogenic and may result in neurotube defects. Hyperthermia-induced dehydration may also precipitate premature labor and should be avoided.

There is also evidence to suggest that strenuous exercise during pregnancy may be linked to intrauterine growth retardation.[18,20] Working mothers tend to have babies with birth weights as much as 400 grams lower than babies of non-working mothers.[18]

Maternal hormonal changes during exercise are transitory, reversible, and have no marked effects. Prolactin has a role in water electrolyte balance, which, in turn, has an effect on energy. It has been found that submaximal exercise during pregnancy will elevate serum prolactin levels significantly for 1 hour. Estradiol and progesterone, the ovarian hormones, will increase during exercise, especially strenuous activity.[20] Low values of estriol reflect fetal distress. After submaximal exercise there is a significant brief rise in estriol, which may indicate fetal well-being, or an increased flow of estriol rich, uteroplacental blood.

Various endocrine adaptations occur during maternal exercise, however. Glucose utilization and production increase during exercise. During mild exercise glycogen rises slightly, but insulin level does not. When exercise is more intense, glycogen levels increase significantly, increasing glycogenolysis and gluconeogenesis in the liver. These increases have a primary role in the physiological adaptation to exercise. Increased glucocorticoids induce lipolysis and possess anti-inflammatory properties. Exercise may be used to achieve a normoglycemic state in pregnancy.[20] With medical supervision, pregnant diabetics can capitalize on individually-designed exercise programs. However, hypoglycemia is a major problem in diabetics during and after exercise. Studies suggest that prolonged strenuous exercise may induce hypoglycemia faster in pregnancy. In addition, exercise may cause a rise in norepinephrine, which can act as a stimulant to the uterus and possibly induce uterine activity.[15] There are minor changes in cortisol levels during exercise, because mild exercise produces only a minimal adrenal effect; therefore, it appears that the cortisol level has a limited role during maternal exercise.

The basal energy expenditure or metabolic rate of maternal tissues alone, during pregnancy, cannot be measured. During pregnancy, the increases in resting VO_2 and metabolic rate are related to changes in lean or total body mass.[20] The non-protein respiratory quotient in non-pregnant and near-term women, despite fetal growth, is the same or slightly increased (about 0.85).[20] Similarly, during mild bike exercise the non-protein respiratory quotient is not significantly higher in pregnant women than in non-pregnant controls. Consequently, the ratio of fat-to-carbohydrate used for energy expenditure remains constant. The metabolic rate appears to vary linearly with VO_2.[20]

Artal found, however, that during weightbearing exercise pregnant women used primarily fat, and proportionately less carbohydrate, as a fuel source. He suggests this mechanism may protect the mother from exercising anaerobically and the fetus from hypoxia. However, with some forms of aerobic exercise, for example, pedaling in water, carbohydrate stores were the primary energy source.[19] In cases of moderate non-weightbearing exercise on the ergometer, the calculated metabolic costs are slightly (but not significantly) higher during pregnancy.[20]

There is a decrease in physical work capacity in the first trimester, so women with low physical capacity may be functioning at their limit to perform simple activities of daily living. If, however, the pregnant woman's physical work capacity is high, she will probably be able to tolerate greater demands during the first trimester. Weightbearing exercise, however, requires increasing oxygen uptake as the pregnancy advances. Weightbearing exercise increases respiratory frequency more than during non-weightbearing exercise. Minute ventilation and tidal volume also increase at rest, during, and following exercise.[1,18] Because energy demand with weightbearing exercise increases, and maximum work capacity remains the same or decreases, the absolute intensity of weightbearing exercise should be lowered as the pregnancy advances into the second and third trimesters.

Fetal Response to Maternal Exercise

Typically, the fetal heart rate is used to assess fetal well-being. Changes in fetal heart rate reflect hypoxic and non-hypoxic stress, sympathetic and parasympathetic activity, or asphyxia. However, a 50% reduction in uterine blood flow would have to occur to cause such changes. The healthy fetus can tolerate brief periods of asphyxia, which may occur during maternal exercise (see Figure 4-11). The fetus will respond to this asphyxia with increased blood pressure and tachycardia. In this way, blood circulation is facilitated, followed by an increase in O^2 and a decrease in CO^2 tension. In a summary of published studies on fetal heart rate response to maternal exercise, increases of 10 to 30 beats/minute were recorded. These changes do not vary with increased intensity of maternal exercise or gestational age.[15] In a study by Artal of 354 subjects, 22 had fetal bradycardia during or after exercise (6.2% incidence), 11 of the 22 had abnormal pregnancies (pregnancy-induced hypertension or premature labor), and the other 11 had normal pregnancies.[18]

Maternal exercise is associated with an increase in catecholamines metabolized by the placenta. Only 10% to 15% of these catecholamines reach the fetus, but it has been theorized that they could have a restrictive effect on the umbilical blood flow. The combined effect of possible vasoconstriction from elevated catecholamines and decreased blood to the uterus could lead to fetal asphyxia and result in an initial response of tachycardia and bradycardia with prolonged hypoxia and vagal stimulation. Carpenter and colleagues[23] found that brief submaximal maternal exercise (up to 70% of maximal aerobic power; maternal heart rate less than or equal to 148 beats/minute), on the cycle ergometer, did not affect fetal heart rate. Maximal exertion, however, appears to be followed by fetal bradycardia. Fetal breathing movements are episodic and occur 30% of the time in the last trimester. Hypoxia significantly reduces the frequency of fetal breathing and body movements. Gestation, time of day, catecholamine level, and maternal plasma glucose level affect fetal breathing movements as well. It appears that the frequency of fetal breathing movements may be a more sensitive indicator of fetal well-being than fetal heart rate.[20] Fetal breathing movements appear to increase following maternal exercise but decrease in fetuses suspected to be in distress who are carried by hypertensive mothers. Fetuses who have experienced hypoxia, as well as those enduring labor, exhibit decreased fetal breathing movements. Katz and coworkers24 measured fetal and maternal responses to immersion exercise (ergometer with water level to the xiphoid process). At 60 % VO_2 max at 15, 25, and 35 weeks of pregnancy, they found, with underwater ultrasound, that the fetus demonstrated body limb motion and fetal breathing movements. Fetal heart rates were normal and unchanged from those at rest. Maternal temperature was unchanged during exercise, or recovery, at all gestational stages. The nature of the immersion exercise eliminates the major problems with decreased uterine blood flow, physical discomfort, and elevated core temperature.[24]

Placental Responses to Maternal Exercise

The fetus receives a continuous supply of oxygen, which is necessary for growth and development. This supply averages 8 ml/min/kg and is derived from the maternal circulation by diffusion across the placenta. It is possible that maternal exercise may have an effect on this placental oxygen transfer. Many factors contribute to oxygen transfer across the placenta: maternal and fetal arterial PO_2, maternal and fetal diffusion capacity, maternal and fetal hemoglobin affinities, maternal and fetal hemoglobin flow rates, vascular regulation of maternal and fetal vessels, and the quantity of CO_2 exchange.[18] Unfortunately, because of ethical and technical problems in measuring placental transfer, the only studies are on pregnant ewes. In these animals, 10 minutes of 70% maximal exercise on a treadmill at maximal oxygen consumption caused increased maternal arterial PO_2 by 8%, and hemoglobin concentration by 25%. Uterine blood flow decreased by 21%. Fetal and maternal blood pH increased. By the end of the exercise, however, uteroplacental oxygen delivery was unchanged because of the increase in maternal hemoglobin concentration.[20] It cannot, however, be predicted that the same will occur in humans.

Effect of Exercise on Pregnancy Outcome

Physical activity in the workplace has shown that quiet standing, long hours, protracted ambulation and heavy lifting are associated with an increased incidence of low birth weight and prematurity.[25] It has been postulated that these activities cause an intermittent but protracted reduction in uterine blood flow. Recreational activities have shown that regular exercise in pregnancy improve maternal cardiovascular reserve, maternal mechanisms for heat dissipation and placental growth and function.[25] In addition there is evidence that regular recreational exercise is related to shorter labor and is useful in the treatment for gestational diabetes.[26]

THE PHYSICAL THERAPIST AS AN INSTRUCTOR

These details are included here in the Maternal Physiology Chapter, so the reader can easily refer to original background information in designing classes that contain physiology as the main component. Among the many educational classes that the physical therapist can offer to expectant mothers and their partners are classes for early pregnancy; childbirth preparation; breastfeeding; and prenatal, post-natal, or post-Cesarean exercise. Although much of the background information needed by a physical therapist who wishes to teach these classes can be learned through reading and obstetric observation, experienced instructors usually agree that potential instructors should acquire extra continuing education to teach a specific topic within the general OB/GYN specialty.

Although certification is not required to teach or gain access to OB/GYN clients, it is helpful for physical therapists in some locations to become certified as childbirth educators. There are several organizations, listed in the resource guide in the appendix, that conduct programs leading to certification. Some courses are run weekly for a few months. Others are held intermittently on an intensive basis; the participants often completing most of the instruction over a weekend. More recently, home self-study guides have become part of the teacher instruction arsenal. In addition, obstetric experience, a written or oral test, preparation of a class syllabus, and student teaching may be part of the certification requirements. Continuing education or viewing of labors and deliveries to update knowledge may be required by some organizations to maintain certification. The physical therapist that is

Table 4-12
Sample Course Evaluation

Date:

1. Did this course meet your goals?

2. Did you find the handouts valuable?

3. Would you recommend this course to others?

4. Was the information presented in a clear, understandable manner?

5. Do you have any suggestions or comments?

exploring certification, should examine current and future requirements to evaluate which certification process, if any, fits best into plans for practice and marketing.

The teacher must be able to assess the students' needs by observation and non-verbal and verbal communication, as well as streamline information to the needs of a particular group. Courses for single teenage mothers will most likely require a format different from that for married couples, but the basic content must still be presented to both groups. The childbirth educator who implements a plan formulated from an assessment of the goals, needs, and objectives of the group, as well as from their experiences, will probably have a more successful educational program.[27]

Instructor evaluation is a critical component to a successful program. If the material presented and the manner in which it is presented is not under scrutiny, the program will likely become static. A teacher must be alert and evaluate verbal and non-verbal feedback from class participants. A formal course evaluation is also recommended, not only as a means of self-evaluation, but as a way of gathering feedback for referring physicians, nurses, midwives, child-birth educators and colleagues (Table 4-12).

The teacher should be aware of class participants' emotions that become barriers to their learning. Couples may be anxious because of social issues (eg, an argument before the class or financial problems). Some couples may monopolize a class session by using the instructor as a front for their concerns about the birth of the baby, care of the child, or relationship changes. It is a challenge for the teacher to uncover these issues, draw people out, and assist couples in learning about the events to come, while at the same time, addressing their underlying concerns.

One theory ascribes that groups of people in a classroom setting learn by passing through various phases. Initially, a tuning-in phase may occur when the students and the teacher make observations about the setting and other couples in the room and are generally mindful of the surroundings. In the following contractual phase, the teacher introduces himself or herself, relates background experience, and explains what is expected from the class. The students complete this phase when they introduce themselves. As class content is introduced, the work period begins. During this phase, reinforcement is necessary to provide feedback to the class. The final phase is the ending, during which some students may feel anxious about separating from the instructor. The teacher can reduce anxiety by summarizing the information that was covered by giving homework for the week, and by presenting an overview of the next class. These five phases are part of every class, whether the subject is early pregnancy, childbirth preparation, or exercise.[27]

Table 4-13

Sample Class Registration Form

Class date:_____

Name: _____

Partner: _____

Doctor/midwife: _____

Home phone munber:_____

Work phone number: _____

Address:_____

Contacted:_____

Concerns: _____

Notified of: Time and place- _____
            Fee- _____
            Clothing/pillows/other- _____

Additional Comments:_____

_____

_____

EARLY PREGNANCY CLASSES

A woman should be encouraged to join early pregnancy classes as soon as she knows she is pregnant; the sooner, the better. The typical class introduces anatomy, physiology, nutrition, body mechanics, muscle strengthening, and an understanding of emotional issues. The three goals of early pregnancy classes are to assist women and their partners:

1. To recognize physical and emotional changes that occur during pregnancy
2. To learn appropriate comfort measures
3. To provide a forum for women and their partners to enter the experience together and express their immediate concerns[28]

The classes consist of discussions, audiovisual presentations, handouts, and practical sessions. Using this information, women will be able to make appropriate choices regarding exercise, relaxation, nutrition, body mechanics, and plans for delivery. Usually, women are encouraged to bring a partner, spouse, boyfriend, sibling, parent, or friend. It is particularly helpful for the prospective mother to work with the same person she will bring with her for labor and delivery.

Logistically, the early pregnancy class is geared to the woman 1 to 5 months pregnant and her partner. Three weekly 2-hour classes should provide enough time to cover the necessary material, provided the class is limited to 8 to 10 couples The classroom should be located where the instructor and couples can have some privacy and quiet for teaching and learning relaxation Bathrooms should be easily accessible.

Tables 4-13 and 4-14 illustrate a sample registration form and class outline for early pregnancy education classes. If word-of-mouth doesn't draw participants, the instructor may need to advertise the class in the local newspaper or send letters to local obstetricians and midwives.

If a promotional letter is mailed, a statement of objectives, course outline, goals, and possibly, handouts, as well as the physical therapist's resume, may help encourage referrals. A follow-up phone call to answer any questions may also prove fruitful. It often takes a while to

Table 4-14

Suggested Outline for an Early Pregnancy Class

Class 1   Introduction
              Relaxation instruction
              Immediate concerns of couples
              Break
              Emotional aspects of pregnancy
              Fetal and maternal changes

Class 2   Options for delivery
              Nutrition
              Pelvic floor toning
              Break
              Body mechanics
              Pelvic tilt/Positions of comfort
              Relaxation

Class 3   Continue relaxation
              Continue options and planning for delivery
              Father's role
              Break
              Stretching and toning, body mechanics review
              Discussion, questions
              Course evaluation

increase the size of the class, depending on whether it's private-based or hospital-based. Classes taught in a hospital or clinic tend to receive instant approval by both physicians and clients.

A comfortable way to start the class is for the instructor to discuss personal obstetric experience and rationale for attending early pregnancy classes. The participants can then introduce themselves, name their physician or midwife, share their due date, and explain why they are attending the class. This goes for both the woman and her partner. It's often fun to tell husbands it's okay to say their wives made them come. This discussion often breaks the ice and facilitates group interaction.

After introductions are made is a good time for the instructor to go over the contents of any handout packet, which can be added to every week. It is probably a good idea to include in the initial packet, or even with paid registration, a bibliography of suggested reading for pregnancy and childbirth, nutrition, breastfeeding, parenting, and post-partum. It is also helpful to give referral numbers, such as the number for the La Leche League, a nursing mothers' support service, or for labor and delivery classes that require early registration. Packets may also include prepared statements available for purchase, such as the "Pregnant Patient's Bill of Rights" and the "Pregnant Patient's Responsibilities" available from the International Childbirth Association (see Appendix).

Teaching Relaxation: Why it is Important

Many physiologic changes of pregnancy cannot be controlled and may affect a woman's psychological state. For instance, she may have physical discomfort, bizarre dreams, concerns over safety of the baby, or anxiety over birth and parenting. These are normal responses to pregnancy, and fathers may experience similar feelings. This increased anxiety can be stress-producing, but even more stress can occur during labor and delivery. The uterine contractions of labor and delivery occur without voluntary control and can be quite painful. This pain can in turn lead to increased muscular tension as a response to pain. To decrease pain associated with increased muscular tension, relaxation is often the key. However, to relax her body, the laboring woman must be able to relax her mind. Education often provides the answers to stress-inducing questions, thereby decreasing anxiety. Through active relaxation exercises, men and women can not only learn to relax tense musculature, but can develop an awareness of tense musculature. The woman who is able to release tense muscles during labor and delivery will avoid working against herself and, theoretically, will experience less discomfort.

The man or woman who practices relaxation techniques will experience an increased awareness and ability to selectively let go. Relaxation can be helpful in other situations to increase energy and decrease stress, and would certainly be useful to remember when meeting the demands of parenting. Relaxation instruction can take several forms, but only two will be discussed for use in early pregnancy: passive-a meditation-type relaxation in which a person temporarily withdraws from the surrounding environment as a way of breaking from the stress in a state of restful alertness; and active-a conscious recognition and release of tension, which deals with stress by helping the person focus calmly. In the latter type, the person is actively involved in the environment and has an awareness and ability to selectively relax without undue tension and muscle energy expenditure.

In the initial early pregnancy class, the instructor might explain the reasons for relaxation and diaphragmatic breathing and begin relaxation techniques. An effective way to begin relaxation instruction is to first teach class members comfort positions. Both may participate in the exercise. Some women may be comfortable lying on their sides, propped on pillows brought from home, or some may prefer to semi-recline, perhaps against the body of their partner. Playing a tape of music or environmental sounds may be helpful to decrease stress. Jacksonian-type relaxation, in which various body parts are contracted and let go, coupled with deep breathing techniques, can be introduced as a way to bring about total body relaxation. A sample progression would be contractions of the muscles of the forehead, face, jaw, tongue (pushed against the roof of the mouth), shoulders, biceps, fists, abdomen, buttocks, quadriceps, heels (pushing into the ground) and feet (dorsiflexing). A sample command would be, "Tighten the forehead and hold-2, 3, 4-feel the tension in your forehead ... take a deep breath in through your nose, and as you blow out through your mouth, let the tension go ... and, relax..." This sequence should be repeated for each selected body part. It is important to emphasize letting go of muscular tension, rather than simply relaxing. To work at relaxation too hard may defeat its purpose.

The second class in relaxation repeats the first class; however, the partners end their relaxation early for instruction in working with the mothers to check for areas of tension and tightness. This will require specific instruction to focus on tension areas like the forehead, jaw, shoulders, arms, and legs. Mothers can be encouraged to find a focal point as a stimulus for conscious relaxation with their eyes open. The teacher assists each partner in checking for the mother's relaxation.

In the third class, relaxation cards, with a body part written on each, may be handed out to the women indicating the part to keep tense. The partners then lead the women through a relaxation session that encourages concentration on a visual focal point. The partners are then asked to find where the area of tension is located on the mother, and the instructor verifies this.

Teaching About Emotional Changes

A discussion of emotional influences during pregnancy may be facilitated with a flip chart, the instructor listing changes that may have been experienced by the mothers or noted by their support person. After 15 to 20 changes have been listed, the instructor can step back and ask the class to look at the overwhelming number of changes that can occur in such a short time. Such a list may help couples understand that many of their changes are normal and are experienced by others. Many pregnant women have new outlooks on life, changing interests, and different feelings about themselves and their bodies. They may laugh, cry, or become upset easily. They may be more self-confident or more insecure. Some women are unsure whether they really want to change their life are unsure of their capacity to care for a newborn, and wonder how this child will affect their relationships. Others worry if they will be able to adjust financially if one parent has to stop working. They may also be concerned about the baby's well-being, as well as the progress of labor and delivery. All these factors can cause deep-seated stress in a relationship. The partners need to be aware of these changes; they can help each other by listening when feelings are expressed.

Sexual interest changes in both men and women during pregnancy. In the first trimester, there may be a decrease in interest, if the mother experiences nausea and fatigue. Her partner may believe he will hurt the baby. However, this imagined harm is virtually impossible with the protection afforded by the amniotic fluid and membranes surrounding the fetus as well as by the mucus plug at the opening of the cervix. The muscular abdominal wall and bony pelvis additionally serve to protect the fetus. In the second trimester, there may be renewed sexual interest, but in the third, the mother may be less interested because of discomfort, fatigue, and difficulty in the mechanics. Position changes may be a solution. It is important to realize that these changes may be a variation from what the couple is used to; a discussion of concerns and feelings for each other may help ease tension.

Another well received educational tool is a slide/tape of an uncomplicated vaginal delivery. Couples may find it reassuring to watch another couple go through a delivery. A video such as this may also be a good introduction to a discussion of delivery options, many of which will be unfamiliar to most of the couples. For instance, couples these days need to consider whether they prefer hospital labor and delivery rooms, hospital birthing rooms, birthing centers, or home deliveries. Once this matter is settled, it becomes easier to think about the things or people they wish to take with them to increase their comfort during labor and delivery. There might be a favorite object, music, focal point, or backup support person. Whatever they decide, the mothers and their partners should write down questions about their concerns for labor and delivery to facilitate communication at their next health check. Homework for the week includes practice of relaxation daily for 15 to 20 minutes, to talk over their expectations and list what is important to each for labor and delivery.

Teaching Fetal and Maternal Changes

Fetal and maternal changes can be handled with charts or handouts based on the material presented in this chapter, and Chapter 8. Additional maternal changes are presented in Table 4-15. The film "When Life Begins" by McGraw Hill or a similar one is a good overview of ovulation, fertilization, migration, and implantation of an early embryo. The film also shows the development of the embryo; accompanying changes in the maternal reproductive organs, placenta, and umbilical cord; and the relationship of the fetus to the amniotic sac and fetal membranes. The in utero shots are fiberoptic pictures of a live fetus who is later shown being delivered without obstetric intervention.

Teaching Nutrition

The discussion of nutrition and weight gain is particularly appropriate for early pregnancy classes. Most physicians no longer put mothers on restricted weight gain.[30]

Table 4-15

Maternal Changes in Pregnancy[29]

Maternal Changes by Month	Physiologic Changes
1. Rise in temperature, vomiting, fatigue, tingling breasts, end of menses	Ovulation, fertilization, implantation of ovum, and thickening of uterine lining due to increased estrogen and progesterone
2. Positive pregnancy test; pressure on bladder with frequency of urination; nausea subsiding; profuse, thick vaginal discharge; breasts enlarge	Mucus plug forming in cervix
3. Colostrum leaking from breasts; nausea subsiding; bladder pressure less	Placenta completely formed and secreting estrogen; uterine cavity filled; uterus rising from pelvic cavity into abdomen
4. Abdominal appearance of pregnancy	Blood volume increasing; fundus half way between symphysis and umbilicus
5. Quickening-fetal movement	Placenta covers half of uterine wall
6. Stretch marks; linea nigra appears; possible chloasma (around eyes); period of greatest weight gain starts.	Height of fundus at umbilicus; period of lowest hemoglobin
7. Braxton Hicks contractions palpable-intermittent uterine contractions	Blood volume highest
8. 2-3 pound weight gain, Braxton Hicks contractions stronger; stretch marks more pronounced; backache possibly	Longitudinal stretching of uterus
9. Umbilicus protrudes; shortness of breath, varicosities, ankle swelling; descent of head; lightening (primip), baby drops; easier breathing; urinary frequency	Fundus just under diaphragm (before lightening); lightening more common in primipares; can occur in multiparas; may drop just before birth

It is important to point out that it is never too late to start eating right. There are four major reasons for proper nutrition: to monitor proper weight gain (should gain at least 22 pounds); to ingest adequate high-quality protein to meet the needs of the mother and fetus; to ingest adequate caloric intake to metabolize the protein for use by the body; and to assess the selection of a balanced and varied diet that includes items from all basic food groups. On an allowance of 2000 calories/day, 40% should be from high-quality protein, such as meat, fish, poultry, or eggs; 30% from fats or oils; and 30% from fruits, vegetables, cereals, and breads.

The five food groups are dairy products, protein, vegetables and fruit, breads and cereals, and fats. Dairy products supply calcium, protein, and riboflavin. Mothers need about 4 or more servings a day, 6 or more when lactating. An example of a serving would be 1 ounce of cheese, 1 cup of milk, 1/2 cup of cottage cheese, 1/2 cup of ice cream, or 3/4 cup of plain yogurt.[31,32] (See Table 4-16 for further information on calcium-rich foods.)

Protein sources supply iron and B vitamins. These include lean meats, poultry, eggs, peanut butter, dried beans, lentils, and tofu. Generally, during pregnancy, 75 to 100 gm of protein are needed as compared to the 45 to 50 gm needed when not pregnant. Calories may vary between different meat sources. For example, an ounce of beef has 65 calories, whereas an ounce of fish, delivering the same amount of protein, has 35.

Table 4-16
Calcium Content of Selected Foods*

Average Portion	Calcium (mg)
Milk, whole fresh	1 cup 288
Milk, non-fat	1 cup 298
Buttermilk, whole	1 cup 293
Buttermilk, skim	1 cup 296
Yogurt, plain whole	1 cup 271
Yogurt, plain skim	1 cup 293
Cheese spread	1 ounce 158
Cheese, American	1 ounce 195
Cheese, Swiss	1 ounce 248
Cream cheese	1 ounce 17
Cottage cheese, creamed	1 cup 211
Cheese, cheddar	1 ounce 211
Ice cream	2/3 cup 131
Ice milk	2/3 cup 140
Non-fat dry powdered milk	1 cup (dry) 220
Sardines, canned	3 1/2 ounces 409
Shrimp, canned	3 1/2 ounces 115
Bread: whole wheat	2 slices 57
white	2 slices 48
cracked wheat	2 slices 50
rye	2 slices 46
Beans, common white	1/2 cups 57
Beans, common red	1/2 cups 44
Beans, lima	1/2 cups 54
Beans, snap, yellow	1/2 cups 57
Collards, cooked	1/2 cups 215
Kale, cooked	1/2 cups 214
Lettuce, iceberg	4 ounces 78
Onion, raw	1 large 180
Parsnips, cooked	1/2 cups 52
Okra, cooked	1/2 cups 105
Sweet potato (with skin)	1/2 cups 46
Broccoli, cooked	1/2 cup 101
Molasses, light	2 T 50
medium	2 T 87
blackstrap	2 T 205
Figs, dried	2 ounces 66

*United States Department of Agriculture. Protein sources supply iron and B vitamins. In: Composition of Foods, Handbook No. 8. 1975.

Vegetables and fruits provide Vitamins A and C and roughage. A pregnant woman needs 4 or 5 servings per day of dark green and yellow vegetables and citrus fruits and juices. Raw fruits and vegetables retain more vitamins. The longer a fruit or vegetable has been cooked, the more the vitamins and roughage have been removed.[31,32]

Complex carbohydrates, grown from the ground as opposed to man-made refined carbohydrates, stripped of vitamins and minerals, are utilized better by the body and require the body to use less B vitamins to synthesize their products. Breads and cereals supply B vitamins, carbohydrates and iron. Four servings a day of whole grain products (corn, barley, oats, rice, wheat, or millet) are recommended.

A suggested serving of fats is 2 tablespoons per day to aid the function of the hormones of the adrenal cortex, and for the valuable bacteria in the intestinal tract. Unsaturated fats, found in vegetable oil such as safflower, sesame, and canola oils are suggested. Hydrogenated, partially hydrogenated, processed cheeses, solid cooking fats, fried animal fats, and coconut or palm oils should be avoided. Also recommended are unrefined or cold pressed oils that need to be refrigerated, because they do not have preservatives.

Because the daily caloric requirement is already increased, pregnant woman cannot afford to indulge in nutritionally-poor, highly-refined sweets and starches. It must be emphasized that they should get the most from what they eat. All these foods work in combination, so women need to be taught not to eat all their protein at one meal, or all fats at another. Certain foods must be eaten together to get the most out of each calorie. Because the smooth muscle in the colon slows down in pregnancy, women should consume more bulk, water, and raw bran products in their diet. This may also help them avoid hemorrhoids, which may result from the increased vascularity, pressure of the fetus, and constipation caused by ingestion of prenatal vitamins.[31,32]

So much iron is needed during pregnancy that the National Research Council has advised that supplements be given to expectant mothers. The greatest amount of iron is needed during the last three months of pregnancy when the mother is building iron stores that will be transferred to the baby at birth. Additionally, she will need a supply of iron following delivery to replenish the iron in her own blood. It is wise, therefore, to encourage participants in the early pregnancy class to choose iron-rich foods, such as dried fruits, wheat germ, dried beans, and blackstrap molasses. Couples may benefit from a handout with a list of iron rich foods (Table 4-17).

Although salt restriction was previously prescribed to pregnant women to prevent preeclampsia, the American College of Obstetrics and Gynecology now states that salt restriction in pregnancy is unnecessary.[32] Sodium ingestion is needed to maintain normal salt levels in bone, muscles, and brain to balance the growth of blood plasma and tissue fluids that are a natural outgrowth of pregnancy. Iodine, a natural mineral sometimes added to common salt, is vital for the proper functioning of the thyroid gland. Therefore, physicians recommend mothers salt to taste, or season as they usually do.[32]

It may be helpful for the class to go through an exercise of filling out a menu sheet for the week to see when and what they eat and if they are getting all the necessary nutrients (see Table 4-18). Partners often wish to fill out a menu sheet as well. Excellent nutrition guides during pregnancy are available and are a welcome addition to class handouts (see resources in the Appendix).

It is important to talk to parents about alcohol, smoking, and caffeine use and abuse. The National Institute on Alcohol Abuse and Alcoholism has said that 3 ounces of absolute alcohol are equivalent to 6 average size drinks. Based on that institute's research, a pregnant woman who drinks 3 ounces of alcohol, clearly risks harm to her baby.[33] The blood alcohol level will increase in the mother and in the fetus because of transfer through the placenta. In the first trimester, most of the initial growth and development of fetal organs is taking place. It is at this time, therefore, when utmost caution should be used. In some cases, however, the mother may be already addicted to alcohol or drugs, and there is considerable risk that this addiction can be transmitted to the unborn child. Newborn addicts must then cope with withdrawal symptoms in addition to the normal adjustments to the environment at birth.

It is unknown whether there is a safe amount to drink below 3 ounces of absolute alcohol; but risk has been associated with ingestion of 1 to 3 ounces of alcohol, and caution should be advised.[33] Newborns with fetal alcohol syndrome[33,34] may have low IQs, abnormal facial features, narrow eyes, low nasal bridges, or heart defects. There is also concern that binge drinking, consuming large quantities on an occasional basis, may also prove harmful to the growing fetus.

Table 4-17

Foods High in Iron*
(*more than 1.5 mg of iron per listed serving size)

Food	Serving	Food	Serving
Apricots dried	5 halves	Liver sausage	1 ounce
Beans	1/2cup	Maple syrup	3 T
Beef, cooked	2 ounces	Molasses	2T
Beet greens, cooked	112 cup	Oysters	1 ounce
Brazil nuts	6 medium	Peaches, dried	3 halves
Cereals#	1 ounce	Pork (cooked)	2 ounces
Chard, cooked	1/2 cup	Prunes, dried	4 medium
Chicken, cooked	1/2 cup	Prune juice	1/4 cup
Cider, sweet	10 ounces	Raisins, dried	1-1/2 oz
Clams	1 ounce	Sardines	2 ounces
Corn syrup	2 T	Scallops	2 ounces
Dandelion greens	1/2 cup	Shrimp	8 ounces
Dried beef	1 ounce	Spinach, cooked	1/2 cup
Egg, whole	2	Strawberries	1 cup
Ham, cooked	2 ounces	Tomato juice	3/4 cup
Heart, cooked	Bounces	Tongue, cooked	Bounces
Instant breakfast	1 serving	Tuna	1/2 cup
Kidney, cooked	1 ounce	Turkey, cooked	1 ounce
Lamb, cooked	2 ounces	Veal, cooked	1 ounce
Liver, cooked	1 ounce	Watermelon	6" diameter, 1-1/2 slices

#15% NDR of iron or more per serving. United States Department of Agriculture. Composition of Food, Agriculture Handbook No. 8. 1975.

Table 4-18

Weekly Menu Sheet

Day	Breakfast	Snack	Lunch	Snack	Dinner	Snack	Calories
							(Total)
Monday							
Tuesday							
Wednesday							
Thursday							
Friday							
Saturday							
Sunday							

It may be important to point out alternatives to alcohol, whether they be creative non-alcoholic drinks, or expressive, creative outlets.[35] The physical therapist with a client suspected of alcohol abuse may seek help from the local Alcoholics Anonymous Council. Studies suggest that heavy alcohol drinkers who receive counseling are able to abstain, or significantly moderate, their consumption before the third trimester.[36] This reduction of alcohol was associated with a more normal fetal weight, head circumference, and length.[36]

Smoke also crosses the placenta and can restrict a baby's normal growth in the uterus. Statistics show a direct correlation between smoking during pregnancy and an increased incidence of spontaneous abortion and stillbirths. Pregnant women who smoke a pack or more of cigarettes a day put their fetuses at 50% greater risk of infant mortality.[35] The American Cancer Institute states that babies of women who smoke usually average a birth weight of 6 ounces less than babies of non-smoking women. Nicotine is believed to restrict blood vessels and fetal breathing movements, and carbon monoxide reduces the oxygen available in the fetal circulation.

In addition, vitamin metabolism is also disturbed by smoking. A 1976 study by the U.S. Department of Health, Education and Welfare found that 7-year-old children of mothers who smoked were shorter in average stature, tended to have retarded reading ability, and rated lower in social adjustment than children of mothers who did not smoke.[35] For mothers who smoke then, the risks include: underdeveloped and underweight babies at birth, babies more prone to illness in the first critical weeks of life (related to low birth weight), a greater risk of miscarriage, and babies who have a 20% to 25% greater chance of dying within the first 24 hours after birth.[35]

Caffeine also crosses the placenta, and has been known, when used in excessive amounts, to cause fetal growth retardation and fetal loss. The half-life of caffeine is 2 to 3 times longer in pregnant women than in non-pregnant women. Caffeine may be transported across the placenta and membranes to the fetus and amniotic fluid where concentrations may be greater than those of the mother. Studies suggest that caffeine has the effect of reducing placental blood supply in animals, but the human fetus appears capable of maintaining its umbilical vein blood flow at normal levels.[37]

Caffeine increases catecholamines in the circulation, especially epinephrine. There are known cardiovascular effects, linked to the rise in catecholamine levels; however, further investigation is hampered by the lack of non-invasive methods available in studying human fetal placental blood flow. Physicians, midwives, and maternal health educators may offer guidelines to reduce caffeine intake (Table 4-19).

Teaching Pelvic Floor Toning

It is important for the instructor to show a chart to the class when discussing the pelvic floor. Most men and women have never heard of the pelvic floor, and anatomic diagrams that show the layers of muscles suspended like a hammock running anteriorly from the pubis posteriorly to the sacrococcygeal area are helpful. A perineal view will provide an added dimension to the location of the pubococcygeal muscle. The importance for pelvic floor toning should be explained:

1. It supports the uterus and pelvic contents
2. It may help mother develop an awareness of several degrees of contraction and relaxation, which may be helpful for relaxing the pelvic floor during delivery
3. A healthy, toned pelvic floor may repair more quickly after delivery
4. Adequate muscle tone and the ability to relax pelvic floor muscles may help avoid episiotomy

Table 4-19

Caffeine Content of Various Beverages

	Mg Caffeine per 5 oz. Cup
Coffee instant	66
percolated	110
drip	146
Bagged tea	
black 1-minutebrew	28
black 5-minute brew	46
Loose tea	
green, Japan, 5-minute	20
green, 5-minute brew	35
black, 5-minute brew	40
Cocoa	
2 heaping tsp. instant	13
	Mg Caffeine per 12 oz. Can
Diet Rite	32
Diet RC	33
RC cola	34
Pepsi-Cola	43
Tab	49
Diet Dr. Pepper	54
Mountain Dew	55
Dr. Pepper	61
Coca-Cola	65

Adapted from: Harvard Community Health Plan, *Boston, Massachusetts*

5. A toned pelvic floor may cause greater voluntary contractions of the pubococcygeus muscle and possibly stimulate pubococcygeal nerve endings through the vaginal walls, resulting in enhanced sexual satisfaction

During delivery, the passage of the baby's head through the untoned pelvic floor may cause tissue injury.[38] Pelvic floor toning should be a component of any general conditioning program (Table 4-20).

Teaching Body Mechanics and Center of Gravity

Instruction in body mechanics includes a chart of the center of gravity showing the non-pregnant state versus the pregnant state, and how the center of gravity is measured through the ear, shoulder, iliac crest, knee, and ankle (refer to Chapter 7, Figure 7-2 and 7-3). The additional weight of pregnancy, added breast tissue, and other possible physiologic changes, increase the lumbar lordosis. Postural adaptations may cause a woman to stand with her head forward and shoulders rounded. As a result of poor posture, stress on the brachial plexus may produce some tingling in the hands. Also, at this time, relaxin, progesterone, and estrogen are released and may loosen various ligaments in the body. The pelvic girdle increases in size in preparation for delivery.

It is crucial that the strength in the low back muscles and abdominal muscles be strong to counteract the changes in the center of gravity and accompanying weight gain. The

Table 4-20
Handout for Pelvic Floor Exercises

Exercise #1: The Stop Test

(*Note:* Advise women not do this first thing in the morning and to do only once a week as a test only.) Women with incontinence may have difficulty contracting the pelvic floor muscles in this gravity-resisted position.)

Position:	Sit on the toilet. Spread legs apart for urination and support feet on a stool if voiding is difficult.
Exercise:	As you urinate, stop and hold the flow of urine. Repeat a few times, breaking off the urine flow smoothly and completely. Try not to allow any dribbling of urine. Hold tightly for 5 seconds before starting urine flow again.
Progression:	Let smaller amounts of urine pass each time. Do not worry if this difficult. Try to always end the voiding with an uplifting contraction of the pelvic floor.

Exercise #2: Long Contractions

Position:	Lie on back or side with legs apart and chest relaxed.
Exercise:	Draw pelvic floor upward. Feel the squeeze as the sphincters are tightened, and the inside passage becomes narrow and tense. Focus on the front portion of the pelvic floor where the master sphincter surrounds the vagina and ure-thra. Initially, hold 10 seconds and then completely relax. Attempt to relax a little bit more, releasing any residual tension. Repeat 2 or 3 times, relaxing and repeating. Always end with a contraction.
Progression:	Try other positions such as sitting, standing, and squatting. Do a total of 50 repetitions a day: 10 repetitions at a time, 5 sessions per day, holding each repetitions for 10 seconds. Relax between each contraction.

Exercise #3: Quick Contraction

Position:	Lie on back or side with legs apart and chest relaxed.
Exercise:	Draw pelvic floor upward. Feel the squeeze as the sphincters are tightened, and the inside passage becomes narrow and tense. Focus on the front portion of the pelvic floor where the master sphincter surrounds the vagina and ure-thra. Initially, hold 2-3 seconds and then completely relax. Attempt to relax a little bit more, releasing any residual tension. Repeat 2 or 3 times, relaxing and repeating. Always end with a contraction.
Progression:	Try other positions such as sitting, standing, and squatting. Do a total of 50 repetitions a day: 10 repetitions at a time, 5 sessions per day, holding each repetitions for 3 seconds. Relax between each contraction.

Exercise #4: The Elevator

Position:	Assume any position, although lying down is easier at first.
Exercise:	Imagine you are in an elevator on the first floor. As you ascend to each floor, draw up the pelvic floor muscles a little bit more. When you reach your limit, do not let go, but descend floor by floor, gradually relaxing the pelvic floor in stages. When you have reached the first floor, think about releasing, and con tinue to the basement. Do not hold your breath, blow out through pursed lips. Feel the perineal muscles bulge. Complete this exercise by bringing the pelvic floor back up to the ground floor.

Exercise #5: The Sexercise

Position:	Assume any position of coitus with the legs spread apart and relaxed.
Exercise:	Grip the penis as firmly as you can with your vagina, holding for 5 seconds before you relax. Try to avoid tensing the buttocks and the abdominal mus-cles. Repeat a few times until your partner tells you the strength of the con-tractions has diminished. Rest and repeat in a few minutes.
Progression:	Your muscle strength will increase as you learn to make the contractions stronger, more consistent and more numerous.

[Adapted from E. Noble. Essential Exercises for the Childbearing Year[38]]

instructor should demonstrate the pelvic tilt both in the supine and hands and knees positions. Participants should be encouraged to avoid positions of discomfort, such as bending straight from the waist, sitting for long periods of time, or holding objects far away from their center of gravity as opposed to close to their body. The instructor should also present comfort positions for resting or sleeping. Finding a comfortable position for a woman in later stages of pregnancy can be quite challenging, but the instructor can encourage left-side lying (to relieve pressure from the fetus on abdominal blood vessels), with a pillow under the abdomen, between the knees, and under the head.

The instructor can then talk about additional supports that may be needed in pregnancy corsets, bras, binders, and support elastic stockings. Sacroiliac corsets may be helpful for women who have chronic sacroiliac irritation, and bras are strongly recommended to support the increased weight of the breast tissue. A well-fitting bra improves posture and may minimize upper backache. Some women may also find wearing a bra to bed comfortable. Broad, non-elastic straps with stability and support are preferable. Mothers should also be encouraged to buy nursing bras with the best support and fit.

Although it is best to assist venous return from the legs by using the pumping action of the muscles, some women, because of the increased blood volume of pregnancy, find that their legs ache and are susceptible to varicose veins. These women may benefit from elastic stockings (examples listed in the Appendix). They should not be too tight or have bands that interfere with blood circulation.

Teaching About Partner's Role

It is important to talk about a partner's role and how it changes over the first, second, and third trimesters, and during labor and delivery. In the first trimester, the partner's identity is changing, and each of the couple is exploring new roles. He is becoming involved in the pregnancy and is preparing for the labor and delivery process. He may have unresolved feelings about having a child or may need to reevaluate what it will be like to be a parent again, if he has other children. This may be a time when he reassesses his job, whether or not it is secure; if he has enough salary; and if he has enough life and health insurance. Often, financial matters are the focus.

The partner may notice emotional changes in the mother and can be very supportive at this time by helping with diet, exercises, and emotional issues, and by offering love and companionship. In the second trimester, the movement of the baby at 16 to 20 weeks confirms the pregnancy for the father. The mother may not have physically changed much up to this point, but now she is definitely showing signs of pregnancy. This milestone may plunge the father into thoughts about parenthood, and he may spend time feeling for movements of the baby and listening to hear its heartbeat. The couple may experience sexual freedom and feel generally good about their relationship. At this time, women may look to their partners for help, when ordinarily they would have accomplished tasks independently. A woman may also express unusual anxiety about her partner's safety. It is necessary for the partner to recognize these signs and to participate in his own way. He is definitely needed and can be a very positive support.

In the third trimester, the partner has worked through some of the psychological issues raised by the pregnancy. For example, the changing environment, his role, financial issues, and his changing relationship to his wife have been confronted and handled. He has seen how he has been needed, and, hopefully, he becomes involved by attending early pregnancy and then childbirth preparation classes. If so, he has helped with practicing relaxation, breathing, and exercise techniques, and pregnancy has become a time of real sharing. The reality of the baby increases, and the father may find himself dreaming of his new child in a real situation with himself.

During labor and delivery, partners are allowed to be more involved than they were in the past. There have been stories of men in the late 1960s who would handcuff themselves to their wives as they were wheeled to the delivery room so that they could participate in the birth! Although some cultures used to believe a man would die if he saw his wife in labor, that mystique is changing as fathers see they do have a role as comforter, supporter, and motivator in labor and delivery. Partners today are sometimes allowed to cut the umbilical cord post-delivery and, often, to be in the delivery room if their wives undergo Cesarean sections. It is a very special time for fathers to see the baby they helped create emerge into the world. It is rare for a man to return to a non-participatory role once he has experienced such direct involvement through pregnancy classes, labor, and delivery.

Teaching Exercises

The rationale for exercise needs to be made clear so that the couple will understand the advantages of muscle strengthening, breathing, and relaxation, as well as how the exercised muscles are relevant to childbirth. Rationale includes relief of low back pain and preparation for labor and delivery by increasing strength, stamina, endurance, and tolerance for the physical and mental stress. Exercise also produces a psychological boost, and posture may be improved. If the mother exercises throughout pregnancy, post-partum recovery may be easier and faster. Exercise gives the body strength, muscle tone, and flexibility. It also helps develop new powers of concentration and relaxation.

The instructor can safely recommend that 15 to 20 minutes a day be devoted to light exercise during pregnancy. Each woman must perform at her exercise level and should be challenged to perform additional exercises in a gradually increasing manner. Keeping these factors in mind, it is better to design a simple program that has some flexibility and variability in it to decrease the possibility of boredom and increase the chances of compliance.[24,34-37]

Several cautionary notes must be added here. Pre- and post-natal patients must get clearance from their physicians before participating in an exercise program. They must be screened for conditions that would limit their medical, cardiovascular, musculoskeletal, or pregnancy-related complications.

Early pregnancy is a good time to teach how to check for diastasis recti abdominis (as described in Chapter 7). If there is a rectus separation, exercise can be modified to maintain tone and to discourage further separation. The patient can be instructed to lie supine (less than 3 minutes) with hands crossed over the lower abdomen in a corset-type of arrangement, breathe in, then breathe out as she raises her head up, and simultaneously approximate the abdominal muscles with her hands. This can be done several times throughout the day.

Exercises for the prenatal period may be individually tailored by the therapist, working with each woman independently to meet unique needs. There are numerous exercises that are appropriate for this population, but there are guidelines that are important to understand before designing an exercise program. General guide lines for clients include: exercise regularly and do not attempt to make up for lost time by pushing too hard, exercise sessions should be no more than 2 1/2 days apart; finish eating at least 1 to 1 and a 1/2 hours before working out to avoid gastrointestinal discomfort; Do not diet during pregnancy; Stop exercising if any dizziness, pain, or persistent discomfort is experienced; Drink water before and after a workout (Figure 4-13a and b).

Specific exercise guidelines and contraindications that should be followed by physical therapists include:[40,41,43]

1. After 4 months of gestation, avoid exercises requiring women to lie supine for longer than 3 minutes to prevent compression on the inferior vena cave.

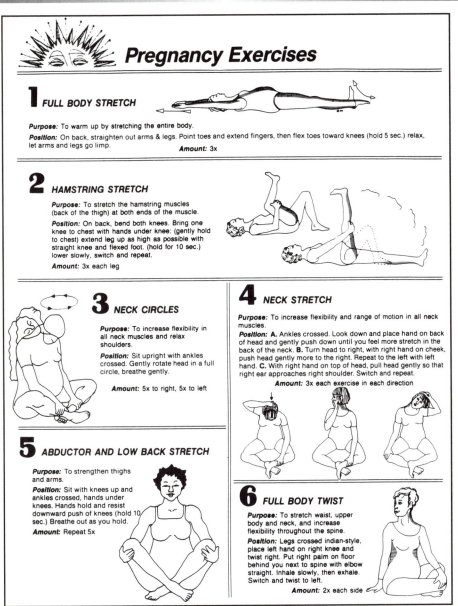

Pregnancy Exercises

1 FULL BODY STRETCH

Purpose: To warm up by stretching the entire body.

Position: On back, straighten out arms & legs. Point toes and extend fingers, then flex toes toward knees (hold 5 sec.) relax, let arms and legs go limp.

Amount: 3x

2 HAMSTRING STRETCH

Purpose: To stretch the hamstring muscles (back of the thigh) at both ends of the muscle.

Position: On back, bend both knees. Bring one knee to chest with hands under knee: (gently hold to chest) extend leg up as high as possible with straight knee and flexed foot. (hold for 10 sec.) lower slowly, switch and repeat.

Amount: 3x each leg

3 NECK CIRCLES

Purpose: To increase flexibility in all neck muscles and relax shoulders.

Position: Sit upright with ankles crossed. Gently rotate head in a full circle, breathe gently.

Amount: 5x to right, 5x to left

4 NECK STRETCH

Purpose: To increase flexibility and range of motion in all neck muscles.

Position: A. Ankles crossed. Look down and place hand on back of head and gently push down until you feel more stretch in the back of the neck. **B.** Turn head to right, with right hand on cheek, push head gently more to the right. Repeat to the left with left hand. **C.** With right hand on top of head, pull head gently so that right ear approaches right shoulder. Switch and repeat.

Amount: 3x each exercise in each direction

5 ABDUCTOR AND LOW BACK STRETCH

Purpose: To strengthen thighs and arms.

Position: Sit with knees up and ankles crossed, hands under knees. Hands hold and resist downward push of knees (hold 10 sec.) Breathe out as you hold.

Amount: Repeat 5x

6 FULL BODY TWIST

Purpose: To stretch waist, upper body and neck, and increase flexibility throughout the spine.

Position: Legs crossed indian-style, place left hand on right knee and twist right. Put right palm on floor behind you next to spine with elbow straight. Inhale slowly, then exhale. Switch and twist to left.

Amount: 2x each side

Figure 4-13a. Illustrates a suggested exercise series for an early pregnancy class.[42]

7 SHOULDER, ARM AND UPPER BACK STRETCH

Purpose: To increase range of motion and flexibility in shoulders, arms and upper back muscles.

Position: Sitting with back against wall, legs out straight. Start with straight arms, palms up at shoulder level. Drag arms slowly up wall maintaining contact with wall. Hold at point where arms want to push away from wall, (hold for 10 sec.), lower slowly. **Amount:** 3x

8 CAT EXERCISE

Purpose: To relieve back pain and increase flexibility in low back muscles.

Position: On hands and knees, arch the back up and drop head down. Reverse the action, to head up and back raised to flat position. **Amount:** 10x

9 BUDDHA

Purpose: To stretch upper back, arms, wrists, and low back muscles.

Position: Sitting on heels with knees a comfortable distance apart, place hands on thighs. Keeping knees bent slide hands forward (on floor) until arms and back are stretched forward, breathe out, stretch. (hold position, breathing easily, for 10 sec.) **Amount:** 5x

10 SQUATTING

Purpose: To stretch hip muscles and increase endurance in the squatting position.

Position: Feet shoulder-width apart and knees pointed out to side, heels on ground, squat holding onto partner or table for support, (hold for 10 sec.), stand, repeat. **Amount:** 4x

11 HIP STRETCH

Purpose: To stretch front of thigh and increase flexibility in legs.

Position: Squat on floor. Place one leg behind and shift weight to bent leg keeping hands on floor. Pull self forward until knee of bent leg is directly over ankle, (hold for 10 sec.). Switch and stretch.

Amount: Alternate 3x each leg

12 SIDE BENDS

Purpose: To stretch arms and trunk.

Position: Feet shoulder width apart. Hold elbow of right arm with left hand. Gently pull right elbow behind head as you bend to the left, (hold 10 sec.). Switch to left. Hold left elbow with right hand.

Amount: 3x each side

13 CALF STRETCH

Purpose: To stretch calf muscles and front of thighs.

Position: Hands on wall, straighten left leg behind. Feet pointing straight forward, lean into wall until stretching is felt in calf muscles (hold 10 sec.). Same position, bend the back knee (hold 10 sec.). Switch and stretch opposite leg. **Amount:** 3x each leg

©Rebecca J. Gourley, R.P.T., Dedham Medical Associates, 1 Lyons St., Dedham, MA 02026
Illustrations by Dawn Martin ©1985. Revised 1989

Figure 4-13 continued. Illustrates a suggested exercise series for an early pregnancy class.[42]

Table 4-21

Target Heart Rate Zones for Pregnant Women and New Mothers

Fit Age	Beginners (60%-70% of SHR*)	Before Pregnancy (70%-75% of SHR)
20	120-140	140-150
21	119-139	139-149
22	118-138	138-148
23	117-137	137-147
24	117-137	137-147
25	116-136	136-146
26	115-135	135-145
27	115-135	135-145
28	114-134	134 144
29	113-133	133-143
30	113-133	133 143
31	112-132	132-142
32	111-131	131-141
33	110-130	130-140
34	110-130	130 140
35	109-129	129-139
36	108-128	128-138
37	108-128	128-138
38	107-127	127-137
39	106 126	126-136
40	106 126	126-136
41	105-125	125-135
42	104-124	124-134

*SHR-safe, maximal attainable heart rate
Adapted from White R. Fitness in Pregnancy. Seattle, Wash: Pennypress; 1984.[39]

2. Avoid exercises that promote straining of the pelvic floor or abdominal muscles.

3. Avoid exercises that excessively stretch hip adductors, which may cause strain and possible trauma to the symphysis pubis.

4. Avoid exercises that involve sharp twists, rapid or uncontrolled swinging or bouncing movements.

5. Avoid exercises that utilize positions in which the buttocks are higher than the head, as in bridging, supine bicycling motions, or modified quadruped position because of potential air embolus introduced through the vagina.

6. Avoid inversion activities.

7. Avoid trhe use of deep heat modalities or electrical stimulation.

Questions will undoubtedly arise regarding the safety of aerobic exercise during pregnancy. Aerobic conditioning in pregnancy still involves strengthening the cardiopulmonary system by making the heart work over a 20 to 30 minute period to create a demand for oxygen met by increased breathing. The types of aerobic conditioning best suited for pregnancy are walking or swimming. A program in which the mother exercises a minimum of 3 times a week, possibly increasing the frequency to 4 to 6 times, should be beneficial.

To have true aerobic conditioning, the heart rate should fall within the target zone. The recommended target zone in pregnancy, and until 12 weeks post-partum, is 60% to 70% of the safe, maximum, attainable heart rate. To determine what that safe heart rate is, the formula is 220 multiplied by 60% to 70% (Table 4-21).[39] Mothers should be taught how to take an accurate pulse, using the carotid or radial artery.

The aerobic program should start with a 5-minute warm-up to prevent injury and to increase flexibility Stretches should include hamstrings; quadriceps; gastrocnemius-soleus groups; and arm, neck, and shoulder muscles (see Figure 4-13a and b). The heart rate should range in the target zone a minimum of 12 minutes, but 20 to 30 minutes is better. The aerobic program should end with a 5-minute cool-down phase. After delivery, the mother who wishes to continue her aerobic walking or swimming program should decrease the total time slightly from the amount she was exercising prior to delivery, and then slowly increase the challenge of her program as tolerated.

SELF-ASSESSMENT REVIEW

1. Pregnant women compensate for physiologic and anatomic respiratory changes by _____.
2. During mild and moderate exercise, cardiac output _____.
3. Exercise in pregnant women with impaired cardiovascular function is _____.
4. The vena cava syndrome is _____.
5. Maternal core body temperature over _____ has resulted in _____ and _____ defects.
6. In the first trimester, there is a _____ in physical work capacity.
7. The fetus responds to brief periods of asphyxia with _____ and _____.
8. The cervix is made up of _____ muscle.
9. The corpus luteum is located in the _____ and produces _____ in pregnancy.
10. Chloasma results in increased _____ around the _____ and _____.
11. Oxygen consumption increases ____% in pregnancy.
12. _____ means absence of menstruation
13. What are two types of relaxation and how do they differ?
14. How many calories should be added to a pregnant woman's diet to insure adequate caloric intake, given that she is maintaining a good diet?
15. It is recommended that a pregnant woman (with a singleton) gains _____ pounds in the first trimester and _____ pounds per week in the second and third trimester.
16. The center of gravity moves _____ during pregnancy with added weight gain.

Answers

1. Breathing deeply. 2. Increases slightly. 3. Contraindicated. 4. Reduced cardiac output in the supine position, due to compression by the expanding uterus. 5. 39°C, teratogenic, neurotube. 6. Decrease. 7. Increased blood pressure and tachycardia. 8. Smooth. 9. Ovaries, relaxin. 10. Pigmentation, eyes and cheekbones. 11. 14%. 12. Amenorrhea. 13. Active relaxation is a conscious recognition of release and tension: passive relaxation occurs when a person withdraws temporarily from the surrounding environment. 14. An additional 300 calories. 15. 2 to 4 pounds, slightly less than 1 pound. 16. Forward.

REFERENCES

1. Danforth DN. *Obstetrics and Gynecology.* 5th ed. Philadelphia, Pa: JB Lippincott; 1986.

2. Wilson JR, Carrington ER, Ledger WJ. *Obstetrics and Gynecology.* 7th ed. St. Louis, Mo: CV Mosby; 1983.

3. Niswander KR. *Manual of Obstetrics: Diagnosis and Therapy.* 2nd ed. Boston, Mass: Little, Brown & Co; 1987.

4. Freed SZ, Herzig N. *Urology and Pregnancy.* Baltimore, Md: Williams and Wilkins; 1982.

5. Davidson JM. The physiology of the renal tract in pregnancy. *Clin Obstet and Gynecol.* 1985;28(2):257-265.

6. Pauls J. *Therapeutic Approaches to Women's Health.* Gaithersburg, Md: Aspen; 1995.

7. Guyton AC. *Textbook in Medical Physiology.* 7th ed. Philadelphia, Pa: Harper & Row; 1987.

8. Broussard C, Richter J. Nausea and vomiting of pregnancy. *Gastro Clin NA.* 1998;27(1)123-147.

9. Vilar J, Kestler E, Castello A. Improved lactation digestion during pregnancy: a case of physiological adaptation. *Obstet Gynecol.* 71(5):697 700, 1981.

10. Pritchard J, MacDonald P. *Williams Obstetrics.* 17th ed. New York, NY: Appleton-Century-Crofts; 1980.

11. Lantz M, Chez R, Rodriguez A, Porter K. Maternal weight gain patterns and birth weight outcome in twin gestation. *Obstet Gynecol.* 87(4):551-6,1996.

12. Luke B. What is the influence of maternal weight gain on the fetal growth of twins? *Clin Ob Gyn.* 1998;41(1):57-64.

13. Festoon T, Thirst J. Twin pregnancy: the distribution of maternal weight gain of non-smoking normal weight women. *Can J Pub Health.* 1994;85(1):37-40.

14. Luke B, Keith L, Johnson T, Keith D. Pregravid weight, gestational weight gain and current weight of women delivered of twins. *J Perinat Med.* 19(1991):333-340.

15. Norstrom A, Bryman I, Wiqvist N, Sahni S, Lindblom B. Inhibitory action of relaxin on human cervical smooth muscle. *J Clin Endocrinol Metab.* 1984;59(3):379-382.

16. Frankenne F, Closset J, Gomez F, Scippo ML, Hennen G. The physiology of growth hormones (GHs) in pregnant women and partial characterization of the placental GH variant. *J Clin Endocrinol Metab.* 1988;66(6):1171-1180.

17. Wong RC, Ellis. Physiologic skin changes in pregnancy. *J Am Acad Dermatol.* 1984;10(6):929-940.

18. Artal RM, Wiswell RA. *Exercise in Pregnancy.* Baltimore, Md: Williams & Wilkins; 1986.

19. McMurray RG, Katz VL, Berry MJ, Cefalo RC. The effect of pregnancy on metabolic response during rest, immersion and aerobic exercise in the water. *Am J Obstet Gynecol.* 1988;158(3):481-486.

20. Loitering FK, Gilbert RD, Long LD. Maternal and fetal responses to exercise during pregnancy. *Phys Review.* 1985;65(1):1-36.

21. Nisei H, Nisell H, Hjemdahl P, Linde B, Lunell NO. Cardiovascular response to isometric handgrip exercise: an invasive study in pregnancy-induced hypertension. *Obstet Gynecol.* 1987;70(3):339-343.

22. Pomerance J, Gluck L, Lynch V. Physical fitness in pregnancy: Its effect on pregnancy outcome. *Am J Obstet Gynecol.* 1974;119(7):867876.

23. Carpenter MW, Sady SP, Hoegsberg B, et al. Fetal heart rate response to maternal exertion. *JAMA.* 1988,259(20):3006-3009.

24. Katz VL, McMurray R, Berry MJ, Cefalo RC. Fetal and uterine responses to immersion and exercise. *Obstet Gynecol.* 1988;72(2):225-230.

25. Clapp J. Pregnancy outcome: physical activities inside versus outside the workplace. *Sem in Perin.* 1996;20(1):70-76.

26. Sternfeld B. Physical activity and pregnancy outcome. *Sports Med.* 1997;23(1)33-47.

27. Hassid P. *Textbook for Childbirth Educators.* Hagerstown, Md: Harper & Row; 1978.

28. Gourley R, Leland P. *Early Pregnancy-Promotional Packet.* Unpublished; 1980.

29. Gourley R. *Early Pregnancy Education, class handouts.* Unpublished; 1981.

30. Danforth DN, Scott JR, eds. *Obstetrics and Gynecology.* 1st ed. Philadelphia, Pa: JB Lippincott; 1986.

31. BACK. *Handbook in Prepared Childbirth.* Newtonville, Mass, BACK; 1976.

32. Goldbeck N. *As You Eat So Your Baby Grows.* Woodstock, NY: Ceres Press; 1980.

33. American Council on Alcoholism. *Drinking and Pregnancy.* Baltimore, Md: American Council on Alcoholism, 1984.

34. U.S. Department of Health, Education & Welfare. *Alcohol and Your Unborn Baby.* Rockville, Md: No.78-521; 1978.

35. American Cancer Society. *Why Start a Life Under a Cloud?* Washington, DC: ACS; 1984.

36. Rosett HL, Weiner L, Edelin KC. Strategies for prevention of fetal alcohol effects. *Obstet Gynecol.* 1981;57(1):1-7.

37. Kirkinan P, Jouppila P, Koivula A, Vuori J, Puukka M. The effect of caffeine on placental and fetal blood flow in human pregnancy. *Am J Obstet Gynecol.* 1983;147(8):939-942.

38. Noble E. *Essential Exercises for the Childbearing Year.* 2nd ed. Boston, Mass: Houghton-Mifflin; 1982.

39. White R. *Fitness in Pregnancy.* Seattle, Wash: Pennypress; 1984.

40. Perinatal Exercise Guidelines. Alexandria, Va. *Sect. Obstet. Gynecol.* APTA, 1986.

41. O'Connor L. Exercising more ways, enjoying it less. *J Obstet Gynecol Phys Ther.* 1989;13(1):8-9.

42. Gourley R. *Pregnancy stretches.* Dedham, Mass: DMA; 1985, rev. 1989.

43. O'Connor L. Proposed guidelines on perinatal exercise for the physical therapist. *Bull Sect Obstet Gynecol.* APTA 1986;10(1):5-6.

Maternal Disorders and Diseases

The physical therapist must be knowledgeable in the process of disease in order to fully evaluate and treat the pregnant woman safely. This chapter serves as a resource on maternal disorders and diseases and their effect on pregnancy and the fetus.

DEATH AND MORTALITY RATES

Unfortunately, maternal and fetal death are part of any discussion of high-risk pregnancy and complicated pregnancy. To understand the difference between death and mortality rates, the physical therapist must first examine the many terms that define and categorize the time of fetal or infant demise. A *live-born infant* is one who shows signs of life: breathing, cord pulsation, voluntary muscle movement, or heartbeat upon complete expulsion from the vagina, regardless of the duration of the pregnancy. *Fetal death*, or stillbirth, refers to the death (no life signs) of a fetus, 500 gm or more, prior to the complete expulsion from the vagina, again, irrespective of the duration of the pregnancy. *Hebdomadal death* is death of a fetus, 500 gm or more, within the first 7 days of life. *Neonatal death* means death of an infant within the first 28 days of life. This infant must weigh 500 gm or more or have completed 20 weeks' gestation to be considered viable. *Perinatal death* includes both fetal and neonatal death (ie, death of the fetus before or during delivery and death of a liveborn infant within the first 28 days of life).

Mortality rates are actually ratios comparing the number of deaths to a particular number of births. It is also important to note that, in some cases, number of births can mean live and stillborn. *Fetal mortality* describes the number of fetal deaths per 1000 births. *Neonatal mortality* includes the number of deaths per 1000 births of liveborn infants in their first 28 days. *Perinatal mortality* is an inclusive term referring to the number of fetal and neonatal deaths per 1000 births. *Infant mortality* describes the rate between the 28th day and the end of the first year of life.

Maternal death is death from any cause during pregnancy or up to 42 days after its termination. A direct maternal death is one that results from an obstetrical complication, and an indirect death is one that results from a previous illness or disease. The *maternal mortality rate* (usually reported as maternal deaths/10,000 live births) has decreased over the years. (Note that in Figure 5-3, maternal mortality is reported as deaths/100,000 live births.)

Reporting of vital data in the United States has been the legal responsibility of the individual states. It is the responsibility of the person who attends the birth or death to report

Figure 5-1. Still-birth rates. (fetal deaths per 1,000 live births), United States 1930 to 1983. (Vital Statistics of the United States, 1930-1983, Vol 2, Washington, DC, US Department of Health and Human Services.) (Reprinted with permission from O'Connor LJ, Gourley Stephenson RJ. *Obsteric and Gynecologic Care in Physical Therapy.* Thorofare, NJ: SLACK Incorporated; 1990.)

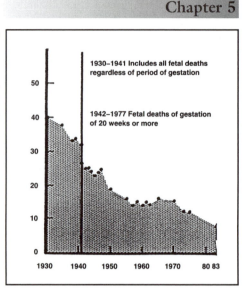

that event to legal authorities. At the time of reporting additional data is required, including age, length of gestation, and cause of death. There is a variability between the states in terms of measuring a gestational period. Some measure by gestational weight and some by gestational age; however, legally, gestations that exceed 20 weeks duration or fetuses of 500 gm in weight are reported as fetal deaths. There are no statistics for total fetal deaths, because most states do not require that deaths from pregnancy of less than 20 weeks be reported. Spontaneous abortions, however, account for 10% to 15% of all pregnancies.

Fetal mortality in the United States has declined to a low of 8.9 in 1981 (Figure 5-1). Antepartum fetal evaluation and intrapartum fetal monitoring are believed to have contributed to the reduction in fetal deaths. Major causes of fetal death are complications of the membranes, cord, or placenta; anoxia; complications of pregnancy; congenital anomalies; gestational growth problems; illness of the mother; and complications of labor and delivery.

Neonatal mortality has also dropped since 1930 (Figure 5-2). In 1983, the United States was at an all-time low of 10/1000 live births. Perinatal centers have contributed to the decrease in neonatal mortality by managing high-risk pregnancies. Most neonatal deaths are associated with high-risk pregnancies- those complicated by diabetes mellitus, hypertensive disorder, multiple fetuses, antepartum bleeding, and hydramnios. The major problems during delivery are abnormal presentations, placenta previa, abruptio placentae, and prolapsed cord. The major cause of neonatal death is impaired oxygenation, which may cause respiratory distress syndrome, hyaline membrane disease, conditions of the placenta, pneumonia, congenital anomalies, and birth injury.

Seven percent of all live-born infants have functional or structural defects. Half of these are diagnosed in the post-natal period. The rest will be diagnosed weeks or years later. Socioeconomic factors do play a part in perinatal mortality, which is higher in poor than in middle and upper class women. Poor women tend to be more malnourished, be more anemic, have less opportunity for good medical care, and have a shorter time between pregnancies.

In 1981, there were 80.5 maternal deaths for each 100,000 live births in the United States (Figure 5-3). Hemorrhage, eclampsia, and preeclampsia are still the most common causes of death among pregnant women. Others include complications of labor and delivery, hypertension, ectopic pregnancy, antepartum hemorrhage, and abortion. Other compli-

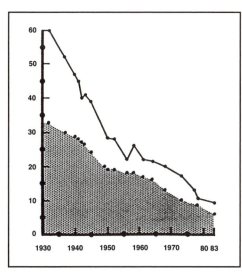

Figure 5-2. Neonatal deaths and infant mortality rates (deaths per 1,000 live births), United States, 1930 to 1983. (Vital Statistics of the US, 1980 to 1983, Vol 2, Washington, D.C., US Department of Health and Human Services.) (Reprinted with permission from O'Connor LJ, Gourley Stephenson RJ. Obsteric and Gynecologic Care in Physical Therapy. Thorofare, NJ: SLACK Incorporated; 1990.)

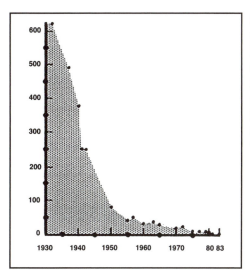

Figure 5-3. Maternal mortality rates. (Deaths per 100,000 live births), United States, 1930 to 1983. (Vital Statistics of the United States, 1930 to 1983, Vol 2, Washington, DC, US Department of Health and Human Services) (Reprinted with permission from O'Connor LJ, Gourley Stephenson RJ. Obsteric and Gynecologic Care in Physical Therapy. Thorofare, NJ: SLACK Incorporated; 1990.)

cations of pregnancy are unknown factors, other medical illness, and hyperemesis. With more sophisticated care offered to pregnant women since the recognition of OB/GYN as a specialty, there has been a decrease in maternal deaths. The use of antibiotics and blood transfusions; improvement in anesthesia and quality of prenatal care; along with the opportunity for safe, legal, abortions have resulted in a significant decrease in maternal deaths.

The physical therapist specializing in obstetrics may either work directly on a ward for mothers with high-risk pregnancies (usually patients are on bed rest or receiving tocolytic therapy), or may work with mothers who may later develop signs of high-risk pregnancy. Therefore, it is important for the physical therapist to be familiar with some of the most common maternal disorders. This chapter does not present every disorder that may occur, but does list and briefly describe in the text and tables[2,3,4] selected problems organized by bodily system and the effects of these problems on pregnancy.

CARDIAC DISEASES AND DISORDERS

One percent of all pregnant women have organic heart disease, half of them being rheumatic in origin. These high-risk patients are having successful pregnancies with the support of careful ante-partum care (see Chapter 6). Here is summary of the effects of cardiac diseases on pregnancy (Table 5-1).

During pregnancy, cardiac surgery is rarely indicated and is avoided, other than in an emergency life-saving measure. Although maternal mortality is not increased significantly, there is a 30 to 50% increase in fetal mortality during open-heart surgery.

Over 150 cases have been reported since 1952 in the literature of women who have undergone cardiac valve replacement surgery prior to their pregnancies. During pregnancy maternal mortality has been low, but management of problems, which are many, has been difficult. Maternal and fetal risk factors depend on what valve has been replaced and the type of replacement used. For instance, pregnancy is not contraindicated for patients with aortic valve replacements. The hemodynamics after aortic valve replacements are different from those occurring after placement of mitral valve prostheses. The fetal mortality rate, however, is increased in mothers with mitral valve prosthesis. Anticoagulants, which may be necessary throughout the pregnancy for the mother's safety, may seriously jeopardize fetal health.

Myocardial infarction (MI) rarely occurs during pregnancy (reported cases total 68 in the period from 1922 to 1987). Continuation of pregnancy depends on the size of the infarct. Small and large infarcts require individual evaluation. Mortality rates range from 30% to 40%. The mortality rate from MI increases the later in pregnancy it occurs. Patients with a history of MI or angina should be have a full cardiac evaluation before beginning pregnancy (see Table 5-1).

PREGNANCY-INDUCED HYPERTENSION

Pregnancy-induced hypertension is symptomatic of various disorders with a common factor of increased mean arterial pressure (MAP). For example, pregnancy-induced hypertension could mean a blood pressure of 140/90 mm Hg during the second half of pregnancy in a usually normotensive woman, which is a 30 mm Hg rise in systolic blood pressure or a 15 mm Hg increase in diastolic pressure over baseline values. To establish the diagnosis, the examiner needs to find increased blood pressure changes on at least two occasions, 6 or more hours apart.

If proteinuria is present, the pregnancy-induced hypertension is reclassified as preeclampsia. There are five classifications of hypertensive disease in pregnancy: gestational hypertension, chronic hypertension, chronic hypertension with superimposed preeclampsia, preeclampsia, and eclampsia.

Gestational hypertension is defined as a rise in the MAP above 106 mm Hg, occurring after 20 weeks of pregnancy, without proteinuria. This hypertension disappears after delivery. Gestational hypertension may be hard to distinguish from chronic hypertension, if the patient is not seen for obstetrical care prior to the 20th week.

Both chronic hypertensive and normotensive women will have a decrease in blood pressure during the middle and early third trimesters of pregnancy. Therefore, if patients with

Table 5-1

Effects of Cardiomyopathies and Other Diseases on Pregnancy

Disease	Symptoms	Effects on Mother	Effects on Fetus
Hypertrophic cardio-myopathy (hypertrophy of the left ventricle; also known as obstructive cardiomyopathy or idiopathic hypertrophic subaortic stenosis; autosomal disorder; mitral regurgitation)	Sudden death at any age from sudden arrhythmias or tachycardia; no specific symptoms before death; pregnancy well-tolerated	Unpredictable occurrence; most patients treated with beta blockers	Fetal growth monitored by ultrasound because beta blockers may cause intrauterine growth retardation
Marfan's syndrome (autosomal dominant disease with abnormal connective tissue due to dysfunctional protein metabolism)	Involvement of any organ; death usually from cardiac complications; mitral valve prolapse common; increased risk of aortic dissection and rupture during pregnancy; joint deformities; weakness of aortic root	Maternal mortality 50%; risk increased if aortic root >4 cm; pregnancy contraindicated; managed by beta blockers; avoidance of bearing-down effort and use forceps delivery	Fetal growth monitored by ultrasound, because beta blockers may cause intrauterine growth retardation
Peripartumcardio-myopathy (rare: 1/1500 to 1/4000 pregnancies; etiology unknown; most common in black multiparas; preeclampsia in 7% of patients)	Enlarged heart, development of congestive heart failure during last month of pregnancy (7%), in 1st 3 mo post-partum (82%), in 4th or 5th mo (11%); ECG tracing of ventricular CHF.*	Maternal mortality 10% to 15% if heart returns to normal; 85% if not; future pregnancy contraindicated	None
Primary pulmonary hypertension (rare disease associated with >50% mortality)	Progressive constriction and fibrosis of pulmonary arterioles and muscularization; pulmonary artery pressure high; progressive RVH*; dyspnea, syncope, chest pain; death due to arrhythmia	Death any time, but most often in last mo. of pregnancy and early puerperium from increased blood volume and cardiac output, with RV failure arrhythmias; future pregnancy contraindicated	None

*CHF, congestive heart failure; RVH, right ventricular hypertrophy

unrecognized chronic hypertension are seen for the first time at the 24th week of pregnancy, they may appear normal; but early in the third trimester, the blood pressure may rise to an unrecognized hypertensive level, making it impossible to distinguish between pregnancy-induced hypertension and chronic hypertension. There are, however, clinical findings that can help determine if the disorder is chronic in nature: retinal hemorrhages and exudates;

plasma urea nitrogen concentrates above 20 mg/dl; plasma creatinine concentration above 1 mg/dl; and the presence of renal disease, collagen vascular disease, diabetes mellitus, or other disorders that predispose a woman to chronic hypertension. Chronic hypertension is suspected if blood pressure is above 140/90 mm Hg, if hypertension is detected earlier than 20 weeks, if hypertension dates to prior to the pregnancy, and if hypertension is not accompanied by proteinuria.

Chronic hypertension with superimposed preeclampsia is characterized by hypertension starting before the 20th week of pregnancy with the addition of proteinuria and edema in the latter half of pregnancy. This disorder occurs in 13% of treated chronic hypertensive patients.[3]

Preeclampsia denotes hypertension, proteinuria, and edema, usually occurring in primigravidas after the 20th week of pregnancy. Degrees are mild, moderate, and severe. In the mild form, MAP is less than 106 mm Hg (140/90 mm Hg), diastolic pressure increases more than 15 mm Hg on 2 occasions 6 hours apart with patient at bed rest, and there is proteinuria or edema. In moderate preeclampsia, MAP is 106 mm Hg (140/90 mm Hg) to 126 mm Hg (160/110 mm Hg, or a rise of blood pressure greater than 30 mm Hg systolic or greater than 15 mm Hg diastolic). Increased proteinuria and edema of the lower extremities may also be noted. In severe preeclampsia, MAP is greater than 126 mm Hg (160/110 mm Hg) on two occasions 6 hours apart with the patient at bed rest, proteinuria is greater than 5 gm/24 hours, and the patient complains of headaches and blurred vision. There may also be right upper quadrant pain, oliguria, pulmonary edema, and edema of the face, hands, and lower extremities.[3]

Eclampsia is characterized by generalized seizure activity with hypertension and proteinuria in the pregnant patient. This seizure occurs within the first 24 hours post-partum. No one is able to accurately predict which patients with pregnancy-induced hypertension will develop eclampsia. Its etiology is unknown, although three major theories of causes exist: increased vasoconstrictor tone, abnormal prostaglandin action, and immunological factors. It is likely that the disease process begins with vasospasm and then leads to a reduced blood flow to the uterus and other organs. Reduced intravascular volume and, ultimately, hypertension develop.

VASCULAR DISEASE

There are three causes of venous thrombosis and pulmonary embolism: changes in blood clotting factors, vessel wall damage, and venous stasis. Some blood clotting factors are increased, others decreased, during pregnancy. Vessel wall damage may occur during delivery, especially during Cesarean section. Prolonged use of stirrups for a vaginal delivery may also lead to vessel wall damage in the patient's legs. Pooling of blood in the lower extremities is common in pregnancy: this increased venous distensibility occurs in the first trimester; and by 28 weeks of gestation, the venous pressure in the legs is 2 times non-pregnant values. Additionally, the enlarging uterus interferes with venous return from the legs, thereby reducing the velocity of venous flow by half. Consequently, the incidence of thromboembolitic disease during early pregnancy is only slightly increased, but as pregnancy progresses, and at term, the incidence is about 50% above non-pregnant values. In the early puerperium, the incidence is five to six times higher than it is in a non-pregnant woman.

Varicose veins, often a familial trait, increase 11% to 25% in pregnancy.[1] The cause may relate to the hormonal changes of pregnancy and to the mechanical obstructions to blood flow by the increasing size of the uterus. Varicosities usually become evident at 10 to 12 weeks of pregnancy; and symptoms include a feeling of heaviness or discomfort in the legs, usually after walking, possibly accompanied by incapacitating pain. Stasis and ulceration may accompany the pain. Varicosities occur more frequently with subsequent pregnancies and may predispose the mother to thrombophlebitis. There is no effect on the fetus. Management includes pressure-graded elastic stockings, bed rest with feet elevated, dorsiflexion and plantarflexion exercises performed frequently throughout the day, and avoidance of binding stockings or socks. Hemorrhoids are rectal varicosities that can cause pain, itching, and bleeding during bowel movements. Resolved preexisting hemorrhoids may become symptomatic during labor, and especially after delivery.

One-fifth of pregnant women may develop vulvar varicosities due to a 30-fold increase in the circulation by the third trimester and increased pressure through the iliac vein branches as the weight of the uterus increases. These varicosities are not hazardous to mother or fetus, although maternal discomfort is common and rupture may produce a hematoma. Varices will regress after delivery, and discomfort can sometimes be reduced by pressing pads to the labia. Additionally, the full support of the Baby Hugger (TrennaVentions, Inc., Derry, PA) can decrease the discomfort of vulvar varicosities.

The saphenous veins are frequently affected by superficial venous thrombosis, which is more common than deep vein thrombosis. Superficial venous thrombosis occurs in patients with varicosities. Redness may be present, and pain is evident along the course of the vein. Conservative management, as mentioned above, is helpful. This disorder is rarely associated with embolism, and there is no effect on the fetus. (See Appendix for venous support hose information.)

Pregnant women show an increased susceptibility to deep vein thrombosis. It is difficult to diagnose, and the onset is usually abrupt, occurring more often in the puerperium. On examination, one leg may be at least 2 cm larger in circumference than the other. There may be a temperature difference between legs, as well. A Doppler ultrasound and limited venography will confirm the diagnosis. Treatment consists of bed rest with the bed elevated on 8 inch blocks to decrease the edema and application of heat. Pelvic thrombophlebitis occurs in 0.18% to 0.29% of pregnant women and 0.1 to 1.0% of post-partum women.

Pulmonary embolism occurs in 16% of patients with deep venous thrombosis without coagulation, and in 19% with coagulation. A threat of abortion may occur as the result of iliac vein obstruction, but usually, the fetus is unaffected. Pulmonary embolism is a dangerous complication of venous thrombosis, Cesarean section, forceps delivery, and advanced maternal age. The risk of pulmonary embolism during pregnancy and the puerperium is 5.5 times greater than for non-pregnant women. Without anticoagulation medicine, mortality is extremely high. Pulmonary embolism is the main nonobstetric cause of post-partum death, and maternal hypoxia experienced during pulmonary embolism causes fetal death or impairment.

Few arterial diseases are unique to pregnancy. Raynaud's Phenomenon usually undergoes remission during pregnancy, and medications that can cause arteriospasm are to be avoided. Dissecting aneurysm of the aorta may occur in the last trimester of pregnancy or in the puerperium, as a result of an increase in blood volume and associated with coarctation of the aorta induced by hypertensive stress. There may be a familial history of this disease that causes chest pain, and prognosis for mother and fetus is grave; maternal death is frequent. Management is usually surgical. Splenic artery aneurysm is more frequently associated with grand multiparity and can result in rupture, leading to intraperitoneal hemorrhage. Prognosis for mother and fetus is grave. Management involves blood transfusion and laporotomy to remove the spleen and aneurysm.

ENDOCRINE DISEASE

Perhaps the most devastating diseases of pregnancy can be linked to endocrine dysfunction. The regulation of endocrine function determines fetoplacental influences vital for blood flow, nutrition, and organ differentiation. It may even be true that the fetus, through endocrine mechanisms, signals the start of labor. Diabetes and gestational diabetes are among the most common endocrine diseases influencing pregnancy, but disorders of the thyroid, parathyroid, adrenal, and pituitary glands, described in Table 5-2, can also cause complications.

Niswander describes diabetes mellitus as a "chronic metabolic disorder characterized by relative or absolute lack of circulating insulin resulting in hyperglycemia and glucosuria, increased protein and fat catabolism, and the tendency in some patients to ketoacidosis."[4] Some complications of diabetes mellitus include neuropathy, retinopathy, vascular disease, and polyneuropathy. The etiology of diabetes is unknown. It has been theorized that genetic and acquired mechanisms play a role in this multifaceted disease.

Many advances in the last 12 years have been made to help the pregnant woman with diabetes mellitus. Maternal mortality has been almost eliminated, and maternal morbidity has been reduced significantly. For patients who are insulin-dependent, the perinatal mortality rate has approached the rate for normal gravidas. Traditional management of the pregnant diabetic patient has included an elective, premature delivery date between 36 and 38 weeks gestation,[6] but because of advances in antepartum fetal monitoring, more diabetics can be brought to term with successful outcomes.

The rate of glucose intolerance in pregnant women ranges from 3% to 12%, with 0.1% to 0.5% dependent on insulin.[1] Glucose values are not controlled by diet. Fasting plasma values greater than 100 mg/dl or mean plasma glucose values above 120 mg/dl require insulin treatment.[7] The mother may experience some change in sugar control, such as hyperglycemia, hypoglycemia, and changes in quantity of insulin needed. She may also experience some pregnancy-induced hypertension, increased urinary tract infections, and polyhydramnios (an excess of amniotic fluid). These changes are manageable and do not change the maternal diabetic prognosis. The rate of uterine growth and possible signs of preeclampsia are all monitored throughout pregnancy.

The problems that can complicate a pregnancy when the mother is insulin-dependent are of more concern to the fetus's well-being than the mother's. The infant may develop microsomia, congenital anomalies, respiratory distress syndrome, neonatal hypoglycemia, hypercalcemia, hypomagnesemia, and hyperbilirubinemia; sometimes death occurs. The degree and presence of these problems are related to the maternal glucose levels. To provide the best environment for the fetus, the maternal glucose level should be monitored daily and should be maintained below 120 mg/dl. The status of the fetus should be monitored during pregnancy, its age determined, and all possible efforts to bring it to maturity be made. Delivery of the infant should be early and safe; the infant should then be assessed by a skilled neonatologist. Fetal well being may be monitored by contraction stress test, nonstress test, and daily maternal assessment of fetal activity.

Gestational diabetes is defined as diabetes that first appears during pregnancy. This occurs in about 3% of all pregnancies. All pregnant women should be screened for diabetes with a 50 gm oral glucose load. If blood drawn 1 hour later exceeds 135 mg/dl, then a 3-hour glucose tolerance test is indicated. If it is determined that the pregnant woman does indeed have gestational diabetes, a diabetic diet, and possibly insulin, will be needed. Class A diabetes is the classification given to pregnant women who have an abnormal glucose tolerance

Table 5-2

Effects of Endocrine Diseases on Pregnancy

Disease	Symptoms	Etfects on Mother	Effects on Fetus
Cushing's syndrome (rare in pregnancy; women usually anovulatory; excess glucocorticoids due to adrenal adeno-mas or carcinomas	Weight loss, edema, nausea, vomiting, weakness, hyperten-sign, easy bruisabil-ity, acne, increased hirsutism, carbohy-drate intolerance	Spontaneous abor-tion; premature labor	High perinatal mor-bidity and mortality
Addison's disease (adrenal insuffi-ciency; patients rarely conceive)	Fatigue, anorexia, nausea, vomiting, hypotension, in-creased pigmenta-tion, fasting hypogly-cemia	Dehydration and elec-trolyte imbalance; delivery indicated; with glucocorticoid replacement; good prognosis	Small-for-gestational-age infants; depressed adrenal function at birth
Pheochromocytoma (rare in pregnancy; adrenal medulla tumor; catecho-lamine excess)	Hypertension, head-aches, palpitations, sweating, weakness, weight loss, glycosu-ria, nervousness, tremor	Possible remission between pregnan-cies, but manifesta-tions more severe with each preg-nancy; high mater-nal mortality, usually during or after deliv-ery; Cesarean and concurrent tumor removal indicated	High fetal mortality
Graves' Disease (hyperthyroidism; 0.2% incidence in pregnancy)	Weakness; heat intolerance; tachy-cardia; resting pulse 100 beats/minute	Possibly life-threat-ening; fever; dehy-dration; nausea, vomiting, mental confusion; increased risk of preterm labor	1% to 2% thyrotoxico-sis rate if untreated
Autoimmune thyroid-itis (Hashimoto's thryoiditis; antithy-roid; mxydema; rare in pregnancy)	Fatigue, cold intoler-ance, excessive weight gain, hoarseness, dry skin, coarse hair, constipation, myalgia	Rise of spontaneous abortion; with hor-mone replacement, excellent prognosis for mother and fetus	two-fold stillbirth rate
Thyroid Nodules (incidence same as in nonpregnancy)	Hard nodule, painful gland, enlarged lymph nodes, hoarseness	Possible englargement of thyroid; rule out mal-ignancy, surgery may be indicated	No effect on gestation
Hyperparathyroidism (rare in pregnancy)	Polydipsia, constipa-tion, nausea, vomit-ing, hypercalcemia, fatigue, muscle weakness (may be asymptomatic)	Subperiostial bone resorption; maternal mortality rare; pre-mature labor 20%	Mortality rates 25% 30% (half stillbirth); 15 to 50% develop neonatal tetany
Hypoparathyroidism (secondary to thry-oid or parathryoid	Hypocalcemia, numbness, tingling, weakness, tetany,	Increased need for calcium in preg-nancy and in labor;	If untreated, risk for neonatal hyperpara--thyroidism

Table 5-2 continued

Effects of Endocrine Diseases on Pregnancy

Disease	Symptoms	Effects on Mother	Effects on Fetus
surgery; rare in pregnancy)	carpopedal spasm, mental aberration	breastfeeding not recommended	
Sheehan's syndrome (post-partum pituitary necrosis due to blood loss during delivery)	Rapid breast involution; decreased pigmentation; loss of axillary and pubic hair	Possible failure to lactate; possible amenorrhea	No effect if treated
Diabetes insipidus (inadequate production of antidiuretic hormone by posterior pituitary gland; incidence 1/16,000 1 /80,000)	Polydipsia, polyuria	Possibility of disease worsening in pregnancy; symptoms alleviated by lactation	No effect if treated
Acromegaly (rare in pregnancy)	Possible tumor expansion, visual field loss, severe headaches, nausea, vomiting	No effect on pregnancy	No effect on fetus
Microadenomas (prolactin-secreting tumors)	Possible headaches, visual field disturbances	No effect on pregnancy; treated with bromocriptine, if enlarges	No effect on fetus

test but do not require insulin treatment. This accounts for 90% of all diabetics in pregnancy.[1] These patients' fetuses are at no higher risk for demise than those of nondiabetic obstetrical patients. Their fetuses are not electively delivered early, but their glucose levels are monitored every 2 weeks. If a Class A diabetic pregnant woman has required insulin in a previous pregnancy, has had either a previous stillbirth or previous hypertension, or develops preeclampsia in the current pregnancy, she is managed as an insulin-dependent diabetic. Her classification, however, does not change.[6]

RENAL DISEASE

Pregnancy causes marked changes in renal function. Disorders affecting renal function in pregnancy may be classified as infections, obstructions, acute renal failure, and chronic renal disease. The most common renal complication during pregnancy is urinary tract infection' characterized by ureteral dilation and relative obstruction. A resulting static column of ureteral urine and elevated glucose and amino acids in the urine facilitate bacterial growth. Because asymptomatic bacteriuria occurs in 2% to 10% of all pregnant women, and, if untreated, can lead to pyelonephritis in 25 to 30%, pregnant women should be screened periodically. Cystitis occurs in 1% of pregnant women. Symptoms include urinary frequency, pus, and painful urination.

Pyelonephritis (inflammation of the kidney) occurs in 1% to 2.5% of pregnancies. Symptoms are fever, bacteriuria, pus in the urine, costovertebral angle tenderness, vomiting, nausea, chills, urgency, frequency, and painful urination. The right kidney is more commonly affected. Acute pyelonephritis is often associated with premature labor, and the recurrence rate is high.

Urinary calculi (kidney stones) appear in 0.05% to 0.35% of pregnancies. Pregnancy does not increase the risk of stone formation. Although there is minimal risk of stone formation, urinary infections occur in 20% to 45% of pregnant patients with calculi. Symptoms include blood in urine, loin pain, flank pain, and severe or unresponsive pyelonephritis. Ureteral obstruction is rare in pregnancy. There have been reported about 10 cases in pregnancy of acute renal failure caused by obstruction from a gravid uterus, associated with a single kidney or uterine overdistention.

Incidence of acute renal failure has decreased dramatically in the last several decades. Preexisting renal failure is the cause of most acute renal failure in pregnancy and is related to dehydration, septic shock, or transfusion reaction. Factors in pregnancy that are associated with acute renal failure, most often occurring in the third trimester, include preeclampsia, placenta previa, and abruptio placentae. Severe hepatic dysfunction and jaundice may accompany acute renal failure. Most patients with acute renal suffer from renal insufficiency, and mortality is high.

Idiopathic post-partum renal failure may occur 3 to 10 days post-delivery in otherwise healthy patients. There is a high incidence of morbidity and mortality, dialysis is required, and surviving patients will have renal impairment.

In chronic renal disease, the incidence of fetal loss is 4.1% to 7% in normotensive mothers and 45% in hypertensive mothers. About one quarter of pregnant women with chronic renal disease are hypertensive and moderate decreases in renal function may occur. Pregnancy, in general, however, does not increase progression of renal disease. Pregnancy outcome in women with chronic renal disease varies.

Women with renal complications from collagen disease (eg, systemic lupus erythematosus) can have successful pregnancies, but in chronic glomerular nephritis, the outcome depends on the degree of renal failure and the amount of hypertension. Patients with diabetic nephropathy demonstrate no greater incidence of maternal mortality nor increased renal disease. Polycystic kidney disease and renal tuberculosis also appear to have no adverse effects on progression of disease or pregnancy, and women with one kidney can tolerate pregnancy. On the other hand, women with pelvic kidney (kidney misplaced into the pelvis) run a greater risk of urogenital tract malformation and dystocia delivery.

Women with severe kidney disease who regularly receive renal dialysis rarely conceive; and patients who do get pregnant are at high-risk. A recent study of 56 pregnancies in which the mother had a renal transplant reported 44 live newborns: 31 deliveries were uncomplicated, and of the fetuses, 4 had congenital abnormalities, 4 had respiratory distress, 2 had adrenal insufficiency, 2 septicemia, and 1 seizures. Patients with severe kidney disease are susceptible to infection and fetal anomalies because of immunosuppressive drugs used post-transplant. Criteria for pregnancy, developed by Davidson and Lindheimer, should be met before pregnancy is recommended to renal transplant mothers: (1) general good health 2 years after transplant (2) status compatible with good obstetric outcome (3) no significant proteinuria (4) no evidence of graft rejection (5) no evidence of hypertension (6) no evidence of pelvicalyceal distention on a recent intravenous pyelogram (7) serum creatinine of 2 mg/dl or less (8) therapeutic drug regimen consisting of 15 mg/dl or less of prednisone and 2 mg/kg/d, or less, of azathioprine (immunosuppressant drug).[4]

RESPIRATORY DISORDERS

Upper respiratory infections occur at the same rate in pregnant women as in non-pregnant women. The mother needs to increase fluids and rest, but she should avoid cough suppressants and antihistamines. Half of all pneumonias in pregnancy are preceded by an upper respiratory infection. During the major influenza epidemics of 1918 to 1919 and 1957 to 1958, mortality of pregnant women increased. The cause of death was influenzal pneumonia, rather than subsequent bacterial infection. Other than during those epidemics, there have been no studies to link influenza with an increase in maternal or fetal mortality or associated congenital anomalies. Treatment for the mother is the same as for upper respiratory infection. Interestingly, there are no data to suggest that vaccines from a killed virus for influenza yield any teratogenic effects on the fetus. Indications for a flu vaccine are the same as in a non-pregnant woman; but, nonetheless, the use of the vaccine in pregnancy is controversial.

General treatment for pneumonia includes use of expectorants, percussion and vibration, postural drainage, rest, fever-reducing drugs, avoidance of narcotics and cough suppressants, and correction of hypoxia. Hypoxia is not tolerated by the fetus, and correction of fluid electrolyte imbalances is vital. Bacterial pneumonia is usually treated with penicillin and the above supportive measures. Microplasma pneumonia is often treated with erythromycin, because tetracycline has been linked to fetal teeth staining, inhibition of fetal bone growth, and congenital anomalies, and, therefore, is contraindicated. Viral pneumonia requires the aforementioned supportive measures, but there is no specific drug treatment available for varicella pneumonia. When chicken pox pneumonia is complicated by a bacterial superinfection, it is associated with mortality as high as 41%. Neonatal mortality rate is as high as 34%. Fortunately it is not a common infection during pregnancy, because most mothers are immune from childhood exposure. Aspiration pneumonia in the mother calls for suction by endotracheal tube, and blood gases need to be closely monitored. Drugs are given to reduce bronchospasm.

A catastrophic event that mimics acute respiratory distress is amniotic fluid embolus. This type of embolus most often occurs in the multigravida mother late in the first stage of labor when the membranes have ruptured and the amniotic fluid is forced into the maternal circulation. Often the first sign is a sense of suffocation, dyspnea, general distress, agitation, and unexplained cough. The patient will develop chills and fever, cyanosis, and tachycardia; and pulmonary edema develops quickly. It is estimated that there is an 80% chance of fatality.

Pneumomediastinum tends to be a disorder that occurs during labor, but it may also occur during pregnancy. It involves increased alveolar pressure as a result of forceful expulsions with a closed glottis, accompanied by alveolar rupture and splitting of the air along the perivascular spaces into the mediastinum. The patient senses sudden onset of chest pain with a crackling, crunching sound (Hamman's sign) associated with heartbeat that may increase during systole. There is an increased presence of air in the subcutaneous tissues of the upper chest and neck 25% to 35% of the time. Without infection or increased mediastinal or intrapleural pressure, it is usually benign and resolves spontaneously.

Chronic obstructive lung disease, chronic bronchitis, and emphysema are not usually seen in pregnant women. Treatment is the same as in a non-pregnant woman except to avoid tetracycline. Conduction anesthesia, rather than inhalation anesthesia, is indicated for labor and delivery. The rate of tuberculosis in pregnancy is 1% to 3%. Symptoms include malaise, cough, persistent low-grade fever, weight loss, night sweats, hemoptysis and chest pains, apical rates, cavernous breath sounds, and pleural effusion. Prognosis for the mother is the same as for a non-pregnant woman. If she has active disease, she should be treated.

There is no teratogenic effect with INH (isoniazid), even when given during the first trimester. If the mother is treated, the fetus probably will not develop complications, because congenital tuberculosis is rare; however, if the mother is untreated, there is a 50% chance the child will develop tuberculosis in the first year of life, as well as a significant risk of death. If the mother has inactive disease, treated in the past, no treatment is required. If untreated, a mother should receive INH after delivery. If a mother's symptoms are covert in the previous 24 months, the risk of developing an active disease is 3% to 5%; she should begin INH for 1 year, starting after the first trimester. Breastfeeding is considered safe for women taking antituberculosis drugs.

INFECTIOUS, GASTROINTESTINAL, AND DERMATOLOGY DISEASES AND DISORDERS

Another strong determinant of fetal well-being and infant health is the maternal response to infectious disease, gastrointestinal disturbance, and Dermatologic disorders. Many infectious diseases can be easily contracted by the mother, particularly if she has other children. Sexually-transmitted diseases also can have devastating consequences for the pregnant woman and her baby. Highlights of selected infectious diseases are listed in Table 5-3 and selected gastrointestinal and dermatologic disorders in Tables 5-4 and 5-5.

REPRODUCTIVE TRACT DISORDERS

Alterations in the reproductive tract can occur during pregnancy as a result of uterine pressure on the vessels, tumors, congenital anomalies, and pelvic infections.

Retrodisplacement of the uterus (backward displacement of the uterus) occurs fairly often in the early months of pregnancy. If retrodisplacement occurs at the ninth or tenth week, however, the uterus may become lodged by the hollow of the sacrum, resulting in compression of the urethra and bladder neck. Knee-to-chest position may help dislodge the uterus, or, if that fails, anesthetic procedure may be performed.

Similarly rare is torsion of the uterus, associated with considerable pain and pathology such as myomas, ovarian cysts, adhesions, or uterine anomalies. The uterus rotates on a radial axis of 45% or greater. Cesarean section is often advised, but fetal mortality is high, and maternal mortality occurs in 50% of all cases.

Uterine sacculation, prolapse, and inversion are extremely rare disorders, but can produce pain and premature labor. If the uterus sacculates, it can result in severe anteflexion due to poor abdominal tone in the late third trimester. Most often seen in grand multiparas, this may result in abnormal fetal presentation or lack of engagement. Uterine prolapse however, also usually seen in a multipara, may occur during any trimester. Treatment requires bed rest with a slight Trendelenburg position to avoid premature labor and rupture of membranes. Cesarean section may be necessary. More severe than prolapse is uterine inversion, which may occur immediately following delivery. In this case, the uterus turns inside out and protrudes through the cervix and outside the vagina. This condition can be acute, subacute, or chronic. It happens most often to multiparas with a lax uterus, from fundal pressure following delivery, and from excessive umbilical cord traction.

Table 5-3

Effects of Infectious Diseases on Pregnancy

Disease	Symptoms	Effects on Mother	Effects on Fetus
AIDS (acquired immunodeficiency syndrome;transmitted by blood and body fluids sexually and transplacentally)	Hypergammaglobulinemia, weight loss, lymphadenopathy, hepatosplenomegaly, diarrhea	Spontaneous abortion rate 25%-50%; hypoxia; premature labor; prognosis poor	No fetal malformation noted; transplacentaltransmission; prognosis poor
Coxsackie virus (type A similar to common cold; type B, severe chest wall pain)	Minor respiratory symptoms	Usually self-limiting; no effect on mortality	Type A, no effect on fetus, type B. myocarditis, encephalitis, mortality, tetralogy of fallot
Cytomegalovirus (in U.S., 50% adults seropositive; herpes virus; infects 50%-60% of women in childbearing ages)	Lowgrade fever, malaise, lymphadenopathy, enlarged liver and spleen; may be asymptomatic	Self-limiting infection; no increase in morbidity or mortality in pregnancy	Fetus infected through the placenta or at birth when passing through infected birth canal; possible mental retardation, hearing loss, microcephaly, intracranial calcification, enlarged liver and spleen; stillbirth
Epstein-Barr virus (serologic diagnosis)	Malaise, fatigue, muscle soreness and tightness, fever, infections, swollen glands	Unknown	Unknown
Hepatitis (type A, infectious; B. viral; C, serum; 15-180 day incubation)	Malaise, fever, anorexia, nausea, vomiting; chronic liver disease; jaundice; itching; rash, myalgia, lymphadenopathy	Spontaneous abortion and prematurity	Congenital abnormalities; paralysis, convulsions; jaundice; 34% mortality
Herpes simplex virus 1 and 2	Type 1, cold sores; Type 2, genital blisters	Premature labor; Cesarean section recommended	Transplacental transmission rare; possible fetal contact with infected genital tract in delivery; possible skin lesions, general infection, brain damage, encephalitis
Malaria (transmitted by anopheles mosquito)	High, spiking fever, headache, myalgia	Abortion possible in severe attacks, prematurity, stillbirth	Growth retardation; fever, enlarged liver and spleen, seizures, jaundice, pulmonary edema 48 to 72 hours after delivery
Mumps (vaccine contraindicated in pregnant women; contagious disease; 2-3 week incubation)	Generalized infection; swollen parotid glands; possible aseptic meningitis, meningoencephalitis, adenositis, pancreatitis	Spontaneous abortion first trimester	No increase in congenital malformations; possible endocardial fibroelastosis
Poliomyelitis (rare disease in pregnancy; vaccine should be avoided	Lower motor neuron paralytic motor disease; fever; nausea; vomiting;	Spontaneous abortion	Paralysis, neonatal poliomyelitis; mortality rate 25%

Table 5-3 continued

Effects of Infectious Diseases on Pregnancy

Disease	Symptoms	Effects on Mother	Effects on Fetus
during pregnancy)	nasal inflammation; sore throat; hyperes--thesia; muscle pain		
Rubella (German measles; vaccine decreased number of cases; 15%-20° of childbearing women do not have antibody; 3-mo. wait required before pregnancy after vaccine; highly contagious; incubation period 10-21 days)	Erythematous raised rash; lymphadenopathy; arthralgia; arthritis; fever; cough	Spontaneous abortion and stillbirth 2-4x more frequently	Congenital rubella syndrome; 70% chance of direct infection of fetus in first trimester; risk of fetal malformation or death ranges 10-34%; cataracts, blindness, cardiac anomalies, deafness, mental retardation, cerebral palsy, encephalitis, cleft palate, hemolytic anemia, birthmarks, hepatosplenomegaly, thrombocytopenia purpura
Ptubeola (measles; slight increase recently; attenuated vaccine given 1957-1967, requiring revaccination; highly contagious disease incubation 10-12 days)	Small, irregular red spots on face and extremities; fever; encephalitis in 1/100 cases	Spontaneous abortion rate high; premature delivery	Death within 2 years; congenital malformations
Streptococcal infection (group A, puerperal fever; B. genitaltract)	Symptoms of bacterial infection; treatment with penicillin required	Endometritis, chorioamnionitis, septic abortion, pelvic peritonitis, premature rupture of membranes	25% neonatal sepsis, meningitis; pneumonia
Toxoplasmosis (common worldwide infection, usually from cat feces and poorly cooked infected meat)	Asymptomatic lymphadenopathy; sore throat, myalgias, macular rash; enlarged spleen and liver; pneumonia; meningitis	Morbidity and mortality unaffected; 10%-15% increase in spontaneous abortion in first and second trimesters	First trimester, lowest incidence of congenital infection; highest in third trimeter; possible stillbirth or premature birth; possible mental retardation, hydrocephaly, microcephaly, corioretinitis, convulsions, blindness, deafness
Varicella (chicken pox or later shingles, herpes zoster)	Prodromal symptoms of fever, malaise, rash, possible pneumonia; 1/3 of adults develop pneumonia	Mortality 41%	Mortality 34%; anomalies; neurologic deficit, mental retardation; seizures, paralysis, limb atrophy, cutaneous scars; rudimentary digits; convulsions; cortical atrophy

Table 5-4

Effects of Gastrointestinal Diseases on Pregnancy [2,3,4]

Disease	Symptoms	Effects on Mother	Effects on Fetus
Nausea and vomiting (after first missed period, may last up to 12 weeks)	May be related to elevated levels of steroid hormones and hCG	Usually none	Usually none
Hyperemesis gravidarum(protracted nausea and vomiting occurring throughout pregnancy, any time of day in 3.5/1000 pregnancies)	Weight loss, electrolyte imbalance, dehydration, ketonemia, possible renal or hepatic damage, bleeding from strained throat muscles; increased gastric acid causing gum recession	Endurance may be decreased; nutritional deficiency	No increase in congenital malformations or abortion
Appendicitis (occurs 1/1500 deliveries)	Pain in right lower quadrant in early pregnancy, in right upper quadrant in third trimester; mortality 2% overall; 7% in mid trimester and in general population 1.8%; increased morbidity due to delayed diagnosis from pregnancy-masking signs and symptoms	Possibility of appendix rupture with infection if removed near term; retention sutures used so mothers can push during delivery and not disturb wound	Mortality 97%; increased with generalized peritonitis
Reflux esophagitis (heartburn compliGates up to 25% of pregnancies; associated with reflux secondary to progesterone and relaxation of lower esophageal sphincter)	Substantial burning, worse after eating and lying down or bending over; usually appears at end of second month; most severe at 32 wk gestation	No known complications	No known complications
Intestinal obstruction (uncommon in pregnancy; can be caused by adhesions)	Abdominal pain, steady or colicky; vomiting, nausea, abdominal distention, constipation	Surgical intervention needed if stomach decompression not successful; possible hypoxia or hypertension	Negative effects from complications of surgery
Peptic Dicer disease (pregnancy has beneficial effect on the disease; 45% of patients symptom-free in pregnancy; pregnancy may protect against development of duodenal ulcers; prostaglandins assert	Upper gastrointestinal bleeding, usually worse when the stomach is empty; relieved by food or antacids	High incidence ulcer recurrence during lactation; breastfeeding usually not recommended	

Table 5-4 continued

Effects of Gastrointestinal Diseases on Pregnancy [2,3,4]

Disease	Symptoms	Effects on Mother	Effects on Fetus
protective effect on gastric mucosa)			
Inflammatory bowel disease (chronic re-lapsing and remission disease little affected by pregnancy; inclu-des ulcerative colitis and Crohn's disease)	Decreased fertility rate; weight loss, abdominal pain, diarrhea, fever	Relapse common in pregnancy	No increase in prenatal mortality, anomalies or abortion
Pancreatitis (related to gallstone in 2/3 of cases)	24-48 attack of right upper quadrant and abdominal pain, nau-sea and vomiting, pain radiating to back	37% mortality	Perinatal mortality 37.9%
Cholecystitis (gall bladder emptying time may be slowed)	Pain in the midepigas-trum, right scapular and shoulder pain, nausea, vomiting, right upper quadrant pain, jaundice	Surgical treatment, if medical therapy doesn't respond in 4 days	Negative effects only from complications of surgery
Intrahepatic choler-tasis (estrogen-related defect in hepatic bile excre-tion)	Develops late in preg-nancy with itching of hands and feet as early as the 6th wk; jaundice if severe	No serious maternal effects; symptoms resolve within few wk of delivery	Perinatal mortality is 4x that of controls; fetal distress present in 40%; increase of preterm labor labor, still-births, meco-nium staining
Acute fatty liver of pregnancy (rare, leth-al disorder of un-known etiology; occurs between 30 and 38 wks of pregnancy; more common in twin twin and male births and in primigravidas)	Repeated vomiting, abdominal pain, nau-sea, jaundice; in severe cases, hepatio enceph-alopathy, renal failure, and hemorrhage; may not occur in subse-quent prenancies	Prognosis for the fetus and mother 75%-80% mortality Early delivery when lung maturity reached may reduce infant mortality	
Chronic liver disease	Treated with predni-sone and azathio-prine	No affect on maternal survival or number of hepatitis occurrences	Increased incidence of fetal morbidity and mortality
Cirrhosis (rare dis-ease in pregnancy; complications in estrogen metabo-lism may result in infertility)	Increased portal pres-sure due to increased blood volume; eso-phageal varices due to added weight of gravid uterus on vena cava	Possible fatal hemor-hage, deteriorated liver function; complications from bleeding or eso-phageal varices, post-partum hemorrhage	Perinatal mortality increased
Hepatic tumors of pregnancy (ade-noma; associated with prior contracep-tive steroid use)	Highly vascular tumors enlarged in response to estro-gen, may rupture and hemorrhage	Successful pregnancy possible but contra-indicated in patients with an unresected adenoma	

Table 5-5

Effects of Dermatologic Diseases on Pregnancy

Disease	Symptoms	Fetal/Maternal Complications
Pruritus gravidarum (affects 20% of pregnant women; associated with cholestasis)	Severe generalized itching in third trimester	None; disappears after delivery
Pruritic urticarial papules (rash of symmetric, itching papules)	Rash in third trimester in primigravidas	None; disappears after delivery
Herpes gestationis (unrelated to herpes virus; may recur with subsequent pregnancy, menstruation, or from progesterone medications, usually occurs in second or third trimester)	Malaise, chills, fever, headache, nausea, abdominal and trunk lesions, progressing to extremities; polymorphous, blister-like eruptions	Resolves 3 mo after delivery; fetus small for gestational age; occasionally transient blueness noted in newborn mother
Impetigo herpetiforrnis (rare, pustular eruptions; onset third trimester)	Rash in axillae and inguinal folds; may become widespread; malaise, chills, vomiting, diarrhea, sometimes tetany	Remission post-partum; may recur in subsequent pregnancies; treated with corticosteroids; may result in still-birth or placental insufficiency

Myoma uteri is a benign tumor of the uterine muscle, occurring in some 40% to 50% of women, as determined by autopsy. These tumors may enlarge during the first 12 weeks of pregnancy, but are usually stable after that time. There is a slight chance of late abortion, premature birth, or fetal death in utero. Symptoms include pain in the right lower quadrant on the side of the myoma. Ultra sound confirms diagnosis and placement to determine if the myoma overlies the placenta. If they do overlap, there is a 75% complication rate and a two-fold increase in limb anomalies. Cesarean section may be indicated.

Ovarian tumors may occur in the first trimester, and 35% of women will spontaneously abort. This type of tumor is best removed between 16 to 18 weeks of gestation to decrease the chance of spontaneous abortion. Malignant ovarian tumors occur once in every 9000 to 25,000 deliveries.

One to 1.5 million women were exposed to diethylstilbestrol (DES) between 1940 and 1970. Exposure in utero has increased the incidence of spontaneous abortion in the first and second trimesters, related to incompetent cervix in the daughters of DES-exposed women. Other anomalies in the female reproductive tract have been linked to DES exposure as well. Thirty-five percent have intrauterine defects, irregular margins, T-shaped uteri, and narrow cavities; 35% have increased incidence of clear cell adenocarcinoma of the vagina; and 24% have cervical structural changes. There appears to be a 20-fold increase in ectopic pregnancies.

DES is also believed responsible for 90% of Mullerian duct anomalies, including divided uteri, two uteri and two vaginas, and an unfused or bifurcated uterus in the vagina. Problems arise with pregnancy. Multiple anomalies of urinary and reproductive tract are the most complex: persistent cloacae when the urorectal septum fails to form, exstrophy of the bladder, and anomalies of the external genitalia due to defective closure of the abdominal wall.

Pelvic infections are yet another reproductive tract dysfunction that the practitioner needs to be aware of when treating patients. These diseases and their effects on the pregnancy are summarized in Table 5-6.

NEUROLOGIC DISEASES AND DISORDERS

Neurologic diseases and disorders may be divided into three major categories: disorders of the peripheral nervous system (Table 5-7), disorders of the central nervous system (Table 5-8), and neuromuscular diseases (Table 5-9). Obstetric palsies occur once in every 2600 deliveries. The nerves most commonly injured during delivery include: the obturator (L3-4), caused by compression by the fetal head antepartum or during delivery and resulting in weakness of the thigh abductors with minimal sensory deficit over the medial aspect of the thigh; the femoral (L2-3), caused by psoas muscle hemorrhage, pelvic trauma, or compression in the pelvic cavity and resulting in weakness of the quadriceps or psoas muscles with minimal sensory loss in the anteromedial thigh; and the peroneal nerve (L4-5), caused by compression by stirrups and resulting in weakness of toe extensors and foot aversion with sensory loss over the anterolateral leg and dorsal foot. In all of the above cases, physical therapy is indicated to increase strength and mobility and to instruct in the use of assistive devices or orthoses.

In addition to injuries during delivery, peripheral nerves may become irritated during pregnancy from mechanical disturbance or compression from increased fluid volume.

Some studies show a three-fold increase during pregnancy of Bell's palsy, although this disorder is not associated with parity or preeclampsia. Pregnancy does not alter the prognosis for multiple sclerosis patients, but the frequency of exacerbation is most profoundly decreased in the third trimester.[1]

MUSCULOSKELETAL DISORDERS

Disorders of the musculoskeletal system are of major interest to physical therapists. Here, our skills are utilized most appropriately in diagnosis and treatment. The multiple musculoskeletal pains of pregnancy in the back, arms, and legs are so commonplace that concern and treatment may be overlooked. Simple, conservative, noninvasive measures minimize and eliminate these pains. Etiology is the focus of this chapter. Evaluation and treatment methods for these disorders are fully examined in Chapter 7.

Low back pain may be caused by sacroiliac pain, ruptured disk, symphysial separation, and dislocation of the coccyx. Muscular pain often occurs in the second and third trimester of pregnancy due to the increased weight of the uterus and the body's center of gravity shifting forward with resulting increased lumbar lordosis, a weakening of abdominal muscles, and relaxation of the sacroiliac ligaments. Excessive stress is placed on the facet joints and posterior ligaments of the lumbar spine. Pregnant women complain of pain in the lower lumbar area, usually aggravated by standing, walking, and lifting and relieved by recumbent or side-lying positions.[10] This lower lumbar pain occurs frequently and is the major cause of back pain in pregnancy. Relaxation of the symphysis pubis and dislocation of the coccyx may also be responsible for referred low back pain.

Table 5-6

Effects of Pelvic Infections on Pregnancy

Disease	Symptoms	Effects on Mother	Effects on Fetus
Syhphilis (bacterial; transmitted through sexual contact; 25,000 cases/yr. in U.S.)	Primary oral and anal cankers extra-genitally; secondary symptoms of skin rashes on palms, soles and perigenitally; general adenopathy and low-grade fever	Morbidity same as in non-pregnant women	Risk of infection 80% to 95% if mother untreated; 25% of fetal death in utero; 25% to 30% fetal death shortly after birth; syphilitic symptoms in 40% of survivors after third week of life
Gonorrhea (basterial; asymptomatic in 80%; affects urethra, cervix, fallopian tubes, Bartholin's gland)	Pain and tenderness in the pelvic region; cervical discharge; fever and painful urination	Affected in the last 20 wk of gestation of puerperium; increased chance of gonococcalarthritis; abortion possible from premature membrane rupture	Neonatal gonorrhea higher in utero and during delivery; infections, including conjunctivitis, otitis externa; vulvovaginitis
Chlamydia (increased incidence of intracellular bacteria	Same as for gonerrhea	Morbidity and mortality same as in non-pregnant women	Transplacental infection occurs; 40% to 50% will have inclusion conjunctivitis
Trichomonissis vaginitis (50% asymptomatic; venereally transmitted)	Itching, painful urination	Discomfort	Drugs to be avoided in early pregnancy
Candidissis vaginitis (causes more than 90% of vaginal yeast infections)	Itching, burning, red vulva; cottage cheese-type discharge; frothy, yellow-green discharge	Risk for developing candida vulvovaginitis; discomfort	Drug not to be used during the first 20 weeks
Gardnerella vaginitis (bacteria may be sexually transmitted)	Slight yellow-gray discharge	Discomfort	Drugs to be avoided in early pregnancy

Table 5-7

Effects of Peripheral Nerve Disorders on Pregnancy

Disease	Symptoms	Effects on Mother	Effects on Fetus
Carpal tunnel syndrome (occurs in 1%-10% of pregnancies; compression of the median nerve or retinaculum; symptoms appear in third trimester and may persist up to 12 wks post-partum)[9]	Pain and paresthe-sia along median nerve distribution; pain worse at night, weakness, thenar atrophy; sensory loss	Impaired hand strength requires decrease in activities requiring heavy use of hands; possible steroid injec-tions may require sur-gical decompression after pregnancy	None
Guillain-Barre syn-drome (acute polyra-diculoneuritis; rare during pregnancy; usually follows a viral illness; accom-panted by ascending paralysis in cranial nerves; tendon reflexes absent)	Paresthesias and muscle pain; all muscles possibly involved; maybe respiratory depres-sion	Onset during third tri-mester, may increase chance of premature labor; assistance possi-bly needed curing 2nd stage of labor due to weak-ness of the voluntary abdo-minal muscles; uterine musculature normal; phy-ical therapy treatment for rehabilitation imperative in recovery phase; recovery rate high with appropriate support and therapies	Possible risk of pre-mature labor during 3rd trimester
Radiculopathy (involves interverte-bral disk bulge, herniation, or nerve root lesion)	Severe back pain rad-iating into leg; pares-thesias, sensory loss, reflex impairment, weak distribution of nerve root lesion	Extreme discomfort; conservative treat-ment usually at-tempted first, involv-ing rest, physical therapy, and support	None
Sciatic neuritis (pain and tenderness over the scia-tic and femoral nerve distributions from relax-ation of the sacroiliac joints, subsequent rota-tions of the pelvis or trauma to the nerves)	Irritation along sciatic nerve and, occasionally, femo-ral nerve	Discomfort, difficulty in getting around; physical therapy need-ed to instruct on com-fort positions, orthoses use, activities of daily living	None
Polyneurites (related to thiamine deficiency from hyperemesis gravidarum; degener-ative nerve changes)	Diminished sensa-tion, paralysis, muscular atrophy; may involve single nerve or more	Discomfort depends on degree of disorder; decreased muscular coordination, strength; possibly fatal	Varies according to degree of disease
Myalgia paresthetica (co-mmon disorder in preg-nancy from compression of lateral femoral cuta-neous nerve at inguinal ligament or where ante-rior branch enters tensor fasciae latae; often appears in 3rd trimester)	Pain, numbness, and tingling in mid-die third of lateral thigh; no motor dysfunction; pain may be excerbated by standing or walking, relieved by sitting or supine	Discomfort, restric-tion in activities; benefits from in-struction in posture correction and modification of activities; resolves after delivery	None

Table 5-8

Effects of Central Nervous System Disorders on Pregnancy

Disease	Symptoms	Effects on Mother	Effects on Fetus
Aneurysm (rupture usually in the angle of bifurcation of vessels in the circle of Willis)	Sudden extreme headache, neck rigidity, nausea and vomiting, hemiplegia, seizures; usually occurs late second or third trimester; rare in delivery or in puerperium	Delivery usually augmented with epidural anesthesia with assisted second stage delivery; morbidity and mortality rate is 47%-70% in patients managed conservatively with bed rest compared to 8% mortality after neurosurgery; possible hemiplegia; physical therapy indicated	Fetal distress and premature labor if hypotension results during neurosurgical procedures
Arteriovenous matformations (AVM) (commonly located in the frontoparietal or temporoparietal region; more common in multiparas; may bleed in first or early second trimester	Severe headache, seizures present in 3096; focal neurological deficits in 20%; hydrocephalus possible	High morbidity and mortality for mother; Cesarean section at 38 wks offers protection; Valsalva manuever contraindicated; low forceps delivery with augmentation	Fetal complications as high as 49%
Intercerebral hemorrhage (primary form is rare in pregnancy; may occur from eclampsia, hypertension, or bleeding from AVM)	Acute onset of headache and alterations in consciousness; other symptoms dependent on location and size of hemorrhage; focal seizures possible	Possibility of hydration, steroid inbalance, ventilatory failure	Unknown
Cerebral artery occasions (preeclampsia possible predisposing factor; increased risk of carotid artery stroke in pregnancy)	Signs and symptoms dependent on location and magnitude of infarct; hemiplegia; hemi- sensory imbalance, visual defects, speech disturbances, headache; seizures	Vaginal delivery favored over Cesarean due to possibility of further infarct brought on by hypotension from hemorrhage or anesthesia; physical therapy crucial	Unknown
Cerebral venous thrombosis (can occur 1-4 wk after delivery; rare in pregnancy)	Headache usually precedes onset of seizures; recurrence of seizures, implying spreading of the thrombus; fever	Morbidity 30%-50%; survivors less disabled than those who have arterial stroke	No effect
Pituitary tumors (may increase during pregnancy; may prevent ovulation)	Decreasing vision and visual field deficits form pressure on optic chiasm	Surgery or radiotherapy indicated for rapidly failing vision; remission usually after delivery	None
Meningiomas (may increase in size during pregnancy; astrocytomas and	Signs and symptoms dependent on size and location of tumor; headaches, visual field	Anesthesia needed in labor to decrease intracranial pressure from Valsalva maneuver	Unknown

Table 5-8 continued

Effects of Central Nervous System Disorders on Pregnancy

Disease	Symptoms	Effects on Mother	Effects on Fetus
spinal angiomas)	defects; focal neurologic deficits possible and progressive		
Choriocarcinoma (occurs after molar pregnancy abortion or sometimes after normal pregnancy)	Usually symptoms appear and progress in the second half of pregnancies; decrease after delivery, but reappear in future pregnancies; metastases, seizures, intracerebral hemorrage, subdural hematoma, subarachnoid hemorrhage	Neurosurgery, if indicated carried out in any stage of pregnancy; therapeutic abortion option for malignant brain tumors; re gional anesthesia important to decrease the possibility of intracranial pressure from Valsalva maneuver	Unknown
Epilepsy (affects 0.3%-0.5% of pregnancies; increased seizure frequency in 37%, decreased in 13%)	Frequency of seizures returns to pregestational level after pregnancy	Risk of seizures if not taking medication or not being properly monitored; after birth, anticonvulsant drugs transported in breast milk, breastfeeding contraindicated	Defects of coagulation rates noted in newborns of mothers who take anticonvulsants; may have hemorrhages shortly after or during birth; congenital malformations in 4%-5% of children with mothers who do not take antiepileptic drugs and 6%-11% in children whose mothers do take antiepileptic drugs; most common malformations- mid line closure- orofacial clefts and cardiac septal defects; 2% increase of seizure activity in children born to mothers having seizure disorders
Migraine(recurrent vascular-type headaches that last hours to days; 30% of women with migraines asymptomatic during pregnancy; 50%,- fewer, or less severe migraines; 20%, worsen or fail to improve)	Usually throbbing, severe headache, may cause photophobia, vomiting, nausea, hemianopsia, or necrologic disturbance	Traditional migraine medicines not suggested during pregnancy; biofeedback and other noninvasive physical measures may be indicated	None
Pseudotremor carebri (benign, intracra-	Headaches; blurred or double vision in	Frequent ophthalmologic examinations	None

Table 5-8 continued
Effects of Central Nervous System Disorders on Pregnancy

Disease	Symptoms	Effects on Mother	Effects on Fetus
nial hypertension that mimics tumor; spontaneous recovery, may occur 12-20 wks gestation; symptoms stop in 1-2 wks but intracranial pressure remains elevated; remission after delivery; recurs in 5%-10% subsequent pregnancies	10% of patients; tinnitus, nausea vomiting, papillar edema, or swelling or optic nerve; present bilaterally, with weakness of the abducens nerve	necessary	
Wemicke's encephalopathy (caused by severe cases of hyperemesis gravidatum, leading to thiamine deficiency)	Ataxia, global confusion, horizontal and vertical nystagmus, ophthalomoplegia; Korsakoff's psychosis possible if untreated	Treatment with thiamine and other B vitamins and fluids; disease may be fatal	Possibly fatal if untreated in mother

Table 5-9
Effects of Neuromuscular Diseases on Pregnancy

Disease	Symptoms	Effects on Mother	Effects on Fetus
Chorea gravidarum (rare disease of pregnancy; form of Sydenham's chorea, may first appear during pregnancy, usually in 1st or 2nd trimester; goes into remission before delivery)	Nonrhythmic movemeets that are rapid, jerky, involuntary of extremities, face or trunk; usually aggra--vated by emotional stress; symptoms decrease during sleep	Maternal mortality greatly decreased since 1930s	Fetal mortality greatly decreased since 1930s
Myasthenia gravis (autoimmune disease characterized by high titers of IgG antibodies against acetylcholine receptors in striated muscle; remission in 30% during pregnancy; 30-40% have exacerbation, esp. in puerperium)	Weakness of muscles innervated by the cranial nerves; visual symptoms, difficulty with speech and swallowing	Uterine smooth muscle unaffected	12% to 20% of offspring develop neonatal myasthenia gravis, mild to severe muscle weakness; symptoms possible first day, persist 2-4 wks
Myotonic dystrophy (autosomal dominant inherited disease)	Progressive musculardystrophywith weakness in limbs, cataracts, myotonia, wasting of the muscles of the neck and limbs, baldness, testicular atrophy, mental retardation, arrhythmias	Spontaneous abortion, premature delivery; involved uterine muscle possibly unable to retain fetus	High rate of fetal loss; increased incidence of hydramnios; weakness; diplegia; foot deformity; arthrygrypolis multiplex congenital hypotonia; difficulty in swallowing, sucking, and breathing[2,3,4]

Cervical spine irritation may result from increased weight gain in the breast tissue, adding strain to the brachial plexus, and causing a change in posture in the neck and upper back positions. The shoulders become naturally rounded and the neck follows. The neck lordosis increases as the eyes look to the horizon. Over time, it may lead to irritation of the cervical nerve roots.

Leg cramps occur in 15% to 30% of all pregnant women usually in the second half of pregnancy,[5] and are painful, tetany-like contractions of the gastrocsoleus groups or occasionally of the thigh muscles. They occur most frequently when women are sleeping and may be strong enough to awaken them. The cramps may last from several seconds to several minutes. The etiology is unknown, but a deficit of calcium or magnesium has been proposed as the cause.

Stretching of the gastrocnemiussoleus group, along with the strengthening of the anterior tibialis, may lead to a reduction in these cramps.

Transient osteoporosis is a rare complication of pregnancy (100 cases described up until 1984). It usually does not develop until the last trimester. Vague pains in the pelvis, hip, thigh, and groin may be mistaken for pelvic instability or simple muscular fatigue. There may be unilateral pain in the hip and groin with radiation to the knee. If untreated, this disorder can precipitate complete stress fracture of the femoral neck. It has been proposed that this is a variant of Sudeck's atrophy or reflex sympathetic dystrophy. Symptoms appear gradually. Low back pain is rarely present, and the symptoms usually become so intense that the woman is unable to bear full weight. These women should avoid full weightbearing and use crutches to decrease the stress on the proximal femur. If a stress fracture does occur, surgical treatment may be necessary, and degenerative change in the hip joint may occur in the future. Hip and groin pain decrease significantly a few months after delivery. Gradually, the proximal femur reconstitutes itself. Four to 6 months after delivery, most women will be asymptomatic and x-rays will appear normal.

Osteogenesis imperfecta is an inherited disorder characterized by bone frailty, blue sclerae, and osteosclerotic deafness. The condition results from hypoplasia of the bone mesenchyme. Usually, patients with this condition have a complicated pregnancy. Previous fractures may have distorted the pelvis, making a vaginal delivery impossible. Weight gain during pregnancy may put additional stress on the pregnant woman's fragile bones, increasing the likelihood of fracture. Uterine labor contractions can be strong enough to cause fractures, if the fetus also has osteogenesis imperfects, making Cesarean section the preferred method of delivery.

There has been no reported increase in the degree of spinal curvature during pregnancy, despite the additional mechanical stresses and influence of relaxin. Deformities and curves may cause greater discomfort during pregnancy and labor, but there seems to be no increase in progression of the curve as compared to before pregnancy. A daily regimen of stretching and strengthening exercises is believed to be the key to avoiding discomfort in the low back area.

Spinal cord-injured patients are able to carry the fetus to term (see Chapter 6). The major problem is that these women are unable to sense the onset of labor. They can have normal contractions but will not feel them. Because of this, second stage may begin before they are able to contact their birth attendant, and they may deliver outside the hospital. During labor and delivery, these patients may suffer from autonomic hyperreflexia. The patient's autonomic nervous system may be stimulated and cause sudden cardiac irregularities, severe hypertension, anxiety, and sweating. These symptoms resolve spontaneously after delivery but should be closely monitored. To avoid this occurrence outside of the hospital or birth facility, due dates should be used to keep a close watch on pregnant women with spinal cord injuries.

Because automobile accidents occur with the same frequency whether a woman is pregnant or not, clients should be advised to wear seatbelts to prevent high-impact skeletal fractures. The lap belt should be worn against the iliac spine, below the enlarged uterus, with the chest strap going across the chest in the normal fashion. If fractures do occur, however, pregnant women have only the traditional treatment options. Surgical fixation may be chosen more often as the stabilization because of the added weight and physical stresses of pregnancy, and, because prolonged skeletal traction for femoral shaft fracture near a pregnant woman's due date would restrict a vaginal delivery. There is also the risk of thrombophlebitis during long periods of bed rest if skeletal traction is considered. If surgery is the answer, procedures are better tolerated by women in their second trimester. X-rays may be taken, if necessary, with careful shielding of the fetus.

Prior pelvic fractures may predispose a pregnant woman to cephalopelvic disproportion, especially as a result of central fracture, dislocation of the hip with residual medial protrusion of the acetabulum and femoral head, and Malgaigne-type fracture dislocations, (ilium on the injured side is displaced in a cephalad direction). Pelvimetry and clinical exam allow the physician to measure the birth canal and predict whether the fetal head will be able to pass. Many women are able to have a normal vaginal delivery following a previous pelvic fracture.

SELF-ASSESSMENT REVIEW

1. Gestational diabetes is defined as _____.
2. Name two reasons why there is an increased possibility of back pain in pregnancy: _____, _____.
3. Pregnant women should not wear seat belts as the belt may exert excessive pressure on the fetus during an accident, true or false?
4. _____ is a benign tumor consisting of muscle tissue.
5. Preeclampsia is characterized by _____, _____ and _____.
6. Eclampsia, if untreated, will lead to _____.
7. Hyperemesis gravidarum is marked by severe and protracted _____.
8. Asthma (acute or chronic) is a disease characterized by _____, _____, and _____.
9. With an acute viral upper respiratory infection (URI), treatment methods do not include _____.
10. A pregnant woman with a prior pelvic fracture may still be able to deliver _____.
11. Cervical spine irritation may occur in pregnancy due to _____, with resulting _____.

Answers

1. Diabetes that first appears during pregnancy. 2. Effects of hormones on pelvis and change in postural positions. 3. False. 4. Myoma. 5. Hypertension, proteinuria, and edema. 6. Seizures. 7. Vomiting. 8. Bronchospasm, increased airway secretions, hyperactive airways. 9. Antihistamines and cough suppressants. 10. Vaginally. 11. Added breast weight, change in upper back posture.

REFERENCES

1. Spellacy WN. *Management of High-Risk Pregnancy*. Baltimore, Md: University Park Press; 1976.

2. Danforth DN. *Obstetrics and Gynecology*. 5th ed. Philadelphia, Pa: JB Lippincott; 1986.

3. Wilson RJ, Carrington ER, Ledger WJ. *Obstetrics and Gynecology*. St. Louis, Mo: CV Mosby; 1983.

4. Niswander KR. *Manual of Obstetrics: Diagnosis and Therapy*. 3rd ed. Boston, Mass: Little, Brown & Co; 1987.

5. Queenan JT, Hubbens JC. *Protocols for High-Risk Pregnancies*. 2nd ed. Oradell, NJ: Medical Economics Books; 1987.

6. Dox T, Melloni BJ, Eisner GM. *Melloni's Illustrated Medical Dictionary*. Baltimore, Md: Williams & Wilkins; 1979.

7. Queenan JT. *Management of High-Risk Pregnancy*. 2nd ed. Oradell, NJ: Medical Economics Books; 1985.

8. Bannister R. *Brain's Clinical Neurology*. 4th ed. London, England: Oxford University Press; 1973.

9. Howell JW, Roseman GF. The evaluation and treatment of carpal tunnel syndrome in pregnancy. *Bull Sect Obstet Gynecol*. 11(2):10-11,1987.

10. Heckman J. Managing musculoskeletal problems in pregnant patients. *Musculoskeletal Medicine*. 7:14-24,1984(Part 1),8:35-40,1984(Part 2).

6

Physical Therapy Care in High-Risk Pregnancies

A high-risk pregnancy has been identified as one in which maternal or fetal factors may adversely affect the outcome. A system to identify these high-risk factors has helped avoid adverse outcomes many times. Some factors, such as diabetes, grand multiparity, need for Rh immunization, preexisting heart conditions, chronic illness, disability or teen pregnancy can be identified before conception or in the first trimester, and management of these risk factors decreases the mortality and morbidity rates of mother and child. However, in other situations, risk factors may develop as the pregnancy advances, such as problems related to multiple fetuses, preeclampsia and hypertension.[1]

Prior to the late 1960s, the management of high-risk pregnancy was by trial and error. Pregnancies were often terminated by induction or Cesarean section at a gestational age that provided the fetus and mother the best chance to survive. To calculate this, an estimate was made, at each week of gestation, to determine the risk of intrauterine demise compared to the subsequent risk of neonatal death if termination was delayed. Danforth explains, for instance, that all pregnancies complicated by diabetes were interrupted at 37 weeks, the point in gestation at which cumulative risk of intrauterine and neonatal death was the lowest. He points out, however, that a great number of otherwise normally developing fetuses were delivered prior to their full maturation, proving beneficial in a reduction of fetal mortality in high-risk patients, but often causing prematurely-induced neonatal morbidity or mortality.[2] When Rh incompatibility was recognized in the 1960s as a risk factor for pregnancy, high-risk pregnancy clinics were developed. In addition to Rh-negative patients being screened for antibodies and being treated by specialists in Rh immunization, methods were devised to perform amniotic fluid analysis and intrauterine transfusions to remedy not only Rh incompatibility, but to analyze maternal and fetal status.

GENERAL CONSIDERATIONS FOR HIGH-RISK PREGNANCIES

There are many categories of pregnancies that fall within this broad definition of high-risk from an obstetrical viewpoint. Many patients have illnesses or disabilities that put them in the high- risk group at the onset, whereas others begin with a normal pregnancy only to suddenly develop risk factors that jeopardize the potential success of the pregnancy. Here we

Limitations of activity	Toileting	Positions for Eating
Strict bed rest-No upright activity	Bedpan for all toileting; bed bath	May prop self up on elbow or elevate head of bed 30-45° for eating
Strict bed rest in the Trendelenburg position-head of bed is 15° lower than foot of bed	No upright activity; bedpan for toileting; bed bath	May roll side to side; may prop on elbow for eating
Bed rest with bathroom privileges	May use toilet; shower in a shower chair.	Limited sitting.
Ad lib	No restrictions.	No restrictions.

Figure 6-1. *Adapted from Frahm J, Welsh RA. Physical therapy management of the high-risk antepartum patient.* Clinical Management. *1989, 9(4)15.*

will consider the physical therapy care of women whose pregnancies are labeled high-risk because of the pregnancy, the unique aspects of teen pregnancies and of women who are pregnant while disabled or coping with a chronic illness.

The obstetrician or midwife determines the level of activity for the high-risk patient and the physical therapist can assist the patient in ways to live within those restrictions. Bed rest is prescribed for 18.2% of high-risk pregnant women.[3] Reasons for bed rest include: preterm labor, premature rupture of membranes, amniotic fluid volume disturbances, placental abnormalities, pregnancy-induced hypertension, pulmonary edema, hyperemesis gravidarium, cardiomyopathy and multifetal pregnancy. Limitations of activity will prolong the pregnancy and decrease the risk to the mother and fetus. Classifications of bed rest are listed in Figure 6-1.[4]

THE ROLE OF PHYSICAL THERAPY IN HIGH-RISK PREGNANCIES

The physical therapist's role in treatment of the high-risk woman is to assess her within her resistrictions, prescribing specific exercises or positions while ensuring that she can complete her regime without danger to herself, the fetus or the pregnancy. The physical therapist can support her in managing the crisis, instruct her in stress-reduction techniques, offer understanding of the family dynamics around her restrictions, creatively outline strategies for coping and products for support. The high-risk client on restrictions will be in the hospital or at home. As insurance pays less for hospitalization, more high-risk women will have their care managed at home. Due to the overwhelming restriction that can be placed on the high-risk pregnant woman, the therapist can be a great adjunct to the woman's adjustment, comfort, and successful outcome.

The physical therapist evaluates the woman on bed rest with more restrictions/contraindications than a regular pregnant woman (see Chapter 7). Often the reason for best rest is to prevent premature labor. Uterine contractions can be set off by too much upright activity, rolling or coming to sitting with too much abdominal contraction. The evaluation has to be tailor-made for the woman and her restrictions. Often the information to be gathered will be obtained while she is in sidelying position.

Table 6-1

Circulation Exercises

Circulation Exercises–20 repetitions–3 sessions/day

Sidelying
- Breathing with abdomen relaxed
- Ankle pumps
- Foot Circles
- Tighten and relax knees
- Roll legs in and out
- Bend one knee at a time-hold-slide down
- One knee bent, slowly drop one knee to side-switch

Adapted from Frahm J, Welsh RA. Physical therapy management of the high-risk antepartum patient. Clinical Management. 1989,9(6)29-31.

The side effects of bed rest may quiet uterine activity but at the same time slow the blood flow to the extremities, which increases the risk of deep-vein thrombosis and muscle atrophy. Physical therapy goals for the mother on bed rest include:[5,6]
- Decrease risk of thrombosis
- Alleviate the physiological effects of bed rest
- Maintain uterine blood flow
- Improve posture
- Instruct in proper body mechanics
- Instruct in positions of comfort
- Instruct in stress reduction techniques
- Avoid increased intrabdominal pressure
- Avoid increased abdominal contractions
- Assess for supports
- Conserve energy
- Improve muscle tone
- Increase her sense of well-being
- Assist in referrals to other health care professionals (ie, nutritionist, psychologist)
- Promote post-partum recovery

A sample of exercises for the high-risk woman are in Table 6-1, 6-2, and 6-3.

Due to the many hours spent in bed, in a sidelying position, the use of supports is critical to the comfort of the high-risk mother. Left sidelying is the preferred position because of the location of the vena cava (see Figure 4-1 and 4-2 and discussion of the vena cava syndrome). This would include two pillows between her knees maintaining the right hip knee and foot in line, and one pillow under the abdomen so that the spine is in alignment with support under her head so that the mother can read, watch TV or converse without straining her neck. Right sidelying is also a possible position for the mother with the same support pillows as in left sidelying (Figure 6-2).

Research on the psychosocial effects of bed rest has shown that high-risk women reported a significantly higher incidence of depression and anxiety than low-risk pregnant women. Fifty-one percent of high-risk women were clinically depressed, versus 24% of the low-risk women.[3] In a study of women who were confined to bed rest for pregnancy-induced hypertension, those who were hospitalized were found to have significantly higher mood disturbance, anxiety, depression, confusion and lack of vigor than those on bed rest at home.[3] This indicates that the location of the bed rest is the major source of stress. Additionally, high-risk women describe feelings of isolation, confinement, boredom, uncertainties, financial stress,

Table 6-2

Upper Body Exercises

Upper Body Exercises–5 repetitions–3 sessions/day

Sidelying
- Chin in and push back into pillow-no holding
- Look up look down
- Turn head right and left
- Circle shoulders forward
- Circle shoulders backward
- One arm stretch toward knees-switch
- Arm from one hip to opposite ear-switch
- Trace large letters in the air
- Open and close fists
- Bend and straighten elbows

Adapted from Frahm J, Welsh RA. Physical therapy management of the high-risk antepartum patient. Clinical Management. 1989,9(6)29-31.

Table 6-3

Mobility

Mobility in Bed
- Roll like a log, head stays on the pillow
- To sit- roll like a log, use arms to push up-back straight, legs over edge
- To use bedpan—keep head on the pillow, bend both knees and lift buttocks, slide bedpan under. Reverse the process to remove it.

Adapted from Frahm J, Welsh RA. Physical therapy management of the high-risk antepartum patient. Clinical Management. 1989,9(6)29-31.

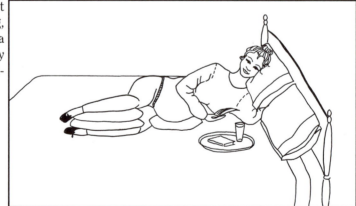

Figure 6-2. Bed rest position, left side lying, for a woman with a high-risk pregnancy whose activity is limited.

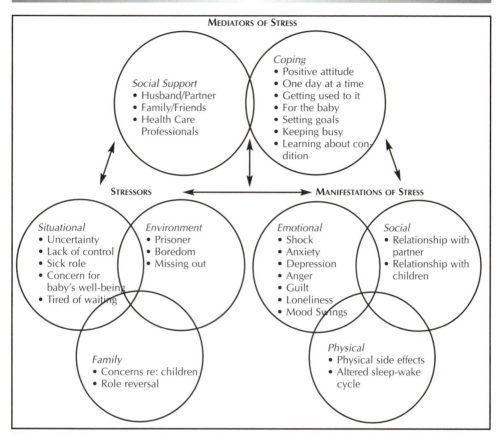

Figure 6-3. Stress process in pregnant woman assigned to bed rest. (Reprinted with permission from Gupton A, Heaman M, Ashcroft T. Bed rest from the perspective of the high-risk pregnant woman. JOGNN. 1997;26(4)426.

and worry about the well being of the baby and the possibility of a preterm birth. The high-risk mother passes through four stages on her way to successful mothering. First she must accept the high-risk status, then accept the uncertainty of the pregnancy, then adapt to the possibility of loss and finally prepare for motherhood.[7] See Figure 6-3, which best shows the interrelation of the stresses that a high-risk pregnant woman experiences.[8]

It may be necessary as in the case of a patient with multiples or with women who have a large rectus diastsis, that she wear a support brace under the abdomen so that she is able to roll with out using her abdominal muscles. This support will assist her in sensory clues and in decreasing the load on the uterus and reduce the possibility of initiating uterine contractions.

TEEN PREGNANCY

Approximately 1 million teenagers become pregnant in the United States each year, of which 51% end in live births, 35% end in induced abortion and 14% result in miscarriage or stillbirth.[9] Historically, in the United States, the highest teenage pregnancy rate was during the 1950s and 1960s before legalized abortion and the development of many forms of contraception. In 1973, when abortion was legalized, the birth rate for US females 15 to 19 years of age, sharply decreased until 1986, when the birth rates rose steadily until 1991.[9] However, there have been decreases every year since 1991.[10] As of 1996, the teenage birth rate was 54.7 live births per 1,000 and 90% of these 15 to 19 year olds describe their pregnancies as unintended.[9]

As of 1995, 56% of girls and 73% of boys have had sexual intercourse before the age of 18.[9] The average age of first intercourse is 17 for girls and 16 for boys and approximately 1/4 of youth report their first intercourse by age 15.[9] The predictors of sexual intercourse during the early adolescent years are; early pubertal development, history of sexual abuse, poverty, lack of attentive and nurturing parents, cultural and family patterns of early sexual experience, lack of school or career goals, poor school performance or dropping out of school.[9] Fifty to 60% of adolescents who become pregnant have a history of childhood sexual or physical abuse and 1/3 of adolescents who become parents are the product of a teenage pregnancy.[9] Delay in the initiation of sexual intercourse include; living with both parents, a stable family environment, regular attendance at places of worship, and increased family income.[9] Physical therapists working with this population must be alert to these findings and should act as a resource for education and referral, especially if physical or sexual abuse is suspected. (see Appendix for sources)

Teen pregnancies are complicated by maternal age, incomplete pelvis ossification (see Chapter 2), lack of prenatal care and inadequate weight gain. The risk for a healthy baby is complicated, as the pregnant teen is still growing herself. During adolescence, teenagers gain 50% of their adult weight, 50% of their skeletal mass and 20% of their adult height. Nutritional surveys show that the highest prevalence of nutritional deficiencies occur during adolescence.[11] Pregnant teens continue to grow but their growth rate is slower than that of their non-pregnant peers. The mother and fetus are competing with each other for nutrients and the growth of each may suffer.[11] Pregnant adolescents have more than twice the mortality rate of adult pregnant women. Infants born to girls younger than 15 years of age are twice as likely to weigh less than 2,500 grams and three times as likely to die within the neonatal period as compared to infants born to adult women.[11] Studies have confirmed the common belief that children of teens do not fare as well as do children born to adult mothers.[11] These children show an increased risk of behavioral disorders, developmental delay, difficulties in school, substance abuse, and an increased chance of becoming adolescent parents themselves.[11]

A usual weight gain of 20 to 30 lbs. is suggested to decrease the risk of a low birth weight baby for a mature woman. In teens, the weight gain should be more in order to decrease the risk of the child having developmental abnormalities. During the second and third trimesters, the pregnant teen requires an additional 300 calories a day. If she is under 15, she needs an additional 500 calories a day. If the pregnant adolescent is already overweight she should gain at least 25 lbs., and if she is underweight she needs to gain 40 lbs. over the course of the entire pregnancy.[11]

Psychosocial problems such as school interruption, limited job opportunities, separation from the baby's father, and repeat pregnancies do not seem to have a long term effect on the mothers. Research shows that two decades after giving birth, most teenage mothers are not on welfare and many have gone on to finish high school and have steady jobs.[11]

The therapist working with this population, as with an adult population, will likely be involved with early pregnancy classes, labor and delivery classes, treatment of muscusketal conditions and post-partum classes. (see Chapters 4, 7, 10, and 11). The physical therapist can assist the pregnant teen to understand the emotional, nutritional, physical, and nurturing changes and needs that she will be facing. Education is key to the healthy outcome of both mother and child. This high-risk client can do a great deal to prevent the possible high-risk outcomes that are possible for this age group. Through repeated exposures, the physical therapist may become a resource as someone she can trust and as a consequence the mother may be receptive to optimal health care and appropriate support.

PREGNANT WOMEN WITH DISABILITIES OR CHRONIC ILLNESS

Pregnant Women with Cardiac Diseases

About 1% of all pregnant women have organic heart disease, about half of it rheumatic in origin. Advances in treatment have decreased the incidence of valvular lesions and the total number of pregnancies affected by heart disease. However, the incidence of congenital malformations has risen and such malformations, plus cardiomyopathies and other cardiac diseases, are responsible for the other half of cardiac-related problems in pregnancy.[12] The New York Heart Association classification system for patients with cardiac disease also applies to pregnant women: Class I, asymptomatic; Class II, symptomatic with heavy exercise; Class III, symptomatic with light exercise; Class IV, symptomatic at rest. Patients of Class III and IV are believed to be at high-risk for complications during pregnancy.

For patients with cardiac disease, the goal of prenatal care is the detection and prevention of major complications of arrhythmia's, embolisms, and congestive failure. Prenatal visits are required more frequently and patients may need extra rest to reduce cardiac work. Diuretics and sodium restriction may be indicated if the patient has a tendency toward congestive heart failure, and patients may be given iron supplements to prevent any kind of anemia. Patients are hospitalized at the first sign of preeclampsia, increased blood pressure, or proteinuria. During labor and delivery, pain relief measures diminish the amount of cardiac work by 20%. Valsalva maneuvers are contraindicated, and the presenting part should descend to the pelvic floor by the force of uterine contractions alone. Forceps are often used to facilitate delivery. It is generally agreed that epidural anesthesia is contraindicated because of risk of hypotension and reduced venous return to the heart. Epidurals are also contraindicated in patients with hypertrophic cardiomyopthy. Cesarean section should only be done for obstetric emergency in patients with cardiac diseases.

Mitral stenosis is present in 90% of the pregnant patients with rheumatic heart disease. Overall morbidity from mitral stenosis is 1% during pregnancy. In severe cases, mortality rates have been as high as 15%. Pregnancy exacerbates mitral stenosis by causing physiologic tachycardia (the increased volume leads to increased pulmonary capillary blood volume) and by causing a need for increased cardiac output, with increased left atrial and pulmonary capillaries. There is also an increased incidence of atrial arrhythmia during pregnancy. A pregnant woman with mitral stenosis of long duration and pulmonary hypertension should avoid pregnancy.

Mitral insufficiency accounts for 6% of pregnant patients with rheumatic heart disease. Women tolerate the pregnancy well as long as there is not a severe mitral regurgitation or atrial fibrillation. Prophylactic antibiotics are indicated during labor and delivery.

Aortic stenosis accounts for 1% of pregnant patients with rheumatic heart disease. Women with mild aortic stenosis will tolerate pregnancy well, but severe aortic stenosis is a threat to maternal life. Mortality is as high as 17%. Venous return of the heart must be maintained by avoiding the supine position and by avoiding excessive blood loss at the time of delivery.

Another 2 to 3% of pregnant patients with rheumatic heart disease have aortic insufficiency. In pregnancy, the shorter diastole reduces the amount of blood regurgitating from the aorta into the left ventricle, and does not increase blood volume as previously believed.

Patent ductus arteriosus used to be a common congenital lesion but it is now a rare maternal complication. Most patients with this lesion tolerate pregnancy well. Shunt reversal is the major pregnancy-associated risk. If shunts totally correct the problem, patients with patent ductus arteriosus have no increased risk during pregnancy.

Tetralogy of Fallot is the most common form of cyanotic congenital heart disease. It is composed of pulmonary stenosis, ventricular septal defect, and dextroposition of the aorta with right ventricular hypertrophy. This tetralogy accounts for 5% of cardiac malformations present at birth. Patients with such a malformation can undergo corrective surgery and have successful pregnancies. In uncorrected cases, cyanosis during pregnancy can lead to intrauterine growth retardation and more complicated outcomes.

Atrial septal defect is the most common congenital lesion seen in pregnant women. Shunting of blood from the left to right atrium leads to an increased load on the right ventricle and increased pulmonary blood flow. Most of these women will demonstrate right ventricular hypertrophy; heart failure is uncommon in persons under 30. Patients with atrial septal defect tolerate pregnancy, but the major risk is shunt reversal during pregnancy, secondary to obstetrical hemorrhage or incorrect use of epidural or spinal anesthesia.

Pregnant patients who have undergone corrective surgery for ventricular septal defects are usually symptom-free, but larger defects may cause shunting of blood from the left to right ventricles with an increase in pulmonary blood flow. There is a significant risk of bacterial endocarditis, and again, the major risk is shunt reversal. However, most of these women do well in pregnancy.

Mitral valve prolapse is a common congenital heart defect that occurs in 6% to 10% of women of childbearing age. The mitral valve tends to prolapse during ventricular systole and leads to mitral regurgitation. A click-murmur syndrome is heard on auscultation. Although most women improve during pregnancy because of the increased blood volume and decreased peripheral vascular resistance, the American Heart Association still advises the use of antibiotics-prophylactically. Symptoms include palpitations, anxiety, fatigue, chest pain, and lightheadedness; but pregnancy is generally well-tolerated.

Cardiomyopathies and other diseases affecting the heart can be acute or chronic, some first diagnosed in pregnancy due to the extra load on the heart. It has been reported that there is an association between antepartum maternal cardiac events and premature labor.[13]

Physical therapy for the high-risk pregnant woman who has heart disease must take into consideration the limitations for exercise and heart rate. This client will need specific goal setting within the confines of her illness and the therapist must carefully coordinate her care with the cardiologist or cardiac surgeon. Exercises that can produce breath-holding or valsalva maneuvers are contraindicated because of the sharp changes that can take place within the valve and in blood pressure. Even if the woman has exercise-induced symptoms as a warning, these symptoms may not be able to predict the ability of the cardiorespiratory system to meet the increased cardiocirculatory demand of pregnancy. This is true in women with pulmonary hypertension, who may be putting their lives at risk if they exercise while pregnant.[14]

Pregnancy-Induced Hypertension

Pregnancy-induced hypertension (see also Chapter 5) is symptomatic of various disorders with a common factor of increased mean arterial pressure (MAP). For example, pregnancy-induced hypertension could mean a blood pressure of 140/90 mm Hg during the second half of pregnancy in a usually normotensive woman, a 30 mm Hg rise in systolic blood pressure, or a 15 mm Hg increase in diastolic pressure over baseline values. To establish the diagnosis, the examiner needs to find increased blood pressure changes on at least two occasions, 6 or more hours apart.

If proteinuria is present, the pregnancy-induced hypertension is reclassified as preeclampsia. There are five classifications of hypertensive disease in pregnancy: gestational hypertension, chronic hypertension, chronic hypertension with superimposed preeclampsia, preeclampsia, and eclampsia.

Gestational hypertension is defined as a rise in the MAP above 106 mm Hg, occurring after 20 weeks of pregnancy, without proteinuria. This hypertension disappears after delivery. Gestational hypertension may be hard to distinguish from chronic hypertension, if the patient is not seen for obstetrical care prior to the 20th week.

Both chronic hypertensive and normotensive women will have a decrease in blood pressure during the middle and early third trimesters of pregnancy. Therefore, if patients with unrecognized chronic hypertension are seen for the first time at the 24th week of pregnancy, they may appear normal; but early in the third trimester, the blood pressure may rise to an unrecognized hypertensive level, making it impossible to distinguish between pregnancy-induced hypertension and chronic hypertension. There are, however, clinical findings that can help determine if the disorder is chronic in nature: retinal hemorrhages and exudates; plasma urea nitrogen concentrates above 20 mg/dl; plasma creatinine concentration above 1 mg/dl; and the presence of renal disease, collagen vascular disease, diabetes mellitus, or other disorders that predispose a woman to chronic hypertension. Chronic hypertension is suspected if blood pressure is above 140/90 mm Hg, if hypertension is detected earlier than 20 weeks, if hypertension dates to prior to the pregnancy, and if hypertension is not accompanied by proteinuria.

Chronic hypertension with superimposed preeclampsia is characterized by hypertension starting before the 20th week of pregnancy with the addition of proteinuria and edema in the latter half of pregnancy. This disorder occurs in 13% of treated chronic hypertensive patients.

Preeclampsia denotes hypertension, proteinuria, and edema, usually occurring in primigravidas after the 20th week of pregnancy. Degrees are mild, moderate, and severe. In the mild form, MAP is less than 106 mm Hg (140/90 mm Hg), diastolic pressure increases more than 15 mm Hg on 2 occasions 6 hours apart with patient at bed rest, and there is proteinuria or edema. In moderate preeclampsia, MAP is 106 mm Hg (140/90 mm Hg) to 126 mm Hg (160/110 mm Hg, or a rise of blood pressure greater than 30 mm Hg systolic or greater than 15 mm Hg diastolic). Increased proteinuria and edema of the lower extremities may also be noted. In severe preeclampsia, MAP is greater than 126 mm Hg (160/110 mm Hg) on two occasions 6 hours apart with the patient at bed rest, proteinuria is greater than 5 gm/24 hours, and the patient complains of headaches and blurred vision. There may also be right upper quadrant pain, oliguria, pulmonary edema, and edema of the face, hands, and lower extremities.[15]

Eclampsia is characterized by generalized seizure activity with hypertension and proteinuria in the pregnant patient. This seizure occurs within the first 24 hours post-partum. No one is able to accurately predict which patients with pregnancy-induced hypertension will develop eclampsia. Its etiology is unknown, although three major theories of causes exist: increased vasoconstrictor tone, abnormal prostaglandin action, and immunological factors. It is likely that the disease process begins with vasospasm and then leads to a reduced blood flow to the uterus and other organs. Reduced intravascular volume and, ultimately, hypertension develop.

The risks to the fetus result from decreased perfusion of the choriodecidual space. This process starts before the clinical manifestations and results in growth retardation. Severe growth retardation ranges from 5% to 13%; with birth weight less than 10th percentile. The risk for premature delivery is 13% to 54% depending on the gestational age when the preeclampsia develops. The overall risk to the fetus depends on the severity of the preeclampsia and how early it starts in gestation.[16]

Women who have preexisting risk factors such as hypertension, renal disease, obesity, diabetes and collagen vascular disease who develop preeclampsia in their first pregnancy have an increased likelihood of doing so in subsequent pregnancies.[16]

Bed rest is the usual prescription for hypertensive disorders with the caveat that the patient must be left side lying so there is no compromise to the venous return due to compression of the inferior vena cava by the enlarged uterus.

Pregnant Women with Respiratory Disease

Asthma is a chronic obstructive lung disease characterized by hyperreactive airways, increased airway secretion, and bronchospasm. Between attacks, the resultant obstruction may be partially or completely reversible with improvement in symptoms. There are two types: extrinsic asthma, an allergic phenomenon; and intrinsic, a nonspecific type. Symptoms are brought about by respiratory infections, emotional stress, exercise, and cold air. There are patients who have mixed types of asthma with both extrinsic and intrinsic characteristics. Asthma is believed to be a disorder of the autonomic nervous system's control of the respiratory system, and affects 1 to 4% of all gestations.[17] Typically, the disease is variable and unpredictable. There seems to be a slight tendency for the disease to improve in the first trimester and get slightly worse in the last trimester.

Women with severe asthma have about an 80% exacerbation rate during the current and subsequent pregnancies. Symptoms include shortness of breath, wheezing, and coughing. On auscultation of the chest, there is an increased expiratory phase and generalized wheezing. Most studies indicate an increased neonatal mortality among infants born to asthmatics; death results from increased frequency of low birth weight, premature labor, and episodes of severe attacks, inducing marked maternal hypoxemia with fetal hypoxia. Treatment during pregnancy is the same as in a non-pregnant state. Bronchodilators or corticosteroids are given for brief episodes. Typical blood gases reveal respiratory alkalosis due to hyperventilation with reduced PCO_2 and elevated arterial pH. This maternal alkalosis brings about a marked reduction in uterine blood flow and hypoxia. In one study, 5.7% of infants with asthmatic mothers developed asthma within the first year of life. Another 18.4% developed severe respiratory disease during the same period. In severe asthmatics, 28% of the pregnancies were associated with perinatal death, 35% produced low birth weight babies, and 12.5% of the infants were neurologically abnormal at one year of age.[18] Asthmatic women might be at an increased risk for hemorrhage during pregnancy and in the post-partum period.[17]

Cystic fibrosis is a congenital, hereditary disease marked by dysfunction of any of the exocrine glands, resulting in an increase in sodium and potassium concentration of sweat and an overproduction of mucus. Women with cystic fibrosis, who conceive and carry pregnancy to term, are generally older than non-pregnant cystic fibrosis patients. Perinatal mortality is 11%, and premature labor occurs in 27%, both 4 times greater than normal. Symptoms include increased sodium and potassium production, sweating, cough of a chronic nature, and production of increased mucus. Cyanosis, dyspnea, and a vital capacity of less than 50% of predicted values are poor prognostic signs. Corpulmonale and pulmonary hypertension in cystic fibrosis patients are absolute contraindications for pregnancy. These patients are more susceptible to bacteriologic pulmonary infection and almost always require chest physical therapy throughout their lives.

Pregnant Women with Arthritis

Pregnancy has a beneficial effect on symptoms of rheumatoid arthritis. Two thirds of pregnant women with rheumatoid arthritis notice a substantial decrease in pain, swelling, and redness, usually immediately after conception, and continuing until 6 weeks post-partum, 5% of patients report that the arthritis is worse with pregnancy.[19] Elevated maternal cortisone levels and a generalized suppression of immune response in pregnancy may account for this remission. There is a mild anemia that accompanies this disease that may be exacerbated by the physiologic anemia of pregnancy. The rheumatoid factor does not cross the placenta, and there are no specific effects of the disease on the fetus.

Physical therapy and occupational therapy measures are helpful in evaluating function, strength, and range of motion of the involved joints. Supportive measures would be splinting, strengthening, and restoration of function coupled with protected daily living activities post-partum. Additional supports may be necessary in the post-partum period to avoid overse hand injuries that can occur in care of the infant. If there is deformity of the pelvis or hips, vaginal delivery may be impaired or impossible. The physical therapist can problem-solve positions for delivery to assist the mother and her health care practitioner explore options for delivery. Consideration must also be given to increased maternal activities involving care of the infant and protection of her joints, strength and energy level.

Systemic lupus erythematosus occurs in 1 of every 1660 pregnancies. Clinically, arthralgia or arthritis affects 90% of women with the disease; dermatologic involvement, 70% to 80%; renal disease, 46%; hematologic abnormalities, 50%; and, cardiovascular disease, 30% to 50%. The disease is characterized by periods of exacerbation and remission. One center reported that although lupus does flare up in pregnancy, most of the symptoms are mild to moderate in intensity and easily treated. They also reported an over 85% pregnancy success rate.[20] If the symptoms have been quiescent for more than one year, the pregnancy has a better outcome. This population has a potential to develop deep vein thrombosis. Aspirin given during pregnancy and heprin after delivery greatly decreases these chances. Maternal complications involve the cardiac and renal systems, spontaneous abortion, premature labor, fetal growth retardation, and stillbirths. Stillbirths are common in these patients. Pregnancy should be considered only after the patient has a complete understanding of the severity of the disease. There should be a coordinated approach between the obstetrician, rheumatologist, and patient.

Scleroderma can cause excessive fibrosis and vascular changes of the skin, gastrointestinal tract, heart, lung, and kidneys. There is a poor prognosis for the pregnancy if there is severe organ involvement. The course of pregnancy is dependent on the function of the kidneys. In a comparative study in 1990, 31% of women with the disease grew worse with pregnancy, and 11% reported a remission.[19] Labor is not affected by scleroderma, and healing from an episiotomy or Cesarean section is normal. There are no known effects on the newborn and no evidence that scleroderma is transmitted to the fetus. Corticosteroids can be of benefit, and treatment of the disease includes strengthening and range of motion exercises for involved joints and muscles. Complications usually appear in the third trimester and can cause premature birth because of maternal needs.[19]

Pregnant Women after Transplant

As transplantation and immunosuppressive regimes improve, women who have liver, kidney, and heart transplants are able to have successful pregnancies. In liver transplant recipients, pregnancies are complicated by hypertension, preeclampsia, anemia, and preterm birth.[22] Outcomes are usually excellent for mother and baby as long there are no other complicating factors such as high blood pressure, diabetes, serum creatinine above 160 umol/l, or if it is less than one year after the transplant.[23]

Pregnant Women with Multiple Sclerosis

Multiple sclerosis (MS) affects 1 in 1000 people in Western countries, mainly affecting childbearing women. The rate of relapse has been shown to decline during pregnancy, mainly in the third trimester. The rate of relapse increases during the first three months post-partum before it then returns to pre-pregnancy levels.[24] Physical therapists working with this population must consider the overall strength, fitness, balance, and coordination of pregnant women with MS and design exercise programs that will support their pregnancy and later mothering, while not exacerbating their neurologic symptoms. Extra care will need to be given to balance training and prevention of falls as the center of gravity changes in pregnancy and that along with MS symptoms can lead to injuries from falls.

Pregnant Women with Spinal Cord Injuries

Spinal cord-injured (SCI) patients are able to carry the fetus to term. Women with SCI are more likely to have complications of urinary tract infections, anemia, spasticity, decubitus ulcers, pulmonary dysfunction and autonomic hyperreflexia. The major problem is that these women are unable to sense the onset of labor. They can have normal contractions but will not feel them. Because of this, second stage may begin before they are able to contact their birth attendant, and they may deliver outside the hospital. During labor and delivery, these patients may suffer from autonomic hyperreflexia. The patient's autonomic nervous system may be stimulated and cause sudden cardiac irregularities, severe hypertension, anxiety, and sweating. These symptoms resolve spontaneously after delivery but should be closely monitored. To avoid this occurrence outside of the hospital or birth facility, due dates should be used to keep a close watch on a pregnant woman with spinal cord injuries so she does not deliver unattended.

The level of the cord injury determines the woman's perception of labor. Active labor to full dilation (first stage) is perceived by pain transmitted by the sympathetic fibers entering the spinal cord at T10-12 and L 1. Full cervical dilation to delivery (second stage) is mitigated by pain and pressure of the perineal tissues and sends signals along the prudendal nerve to the spinal cord at S2-4. Therefore, patients with lesions above T10 may not perceive labor. Those women with lesions above T5-T6 may require anesthesia to prevent autonomic hypereflexia. Women with low lumbar lesions may only perceive the first stage of labor.[25]

Physical therapists who are assisting pregnant women with spinal cord injuries can do much to prevent ulcers, train patients in exercises to reduce spasticity, instruct in adaptation to balance changes as their weight increases as well as offer education on childbirth education.

Women with chronic diseases and physical disabilities need careful assessment and individualized teaching. Principals and implications for perinatal education are:

• Pregnant women with disabilities and chronic illness have the same concerns as all pregnant women and therefore need the same basic information as able-bodied women.

• Women find more similarity among other women with the same degree of disability rather than the same type of disability.

• Women with disabilities and chronic illness are often unsure if the changes that they are experiencing are related to their pregnancy or disability. Therefore the physical therapist becomes a conduit for information on typical changes occurring in pregnancy and assists the pregnant woman to know if she is feeling the changes of pregnancy or her disability.[26]

SELF-ASSESSMENT REVIEW

1. Four reasons for bed rest for a high-risk pregnancy include: _____, _____, _____ and _____.

2. The best rest position for the high-risk patient on bed rest is _____.

3. During adolescence, teens gain____% of adult weight,____% of their skeletal mass and _____% of their adult height.

4. The pregnant teen under 15 years of age, needs at least_____ additional calories a day to best nutritionally support her pregnancy.

5. The five classifications of hypertensive disease in pregnancy are _____, _____, _____, _____ and _____.

6. Pregnant women with arthritis notice a _____ in their symptoms.

7. Active labor to full dilation (first stage) is perceived by pain transmitted by the _____.

8. Women find more similarity among other women with the same degree of disability rather than the same type of disability, true or false.

Answers

1. Pre-term labor, premature rupture of membranes, amniotic fluid volume disturbances, placental abnormalities, pregnancy-induced hypertension, pulmonary edema, cardiomyopathy and multifetal pregnancy. 2. Left sidelying with two pillows between her knees maintaining the right hip, knee and foot in line, and one pillow under the abdomen so that the spine is in alignment with support under her head. 3. Teenagers gain 50% of their adult weight, 50% of their skeletal mass and 20% of their adult height. 4. 500 calories a day. 5. (1) Gestational hypertension (2) chronic hypertension (3) chronic hypertension with superimposed preeclampsia (4) preeclampsia (5) eclampsia. 6. Decrease. 7. Sympathetic fibers entering the spinal cord at T 10-12 and L 1. 8. True.

REFERENCES

1. Spellacy WN. *Management for High-Risk Pregnancy.* Baltimore, Md: University Park Press; 1976.

2. Danforth DN. *Obstetrics and Gynecology.* 5th ed. Philadelphia, Pa: JB Lippincott; 1986.

3. Maloni JA. Bed rest and high-risk pregnancy. *Nursing Clinics of N A.* 1996;31(2)6:313-325.

4. Frahm J, Welsh RA. Physical therapy management of the high-risk antepartum patient. *Clin Manag.* 1989;9(4):14-18.

5. Frahm J, Davis Y, Welch A. Physical therapy management of the high-risk antepartum patient. *Clin Manag.* 1989;9(10):28-33.

6. Appel C. Exercise and the woman with a high-risk pregnancy. *IJCE.* 1997;12(3):40-41.

7. Sather SA, Zwelling E. A *View from the Other Side of the Bed.* 1998;27(3):322-328.

8. Gupton A, Heaman M, Ashcroft T. Bed rest from the perspective of the high-risk pregnant woman. *JOGNN.* 1997;26(4):423-430.

9. Committee on Adolescence: Adolescent pregnancy- current trends and issues: 1998. *Ped.* 1999;103(2):516-520.

10. Kayfmann RB, Spitz AM, Strauss LT, et al. The decline in US teen pregnancy rates, 1990-1995. *Ped* 1998;102(5):1141-1147.

11. Wahl R. Nutrition in the adolescent. *Ped Ann.* 1999;(2):107-111.

12. Queenan JT, Hubbens JC. *Protocols for High-Risk Pregnancies.* 2nd ed. Oradell, NJ: Medical Economics Books; 1987.

13. Siu SC, Sermer M, Harrison DA, et al. Risk and predictors for pregnancy-related complications in women with heart disease. *Circulation.* 1997;96(9):2789-2794.

14. Alahuhta S, Jouppila P. Pregnancy after cardiac surgery in patients with secondary pulmonary hypertension due to a ventricular septal defect. *Acta Obstet Gynecol Scand.* 1994;73:836-838.

15. Wilson RJ, Carrington ER, Ledger WJ. *Obstetrics and Gynecology.* St.Louis, Mo: CV Mosby; 1983.

16. Perloff D. Hypertension and pregnancy-related hypertension. *Cardiology Clinics.* 1998;16(1):79-101.

17. Alexander S, Dodds L, Armson BA. Perinatal outcomes in women with asthma during pregnancy. *Obstet Gynecol.* 1998;92(3):435-440.

18. Queenan JT. *Management of High-Risk Pregnancy.* 2nd ed. Oradell, NJ: Medical Economics Books; 1985.

19. Heyl W, Rath W. Rheumatische erkankungen in der schwangerschaft-probleme aus der sicht des gynakologen. *Weiterbildung.* 1995;55:M121-M124.

20. Petri M. Managing systemic lupus erythematosus in young women. *Women's Health Ortho ed.* 1998;1(5):33-39.

22. Poole J. Liver transplant and pregnancy. *J Perinat Neonat Nurs.* 1998;11(4):25-34.

23. Chevalier P, Poinsignon, Guillemain, Amrein C, Farge D. Grossesse apres greffes d'organe. *Presse Med.* 1996;25(34):1643-1648.

24. Confavreux C, Hutchinson M, Hours MM, et al. Rate of pregnancy-related relapse in multiple sclerosis. *N Engl J Med.* 1998;339(5),285-291.

25. Baker E, Cardenas D. Pregnancy in spinal cord injured women. *Arch Phys Med Rehabil.* 1996;77(5):501-507.

26. Rogers J. Perinatal education for women with physical disabilities. *AWHONNS.* 1993;4(1):141-146.

7

Evaluation and Treatment of Maternal Musculoskeletal Disorders

Certain restrictions apply when planning an evaluation and designing treatment programs for obstetric clients. These restrictions may inhibit standard physical therapy procedures; therefore, accommodation must be made.

CONTRAINDICATIONS

Avoid

1. Positions that involve abdominal compression in mid- to late pregnancy
2. Positions that maintain the supine position longer than 3 minutes after the fourth month of pregnancy
3. Positions that have the buttocks higher than the chest
4. Positions that strain the pelvic floor and abdominal muscles
5. Positions that encourage vigorous stretching of hip adductors
6. Positions that involve rapid, uncontrolled bouncing or swinging movements[1]
7. Positions of inversion
8. The use of deep heat modalities or electrical stimulation[2]

The best place to start is by taking the history. A questionnaire, filled out by the patient before the first meeting, gives the patient time to monitor transient aches and pains, as well as to reduce anxiety about the visit (Figure 7-1).

MUSCULOSKELETAL EVALUATION

Posture

During the course of pregnancy, the posture changes greatly due to possible hormonal action of relaxin on the ligaments, which allows more spinal movement in all directions; increased breast and uterine weight anteriorly; and forward and upward shift of the center of gravity.[3] The spine will adjust to the added weight and change in the center of gravity by increasing the cervical and lumbar curves. As the cervical curve increases, with the increased weight of the breasts, the shoulders round forward. Because the optical righting reflex acts to keep the eyes looking at a horizontal plane, muscles in the posterior neck must work harder to prevent the head from falling forward as the shoulders become rounded. In addition to these spinal changes, the pregnant woman will lean back slightly to allow the weight to shift backwards towards the heels, counteracting the forward influence of the

Name:_____Home phone: _____Business phone: _____
Address: _____
Date of birth:_____Occupation: _____
Responsibilities at home: _____
Level of activity: Sedentary:_____Light: _____Active: _____Very active: _____
Height : _____Weight: _____Due date: _____
Doctor: _____Number of pregnancies: Number of deliveries: _____
Problem: _____

Do you have any history of the same problem? How/when did it happen? _____
_____

Describe the pain: _____
_____

1) Where felt _____

2) When does it start in the day? _____

3) When does it stop? _____

4) What makes it better?_____

5) What makes it worse?_____

6) Do you sleep through the night without interruption from this pain? _____

7) What percentage of the waking day is it felt? _____

8) How many days a week is it felt? _____

9) What intensity is this pain on a scale from 0 to 10 (0 is none, 10 is the worst)? _____

10) Does this pain prevent you from doing activities of daily living, working, recreation or
     assuming sexual positions? _____

11) What self-help measures have you tried? Did they help? _____

Figure 7-1. Patient questionnaire.

enlarging uterus. As she shifts her weight back, and at the same time relaxes her abdominal muscles, she will tend to walk with a waddling gait and may develop back pain (Figure 7-2). The key features of this kyphotic, lordotic posture, as described by Kendall, are weakness in the anterior neck, upper back, and lower abdominal muscles; and often shortness in the hip flexors, pectorals, and low back muscles.

When the body is in good alignment, with the buttocks tucked under, the abdominal muscles support the fundus anteriorly, and the uterine weight rests in the pelvic basin.[4] A plumb line, on side view, will bisect the lobe of the ear, the shoulder joint, the bodies of the lumbar vertebrae, the trunk, the greater trochanter of the femur (anteriorly to the midline of the knee), and slightly through the anterior malleolus at the calcaneocuboid joint[5] (Figure 7-3). Muscle shortness or weakness may cause faulty alignment, and give rise to stretch weakness or adaptive shortening of muscles.[5]

Stretch weakness, from muscles assuming and remaining in a lengthened position beyond neutral, may occur in women with the typical pregnant posture, particularly in the middle and lower trapezius muscle groups, as well as in the lower abdominals. Adaptive shortening of the muscle occurs when it is unable to lengthen in response to relaxation of the antagonist group or to the force of gravity. Consequently, without an outside pull or force, the shortened muscles tend to remain in a shortened position and this is associated with muscle strength.[5] Shortened muscles in the pregnant woman tend to include the low back, anterior shoulder group, and hip flexors. Not all postures will be typical, however, and careful

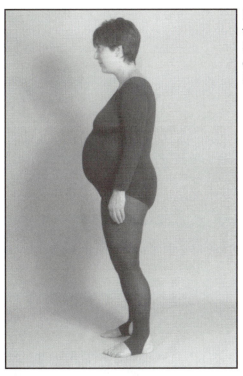

Figure 7-2. Incorrect posture. (Reprinted with permission from O'Connor LJ, Gourley Stephenson RJ. *Obstetric and Gynecologic Care in Physical Therapy.* Thorofare, NJ: SLACK Incorporated; 1990.)

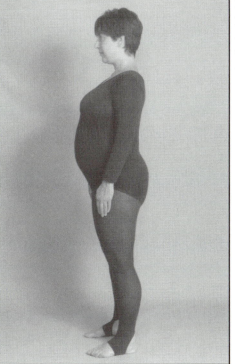

Figure 7-3. Correct posture. (Reprinted with permission from O'Connor LJ, Gourley Stephenson RJ. *Obstetric and Gynecologic Care in Physical Therapy.* Thorofare, NJ: SLACK Incorporated; 1990.)

observation of the body will pick up any deviations from the ideal posture. A Polaroid picture taken from a lateral and anterior point of view may help in treatment design. An extra picture, taken with a plumb line superimposed on it, may help the patient understand her posture deviations and actively change them. A program can then be designed to correct stretch weakness and adaptive shortening. Postural defects may be further intensified during recreation, work, and home activities, and attention should be given to an assessment of posture in these positions as well.

Many of the same excellent evaluation tests used on other patients are indicated for pregnant women: observation; palpation; range of motion; and strength, neurologic, coordination, gait, activities of daily living, and functional assessment. Methods of standard evaluations and treatments not included here can be found in *Physical Examination of the Spine and Extremities* by Hoppenfeld and *Evaluation, Treatment and Prevention of Musculoskeletal Disorders* by Saunders, both excellent references. A musculoskeletal evaluation is included here, however, to highlight a way to evaluate the obstetric client by limiting the number of changes in body position, while at the same time observing pregnancy-related restrictions (Figure 7-4).

Muscle Testing

Because the pregnant woman should avoid the supine position for lengthy periods, as well as avoid positions that compress the abdomen in late pregnancy, some changes are necessary for manual muscle testing positions. Although many of these adaptations do not test the specific muscle in the ideal position against gravity, the therapist is nevertheless able to check for functional strength and substitution. Technically, muscles tested in a nongravity position should not attain a grade better than 2+ out of 5+, but it is believed the experienced practitioner can palpate the strength through these adapted positions. Examination notes should indicate these modifications. An isokinetic testing device may be used as an alternative for some of the positions.

Suggested alternate positions include stabilizing against the wall, a corner, or a backless stationary stool. If frequent positions requiring the supine position are needed, the therapist can direct the patient to turn to left side lying between tests with support at the waist and under the abdomen. However, the pregnant woman with musculoskeletal pain is often extremely uncomfortable during evaluation, and testing positions should be organized in the therapist's mind before asking the patient to make unnecessary position changes.

Suggested adaptations required for Kendall's standard muscle testing positions include the following:

Adapted Manual Muscle Test Positions

- Neck extensors: sitting
- Trapezius: standing facing the wall, arm not being tested is bent at the elbow, forehead resting on it
- Teres major: sitting, therapist stabilizes the anterior shoulder
- Pronator teres and pronator quadratus, supinator and biceps: sitting, arm fixed against a wall
- Triceps: back lying with arm horizontally adducted
- Medial and lateral rotators: sitting, therapist stabilizes shoulder and elbow at 90 degrees of flexion
- Latissimus dorsi: sitting with arm in extension or side lying with the trunk stabilized

1. Standing   Name: _____ Date: _____

   A. Gait

     Head _____

     Arms _____

     Trunk _____

     Pelvis _____

     Legs _____

     Feet _____

   B. Posture

Viewed from	Side	Front	Back
1. Head			
2. Shoulders			
3. Mid/upper back			
4. Abdomen			
5. Low back			
6. Pelvis/hips			
7. Knees			
8. Ankles			

   C. Spinal Movements

       Normal = N

       Pain = X

       Restricted = 1

       Hypermobile = 2

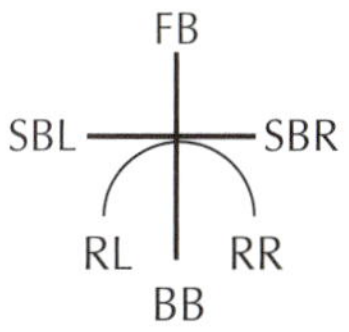

                  FB

           SBL —┼— SBR

              RL   RR

   D. Pelvis   BB

     Level of PSIS and sacral base-

     Active movement of SI joint (Forward bending- landmarks PSISs)

2. Sitting

   A. Neurologic-Strength

Upper Extremities		Lower Extremities	
Right	Left	Right	Left
C1-2 Chin in _____		L-1, 2 Psoas _____	
C1-2 Chin up _____		L-3 Quads _____	
C-3 Lat neck _____		L-4 Tib ant _____	
C4 Shoulder shrug _____		L-5 Ext. H.L. _____	
C-5 Biceps _____		S-1 Flex H.L. _____	
C-6 Wrist extensors _____		S-2 Hams _____	
C-7 Triceps _____			
C-8 Thumb extensors _____		Reflexes	
T-1 Intrinsics _____		L-4 Knee _____	
		S-1 Ankle _____	
		UMN Babinski _____	

    Reflexes

    C-5, 6 Biceps _____

    C-5, 6 Bracorad _____

    C-7 Triceps _____

                    0 = absent

                    1 + diminished

                    2+ normal

                    3+ increased

                    4+ clonus

   B. Trunk motions

   C. Neck

     Range of motion

     Neck strength

     Neck palpation (vertebrae, muscles)

   D. Shoulder/arm:

     Muscle

     Tendon

Figure 7-4. Musculoskeletal evaluation of the obstetric client.

Thoracic outlet
Carpal tunnel
Sensation
3. Supine (No longer than 3 minutes before moving to left sidelying)
    A. Sacroiliac joints
        Anterior and posterior ligaments
        Anterior or posterior rotation of ilium or sacrum
    B. Hamstring length
    C. Rectus diastasis
    D. Hip flexor tightness
    E. Leg lengths
4. Side Lying (with support at waist, under abdomen, and between lenses)
    A. Sacroiliac (test other side as well)
    B. Spinal palpation (thoracic, low back, sacrum)
    C. Leg flexibility (other side as well)
        Hip flexors
        Quad length
        TFL length
Impression
Plan
Goals

Figure 7-4 continued. Musculoskeletal evaluation of the obstetric client. (Reprinted with permission from O'Connor LJ, Gourley RJ. *Obstetric and Gynecologic Care in Physical Therapy.* Thorofare, NJ: SLACK Incorporated; 1990.)

- Quadratus lumborum: standing against the wall stabilizing the leg and abducting the desired leg
- Abdominal muscles: test for rectus diastasis before doing an abdominal test in standard positions
- Back extensors: sitting on a fixed stool
- Hamstrings: standing with the pelvis in neutral position and one knee flexed; semitendinosus and semimembranosus: internal rotation of the flexed knee; biceps femoris: lateral rotation of the flexed knee
- Gluteus maximus: standing on one leg (can be stabilized in corner), therapist pushes the bent leg forward from the posterior position

The chart in Figure 7-5 will assist the therapist in organizing a treatment for the pregnant patient who may have multiple problems.

Additionally refer to Appendix C for suggestions on use of the *Guide to Physical Therapist Practice*[1] for OB/GYN practice in physical therapy. With the publication of the *Guide to Physical Therapist Practice*, clinicians may find it necessary to justify techniques, modalities selected, and number of visits when treating patients with OB/GYN disorders.

Part	Signs and Symptoms	Diagnosis	Treatment	Supports	Home Treatment
Head and neck					
Shoulder, arms and hands					
Abdomen					
Pelvis					
Low Back					
Legs					
Feet					
Other					

Figure 7-5. Summary of evaluation results and outline for treatment.

TREATMENT OF SELECTED MUSCULOSKELETAL CONDITIONS

Neck and Upper Back Strain

Due to changes in posture that often accompany pregnancy, pain may occur in the lateral aspects of the neck and upper back. The trapezius and upper and mid-cervical muscles may frequently be tender or in spasm with trigger points. Lateral flexion and rotation movements are restricted, and neck flexion and extension may be painful at the end of the range. In addition to standard treatment for neck muscle strain,[17] exercises should include pectoralis stretch, head retraction and swallow, upper back stretch at the wall, self-massage, side bending mobilization using the lateral aspect of the hand as a fulcrum, stretching the levator scapulae, and deep cervical muscle isometrics.[11] Posture correction, relaxation exercises, and upper back supports may also be important (Figure 7-6).

Temporomandibular Joint

The temporomandibular joint may be affected in pregnancy, because the laxity of ligaments may allow hypermobility. Usually this is due to an underlying condition that is brought about with the added laxity, allowing the joint to ride over the displaced disk. Problems may also develop from excessive facial muscle tension thrusting the jaw forward during pushing in delivery.[18]

Figure 7-6. Mid back support. From The Saunders Group. (See appendix.) (Reprinted with permission from O'Connor LJ, Gourley Stephenson RJ. *Obstetric and Gynecologic Care in Physical Therapy.* Thorofare, NJ: SLACK Incorporated; 1990.)

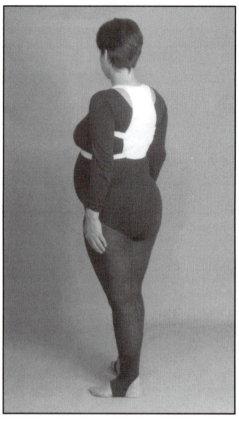

By minimizing the stress on the jaw, the problem may not arise. The patient usually experiences pain in the face and neck muscles and on opening the mouth, and clicking may be felt in the affected joint. There is usually tenderness over the joint and in the upper cervical facial muscles (masseter, temporalis, and pterygoid). Treatment consists of applying heat to the joint followed by mobilization techniques for anterior and lateral glide, plus the Rocobado exercise series to reeducate muscle and jaw movements.

Thoracic Outlet

Symptoms of thoracic outlet syndrome may occur secondary to head and neck postural changes, causing compression of the neurovascular bundle at the cervicothoracic dorsal outlet. This bundle is comprised of brachial plexus nerve fibers and the subclavian artery and vein, usually involving C8 to T1 nerve roots. In the case of *scalenus anticus* and *cervical rib syndrome*, Adson's test is positive. The patient is instructed to take a deep breath, extending the neck fully, turning the chin towards the side being examined. In a positive test, the radial pulse disappears, and pain and other symptoms are reproduced. Treatment consists of exercises to stretch the upper trapezius and levator scapular muscles to bring the shoulder complex upward and backward.[12] If *costoclavicular syndrome* exists, the subclavian artery and brachial plexus are entrapped as they pass between the clavicle and the first rib. To test for this syndrome, the patient takes a deep breath and holds it while retracting and depressing the shoulder. Again, the radial pulse disappears, and symptoms are reproduced in the arm.[12]

Treatment consists of mobilization of the clavicle at the sternoclavicular joint and posture exercises to elevate the shoulder girdle. In the *hyperabduction syndrome*, the subclavian vessel and brachial plexus are entrapped beneath the pectoralis minor tendon and under the coracoid process. To test for this syndrome, the arm is held in a hyperabducted position with the radial pulse diminished and symptoms reproduced. Patients usually complain of pain after sleeping with the arm overhead. Treatment consists of posture correction and stretching of the pectoral muscles.

Carpal Tunnel Syndrome

Carpal tunnel syndrome arises from compression of the median nerve at the wrist usually due to and increase in swelling (see Chapter 5, and Table 3-7). Women will complain of pain over the median nerve distribution, paresthesia, numbness, clumsiness, and atrophy in the hands. Nocturnal awakening may occur secondary to pain or paresthesia. Phalen's test will be positive, (ie, signs will be reproduced by holding wrist firmly in flexion for a minute).[11,12,19] Tinel's sign will also be positive (percussion over the median nerve at the wrist will reproduce tingling in the cutaneous distribution of the median nerve).[11,12,19] Treatment consists of immobilization at the wrist in neutral position with the fingers free to permit activities of daily living.[19] Sometimes only nighttime wearing is required, or alternate splint-wearing time may be needed if both hands are involved. Usually, symptoms resolve post-partum; however, mothers who breast-feed tend to have a longer recovery.[19]

De Quervain's Disease

De Quervain's Disease is tenosynovitis or inflammation of the abductor pollicis longus and extensor pollicus brevis tendon sheaths. This may happen in pregnancy but most often in the post-partum period. This is caused by repeated lifting usually of the infant which results in a repetitive injury. Treatment post-partum is assisted by phonophoresis or iontophoresis, bracing that restrains the thumb, retraining and rest. As the client heals strengthening and stretching are emphasized.

Diastasis Recti Abdominis

Separation of the rectus abdominis muscles occurs at the uniting linea alba. If not during pregnancy, a rectus diastasis can instead develop during the second stage of labor, particularly if there is excessive breath holding during pushing. To check for a diastasis, the woman lies on her back with her knees bent. She raises her head and shoulders until her neck is about 8 inches from the floor. The chin should be tucked and the arms stretched out front. The therapist should check for the presence of a bulge in the central abdominal area, which is evident when the muscles have parted. If so, the numbers of fingers that can be inserted horizontally into the gap at the level of the umbilicus, 2 inches above and 2 inches below, defines the amount of separation between the taut rectus muscles. Any separation of more than two fingers wide constitutes a restriction on any type of curl-up or leg lowering exercises. Trunk rotational exercises should be avoided until there is no separation. Use abdominal support (see Figures 7-20 and 7-21 later in this chapter).

Costal Rib Pain

Costal rib pain is due to normal 10 to 15 cm flaring of ribs usually in last trimester because the fundus is at maximum height. Pain results from stretch on abdominal muscles at their insertion on the ribs. Treatment can decrease the pain through muscle energy techniques to ribs, upper back strengthening exercises, posture correction and self posterior stretches.

Sacroiliac Joint Pain

During pregnancy, the sacroiliac (SI) joints may become a source of pain. This may occur within the first 3 months, possibly related to the circulation of relaxin and the major physiologic and musculoskeletal changes occurring in the woman's body. In addition, some women find that the SI joint becomes symptomatic premenstrually, as well as, post-partum. Joint movement at the SI has been well-documented.[6-13]

The action of the major muscles around the SI joint will greatly influence rotation. Trained and experienced therapists can use mobilization and muscle energy techniques to correct anterior and posterior innominate rotation. Therapists with little training in manual therapy methods should not attempt these techniques on pregnant women, because considerable finesse is required to avoid injuring ligamentous and connective tissue support as well as the joints of the pelvic ring. Indeed, there are many experienced obstetric physical therapists who will not apply these techniques for fear of further injuring the client. Careful assessment of ligamentous stability should be made before carrying out even the most gentle mobilization.

Evaluation of the SI joint includes ligament testing, sacral movement, leg lengths, palpation, and pelvic alignment. After the malposition of the innominate is determined, treatment may involve application of local heat, rest, muscle correction, mobilization, fitting of an orthosis, and a home program to remedy dysfunction. An SI support belt (Figures 7-7a and b) can be applied to assist in maintaining a corrected position. Pregnant clients should also be instructed to avoid widely abducted legs when walking on uneven terrain, frog kicks (as in swimming), certain sexual positions, climbing stairs more than one step at a time, and swinging one leg out of bed when getting up.

Posterior Innominate

The patient with posterior innominate usually demonstrates unilateral buttock pain and well localized pain over the PSIS on the involved side. Some or all of the following signs will be positive: in standing, the PSIS is lower on the side of the involvement with the same side iliac crest and the ASIS higher; in supine, the ASIS on the involved side is higher than on the noninvolved side; in supine-to-sit test, the leg on the involved side will appear longer (patient may need support to sit up and lay back); on side or back bending, pain often increases toward involved side; on forward bending, the PSIS on the involved side will elevate higher than on the noninvolved side; and, on spring test over the sacrum, results will be positive.

The patient with posterior innominate requires an anterior torsion force for correction. For self-correction of a posterior innominate, the iliopsoas is contracted. If the physical therapist feels a need to assist correction, he or she must use extreme caution in attempting to correct the rotation. The practitioner should be extremely familiar with applying these techniques to a variety of non-pregnant women before attempting to work with an unstable pelvis under a lax situation. It is important to know that the symphysis pubis can separate in pregnancy and actually rupture with excessive force.

Figures 7-7a and b. Sacroiliac belt, IEM Orthopedics (see Appendix). (Reprinted with permission from O'Connor LJ, Gourley Stephenson RJ. *Obstetric and Gynecologic Care in Physical Therapy.* Thorofare, NJ: SLACK Incorporated; 1990.)

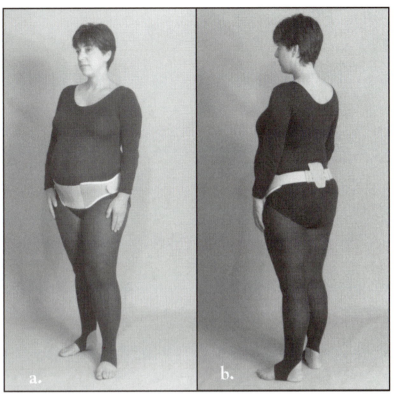

Muscular Correction of Posterior Innominate

Patient: Lies supine with involved leg over side of table.

Therapist: Stands on patient's affected side, stabilizing pelvis on opposite side of body; places one hand on the distal thigh with the hip extended and the knee flexed.

Action: Therapist asks patient to flex the hip against therapist's resistance isometrically and hold for 5 seconds. As the patient relaxes, the therapist gently pushes the hip further into extension by taking up the slack, monitoring the ASIS so that it does not move. Repeats 3 times (reexamines after procedure). Repeats, if necessary (Figure 7-8).

Mobilization for the posterior innominate can be done with the pregnant patient by modifying a technique usually done in prone position.

Mobilization Correction of Posterior Innominate

Patient: Lies on side with the affected side up and supported at the waist and under the abdomen The unaffected leg is flexed forward to stabilize the lumbar spine in flexion and to hold the ilium posteriorly.

Therapist: Stands behind the patient and grasps the thigh above the knee. The hip is abducted 15 to 20 degrees and extended.

Action: Therapist places opposite hand lateral to the PSIS over the ilium and gently thrusts anteriorly, laterally, and superiorly. Repeats 3 times and reexamines after procedure (Figure 7-9).

A home program for a patient with posterior innominate should include, in addition to practice in body mechanics and positioning, the following exercises:

Figure 7-8. Muscular correction of a left posterior innominate. (Reprinted with permission from O'Connor LJ, Gourley Stephenson RJ. *Obstetric and Gynecologic Care in Physical Therapy.* Thorofare, NJ: SLACK Incorporated; 1990.)

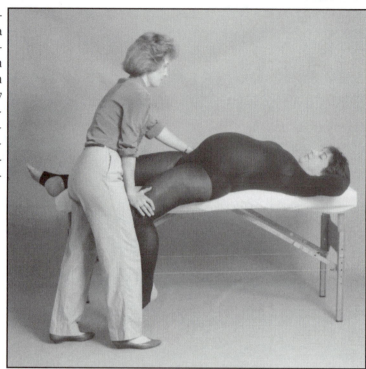

Figure 7-9. Mobilization correction of a left posterior innominate. (Reprinted with permission from O'Connor LJ, Gourley Stephenson RJ. *Obstetric and Gynecologic Care in Physical Therapy.* Thorofare, NJ: SLACK Incorporated; 1990.)

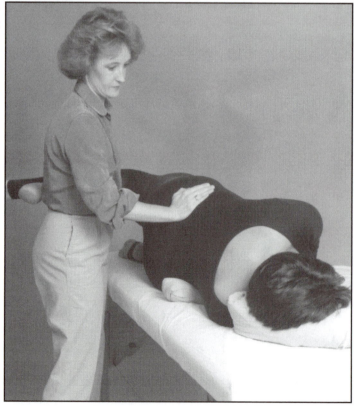

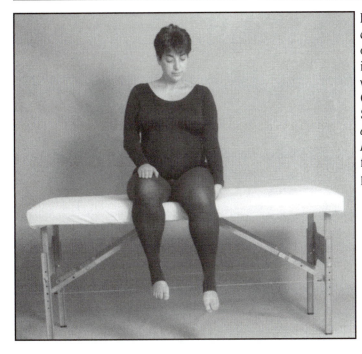

Figure 7-10. Home exercise sitting for correction of a right posterior innominate. (Reprinted with permission from O'Connor LJ, Gourley Stephenson RJ. *Obstetric and Gynecologic Care in Physical Therapy.* Thorofare, NJ: SLACK Incorporated; 1990.)

1. Push-pull isometric exercise for posterior innominate:

a. Sitting or supine, the patient's hand is on top of the involved thigh, which isometrically flexes against the hand. On the non-involved side, the opposite hand is pushing up from behind the thigh, while the hip attempts to extend posteriorly (Figure 7-10 and 7-11).

b. Gluteal stretch: Supine; on involved side, hip is slightly abducted, and patient brings hip and knee into flexion to stretch the buttock muscles (Figure 7-12).

Anterior Innominate

The patient with anterior innominate requires a posterior torsion force for correction. This patient usually has localized pain similar to that of the patient with posterior innominate, but less severe leg pain. Cervical pain may be associated with this disorder. Some or all of the following signs will be positive: in standing, the PSIS will be higher on the involved side; in supine, the ASIS will be lower on the involved side as compared with the noninvolved side; in the supine-to-sit test, the involved side will appear shorter; on forward bending, there will be pain on the involved side, and the PSIS on the involved side will be higher than on the noninvolved side.[13]

Muscular Correction of Anterior Innominate

For self-correction of an anterior innominate, the gluteus maximus is contracted. Other muscle correction may be attempted as follows:

Patient: Lies supine with hip and knee flexed on involved side.

Therapist: Stands on involved side; places most caudal hand under the patient's ischial tuberosity, other hand over ASIS; leans over, takes up slack, and moves patient's hip and knee into further flexion.

Action: Therapist asks patient to extend the hip isometrically against the therapist's chest, hold for 5 seconds, then relaxes, and therapist takes up further slack. Concurrently,

Figure 7-11. Home exercise supine for correction of a right posterior innominate. (Reprinted with permission from O'Connor LJ, Gourley Stephenson RJ. *Obstetric and Gynecologic Care in Physical Therapy.* Thorofare, NJ: SLACK Incorporated; 1990.)

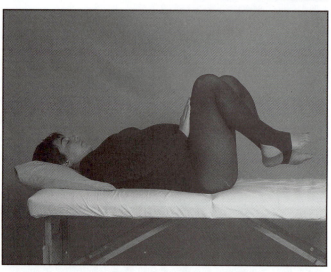

Figure 7-12. Gluteal stretch. Home exercise for correction of a right posterior innominate. (Reprinted with permission from O'Connor LJ, Gourley Stephenson RJ. *Obstetric and Gynecologic Care in Physical Therapy.* Thorofare, NJ: SLACK Incorporated; 1990.)

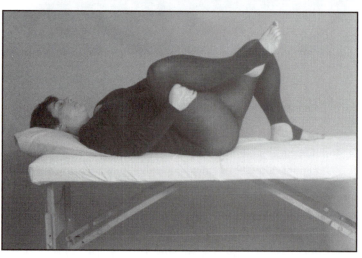

the posterior rotation is produced by downward pressure on the ASIS, as well as an upward pull on the ischial tuberosity (Figure 7-13). Repeats 3 times (reexamines after each).

Mobilization Correction of Anterior Innominate

Mobilization for anterior innominate correction can be performed in different ways. Special caution should be used if the technique is performed as in the first technique listed below:

Patient (supine position #1): lies supine with trunk laterally flexed away from involved side, places hands behind the head, fingers interlocking her fingers behind her head.

Contraindications: If a patient is uncomfortable and unable to tolerate the position, or if there is evidence of lumbar disc disease, try mobilization in a side-lying position or in supine position #2.

Therapist: Stands on the noninvolved side; places one hand on the involved ilium, preventing it from coming up; weaves other hand under the opposite elbow, through the space

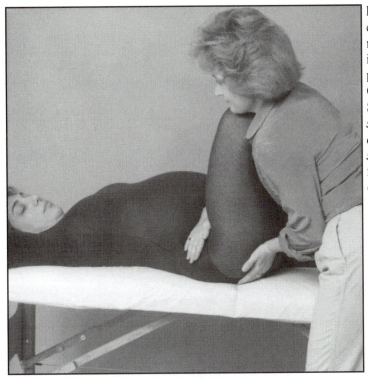

Figure 7-13. Muscular correction of a right anterior innominate. (Reprinted with permission from O'Connor LJ, Gourley Stephenson RJ. *Obstetric and Gynecologic Care in Physical Therapy.* Thorofare, NJ: SLACK Incorporated; 1990.)

made by both the patient's elbows and places flat palm on the treatment table. Position allows firm control of the upper torso with one hand, while the ilium is stabilized with the other.

Action: As therapist's arm weaves through the spaces created by the patient interlocking her fingers behind her head, patient rotates toward the therapist. (Because the opposite hand keeps the ilium on the table, rotation should be performed slowly to avoid pain. Some patients may be unable to rotate completely.) As therapist rotates the upper trunk, the opposite hand gently thrusts on the anterior superior iliac spine in a posterior lateral superior direction (Figure 7-14).

Patient (supine position #2): Lies supine with leg and knee flexed on involved side.

Therapist: Same position but turns to face patient's opposite shoulder.

Action: Therapist applies pressure posteriorly on the ASIS, while pulling forward on the ischial tuberosity with the opposite hand, and repeats in an oscillating fashion 6 to 8 times (reexamines after each- Figure 7-15).

Patient (sidelying): Lies on side with the affected side up, supports under the waist and abdomen, lower hip and knee are flexed; upper leg flexed and wrapped around therapist's waist.

Therapist: Faces patient so that patient's upper leg is ahead of the therapist who places caudal hand over ASIS and other hand over ischial tuberosity.

Action: Therapist gently thrusts both hands together into posterior rotation; repeats in an oscillating fashion 6 to 8 times and reexamines after each (see Figure 7-16).

A home program for the patient with anterior innominate should include, in addition to practice in body mechanics and positioning, the following exercises:

Figure 7-14. Mobilization correction supine #1 of a right anterior innominate. (Reprinted with permission from O'Connor LJ, Gourley Stephenson RJ. *Obstetric and Gynecologic Care in Physical Therapy.* Thorofare, NJ: SLACK Incorporated; 1990.)

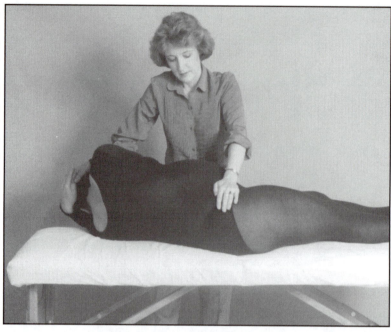

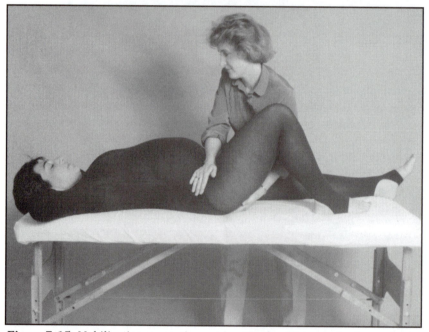

Figure 7-15. Mobilization correction supine #2 of a right anterior innominate. (Reprinted with permission from O'Connor LJ, Gourley Stephenson RJ. *Obstetric and Gynecologic Care in Physical Therapy.* Thorofare, NJ: SLACK Incorporated; 1990.)

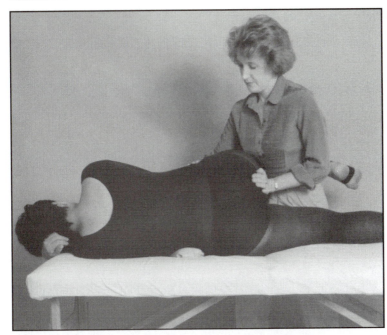

Figure 7-16. Mobilization correction sidelying of a right anterior innominate. (Reprinted with permission from O'Connor LJ, Gourley Stephenson RJ. *Obstetric and Gynecologic Care in Physical Therapy.* Thorofare, NJ: SLACK Incorporated; 1990.)

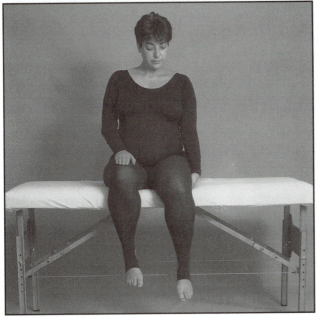

Figure 7-17. Home exercise sitting for correction of a left anterior innominate. (Reprinted with permission from O'Connor LJ, Gourley Stephenson RJ. *Obstetric and Gynecologic Care in Physical Therapy.* Thorofare, NJ: SLACK Incorporated; 1990.)

1. Push-pull isometric exercises for anterior innominate:

   a. Patient sits with knees bent, one hand placed under the thigh of the involved side, against which the hip extends isometrically; the opposite hand is placed on top of the non-involved thigh, against which the hip attempts to flex isometrically 5 seconds. Both push and pull holds are performed simultaneously. The patient breathes easily, relaxes, and repeats 3 times (Figure 7-17).

Figure 7-18. Home exercise supine for correction of a left anterior innominate. (Reprinted with permission from O'Connor LJ, Gourley Stephenson RJ. *Obstetric and Gynecologic Care in Physical Therapy.* Thorofare, NJ: SLACK Incorporated; 1990.)

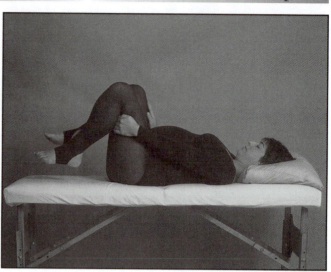

b. Patient is supine with knees bent, hand under the thigh on the involved side, thigh pushes down and is held isometrically; at the same time, the other hand is on top of the noninvolved thigh, and the thigh pushes into flexion; contraction is held isometrically (Figure 7-18).

2. Iliopsoas stretch:

Patient lies on noninvolved side with knee flexed and hip extended on the involved side. Patient holds onto table to stabilize pelvis and actively extends the hip, stretching the iliopsoas (Figure 7-19). If the patient is able to maintain pelvic alignment post-exercise, then pelvic tilt and curl-up exercises (check recti) are added.

Symphysis Pubis

The symphysis pubis may separate a small amount during delivery. With a large baby, or a forceful extraction, more serious injury can result. On examination, the physical therapist may find the following symptoms: Pain: The patient will describe severe pain in the symphysis pubis and SI joints. The urine may be bloody from injury to the bladder neck and urethra. Palpation: The symphysis pubis will be tender, and the ends of the symphysis will be separated. Movement: The bones are usually mobile, and a shift of several centimeters may be felt when the patient shifts weight from one foot to the other.[15]

Treatment may consist of application of heat or cold, a tight binder to immobilize the symphysis pubis, and instruction on performing activities of daily living so the patient's legs are not widely abducted beyond a comfortable resting position. If separation is severe and causes great pain, the patient may require instruction in the use of an assistive device for ambulation.

Low Back

Pregnant clients frequently complain of low back and sciatic pain, which may be caused by the many physical changes of pregnancy: added weight, poor muscle tone, increased lordosis, changes in the center of gravity, and loose pelvic ligaments. Through evaluation, the source of pain must be determined to be mechanical, muscular, joint or discogenic in origin. Uninterrupted pregnancies may predispose women to herniated disks later in life.[14] Pregnant

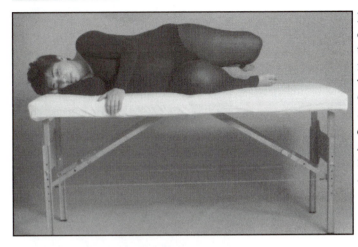

Figure 7-19. Home exercise sidelying for correction of a left anterior innominate. (Reprinted with permission from O'Connor LJ, Gourley Stephenson RJ. *Obstetric and Gynecologic Care in Physical Therapy.* Thorofare, NJ: SLACK Incorporated; 1990.)

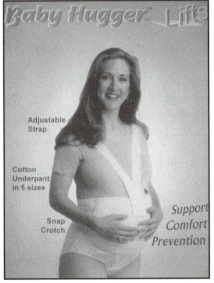

Figure 7-20. Low back support. The Baby Hugger (TrennaVentions, Inc., Derry, PA) (see Appendix B).

women with herniated disks are at a disadvantage, because both evaluation and medications are limited. Evaluations must be performed through clinical exam only, because many imaging techniques and myelograms are contraindicated during pregnancy. Many analgesics and anti-inflammatory medications are ruled as unsafe. The patient should be instructed to monitor radicular signs and adjust activity to avoid reproduction of symptoms. Back supports may be supportive to the expectant mother. (see Figures 7-6, 7-20, and 7-21). Evaluation of patients with herniated disks would be the same as for non-pregnant patients, allowing for restrictions of pregnancy. For treatment see case studies.

Figure 7-21. Low back support. The Dale active lumbosacral support. (Reprinted with permission from O'Connor LJ, Gourley Stephenson RJ. *Obstetric and Gynecologic Care in Physical Therapy.* Thorofare, NJ: SLACK Incorporated; 1990.)

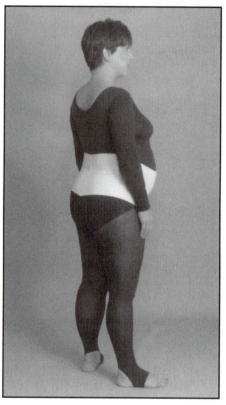

Piriformis

The piriformis may shorten or spasm in pregnancy due to the postural changes and waddling gait. The patient may complain of persistent, severe, radiating low back pain extending from the sacrum to the hip joint over the gluteal region and posterior portion of the upper leg (sciatic nerve distribution).[16] Evaluation may be performed by placing the patient supine with the legs extended. The hip on the involved side will show an increase in external rotation due to the shortened position of the piriformis. On palpation, the buttock on the involved side may be very tender, and the leg on the involved side may appear shorter from contracture of the piriformis. In quadruped position, the sacral base on the involved side may appear to lie anteriorly in relation to the PSIS.[15]

Treatment may consist of heat application in a side-lying position with the affected side up and support at the waist, abdomen, and between the knees. The therapist may attempt to relieve the tightness in the piriformis by applying pressure with the elbow to the affected piriformis near its insertion, while the patient's leg is adducted and internally rotated at the hip, gently stretching along the course of the muscle for 10 seconds and repeating 3 times (Figure 7-22). The patient should experience immediate relief. Deep friction massage to the piriformis muscle may also help, and the physical therapist can instruct the patient's partner on how to apply pressure to the piriformis. The patient may also apply pressure herself by leaning into a tennis ball up against a wall, or by side lying with support, while adducting and internally rotating the hip of the affected side for a self stretch.

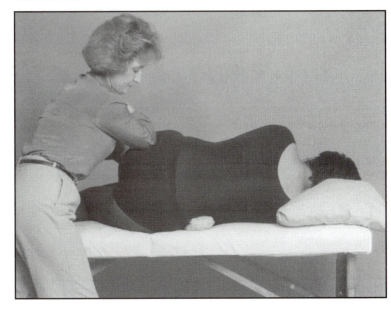

Figure 7-22. Treatment of the piriformis stretch. (Reprinted with permission from O'Connor LJ, Gourley Stephenson RJ. *Obstetric and Gynecologic Care in Physical Therapy.* Thorofare, NJ: SLACK Incorporated; 1990.)

Coccyx

Normally, the coccyx extends in sitting and flexes in standing. Injury to the sacrococcygeal joint may occur during pregnancy or during childbirth. After childbirth, in fact, the coccyx may become subluxed, heal in extension, and become hypomobile.[12] Consequently, the soft tissue over the distal end of the coccyx is quite painful. Treatment includes heat, mobilization of the coccyx, and Thiele's massage (listed below). To mobilize the coccyx, the physical therapist may assist the woman by placing her in a supported side-lying position, inserting a gloved, lubricated index finger into the rectum (patient relaxes sphincter to allow insertion), and placing the thumb externally over the coccyx. An anterior/posterior glide movement and longitudinal traction may be applied to mobilize the joint (Figure 7-23). If the anal canal is too long to get a full glide internally, then the therapist's other gloved hand can be used to additionally mobilize the coccyx externally(with the other hand internally). The patient may be instructed to apply ice externally over the coccygeal area for short periods throughout the day and to use a coccyx pillow for sitting to relieve pressure directly over the coccyx while supporting the rest of the buttocks.

Thiele Massage: a massage technique for treatment of the levator ani and coccygeus muscles
• Massage the muscle fibers along their length from origin to insertion in a sweep motion.
• Use as much pressure as the patient can tolerate .
• At the same time the patient "bears down" to relax these muscles.
• Recommended repeating that this massage 10 to 15 times on each side of the rectum daily for 5 to 6 days. (Thiele. Coccygodynia cause and treatment. *Dis Colon Rectum.* 1963; 6:422-236.)

Knee and Patella Dysfunction

The pregnant woman may have instability and chondromalcia due to effects of relaxin on her knee joints. With the additional weight of pregnancy, the strain may cause knee and patella dysfunctions. After careful evaluation of the knee, if instability is found to be the

Figure 7-23.
Coccyx mobili-
zation.

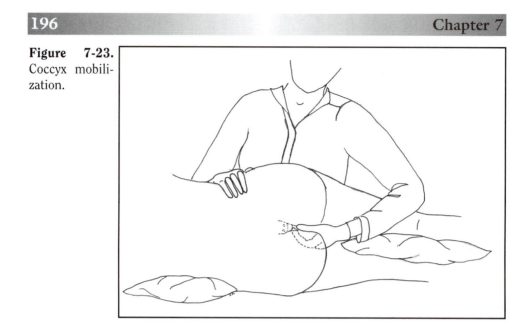

problem, then treatment with taping, and biofeedback to retrain and strengthen surrounding muscles may be indicated. Additionally gait and balance training can decrease the knee pain. To supplement treatment, a knee brace may also be helpful until the pain is resolved and the strength in the knee muscles is restored.

Nerve Palsies

Obstetric nerve palsies occur once in every 2600 deliveries. The most common ones are: *obturator nerve (L3-4)*, *femoral nerve (L2-3)* and *peroneal nerve palsy (L4-5)*. The obturator nerve palsy (L3-4) is caused by compression of the fetal head before birth or during delivery. This pressure results in weakness of the thigh abductors with minimal sensory deficit over the medial aspect of the thigh. Femoral nerve palsy (L2-3) is caused by psoas muscle hemorrhage, pelvic trauma or compression in the pelvic cavity and results in weakness of the quadriceps or psoas muscles with minimal sensory loss in the anteromedial thigh. Peroneal nerve palsy (L4-5) is caused by compression of the stirrups used in delivery which results in weakness of toe extension and foot eversion with sensory loss over the anterolateral leg and dorsal foot. Clear assessment of these palsies will assist the physical therapist in prescribing the correct restorative exercises and any bracing that may be indicated.

Muscle, Tendon Injuries

Because the use of deep heat modalities and electrical stimulation is contraindicated during pregnancy, the treatment of tendon injuries is limited to superficial heat; transverse friction massage across the tendon, muscle, or ligament to break down adhesions;[10] a brace or support[11] and the tendon injury program proposed by Curwin and Sandish:[20]
Tendon Injury Program
1. Warm up the part involved
2. Stretch the part 30 seconds, 3 times
3. Perform eccentric contraction slowly on days 1 and 2, at moderate speed on days 3

through 5, and quickly on days 5 through 7; thereafter, resistance is increased; the patient should be able to do 3 sets of 10 repetitions each at a particular weight, the third set slightly straining the muscle[20]

4. Stretch the involved part (tendon or muscle) using contract/relax techniques

5. Apply ice over the part for 10 minutes

The program is repeated twice daily, increasing the weights so that the third set is always a slight strain to the muscle involved. A support or brace may be helpful, as well.

Table 7-1 is a suggested list of some of the musculoskeletal conditions experienced in pregnancy. This grid is not exhaustive in content and is to be used as a guide to treatment approaches. Each therapist designs a program that is an individual treatment plan for their patient.

CASE STUDIES

Pregnant Client with Back Pain Relating to Posture Changes

Subjective: A 27-year-old primigravida pregnant client was seen in the clinic in her forth month of pregnancy. She complained of severe back pain, level 7 on 0-10 scale, 10 being the worst, and 0 being the least pain. In the morning upon arising she had no back pain and felt progressively worse by the end of the day. She was trying to maintain a walking program but was too tired and in too much pain to walk at the end of the day. She worked full time and drove 45 minutes to work each way.

Objective:

1. Observation: the client stands with a forward head, rounded upper back, increased lordosis, pelvis is tilted anteriorly, with a protruding abdomen

2. Muscle testing: weak upper back and abdominal muscles -3/5

3. Muscle tightness: pectorals, low back muscles, and hip flexors

Assessment: Client had back pain related to postural changes and muscle weakness.

Plan and Goals:

1. Restore full range of motion

2. Increase strength and endurance in weak, target muscles

3. Teach correct posture through serial photographs

4. Increase general fitness level

5. Adapt job, home, and recreational activities to promote proper posture

6. Use upper back support to assist in stretching of pectorals and decrease strain on middle and lower trapezius

7. Suggest car seat that will maximize her comfort for the long drive and problem-solve with her how she can stop and change positions

Treatment:

Exercises:

1. Stretching:

   a. Head retraction: retract head and swallow; hand pushes in on chin

   b. Wall exercise: stand with back resting on wall, feet 12" from wall; bend knees, pelvic tilt, keep shoulders and head back, pull chin in and swallow; hold arms out straight, drag arms up wall (palm-up), hold 10 seconds; when arms start to pull away from wall, stop, lower with control, stand up against wall with aligned posture; rest, repeat

Table 7-1

Musculoskeletal Conditions in Pregnancy.

Dysfunction	Direct Treatment	Education	Supports/Braces	Exercise	Home Treatment
Head & Neck	Myofascial release, Craniosacral	Neck Care positions to avoid, overuse-correct	Supported sleep position, Mid-back support	Stretch the scalenus, pecs + scm strengthen the upper trapezius and levator scapulae muscles	Supine strengthening, Self massage, Heat/ice, ROM, Cervicle isometrics
TMJ	Heat, trigger point releases on face + pterygoids Mobilize TMJ	Relaxation Adjust eating	Night guard if clenching	Rocobado exercise series	Heat, Self massage, Exercises
Thoracic Outlet	Mobilization of clavicle	How to release brachial plexus		Stretch upper trapezius + levator scap-ulae, streng-then neck, upper back extensors, upper extremity	Release brach-ial plexus before sleep
Carpal Tunnel	Heat, trigger point releases	Avoid overuse	Immobilize wrist with splint	Stretch wrist flexors + extensors, Isometrics wrist and hand	Exercises
Diatasis Recti Abdominus	Train to stabilize trunk with ADL's, Standing strength-ening exercises	Avoid sit-ups, Roll with supp-ort	Back and low-er abdominal support	Lumbar stab-ilization	Stabilize in activities
Coastal Rib Pain	Heat, Muscle energy techniques	Upper back strengthening, breathing		Upper back and trunk strengthening	Posture cor-rect in self-stretches
SI Joint Pain	Heat/Ice if acute, Mobilize	Positions to avoid, Rest positions	SI belt	Self correct or with assist-ance, Pelvic/lumbar stabili-zation	Heat/ice if acute
Symphis Pubis	Myofascial release, Pelvic balance , Relieve back dis-comfort, Gait training	Rolling coming to stand, avoid abduction, take small steps side to side up stairs	Lumbo-Pelvic brace, or tight binder over hip and pubis	Pelvic/lumbar stabilization, strengthen abdominals	Rest positions of full support
Back Pain	Heat, Massage, Myofascial release	Avoid back stress, body mechanics	Abdominal support brace	Lumbar stab-ilization, Self mobility of pelvis	Rest, comfort positions, Heat, Exercises
Ruptured Disk	Heat Massage Myofascial release	Avoid disc stress Body mechanics Restrict lifting	Back brace can be individually made	Lumbar stab-ilization	Rest, comfort positions, Heat
Piriformis	Heat, trigger point release, stretch	Tennis ball release	Support pelvis	Strengthen hip internal rotators	Heat

Table 7-1 continued

Musculoskeletal Conditions in Pregnancy.

Dysfunction	Direct Treatment	Education	Supports/ Braces	Exercise	Home Treatment
				Piriformis stretch	
Coccxydnia	External myofascial release, internal mobilization, heat/ ice, Thiele's Massage, Muscle Energy	Correct sitting	Coccyx pillow	Muscle ener- gy with pelvic floor contra- ction	Heat/ice
Knee dysfunc- tion/Patella dysfunction	Train with biofeed- back	Stretch, Strengthen	Patella brace or taping	VMO streng- thening, Closed chain	Taping Ice
Nerve Palsies	Strengthen, Gait correction, Balance training	Strengthen weak ms	Brace if weak	Strengthening	Make home safe from falls
MS/Tendon Injuries	Myofascial Release, Friction massage, Ice	Avoid overuse	Supports: brace	Stretching, Strengthening, progressive	Tendon injury program 2x day

c. Low back stretches: side lying, towel roll under waist, pull single knee to chest; back lying, pull single knee to chest; hands and knees, perform modified buddha and cat exercise (see Chapter 13), long leg stretch with roll underneath knee; slight forward bending to feel stretch in low back and hamstring muscles

d. Iliopsoas stretch: lying near the edge of the bed, pull both knees to chest and hold one knee as other knee drops over side of bed and hold 30 seconds, switch to other side (not longer than 3 minutes on back)

e. Pectoral stretch: stand facing into corner, press arms against wall, hold 30 seconds.

2. Strengthening:

a. Isometric head extensors: later incorporate strengthening of neck rotators, lateral, and forward flexors

b. Trapezius muscle group: standard exercises

c. Abdominal muscles: perform modified curl-ups, leg slides, and active standing abdominal contraction, continuing with wall exercises from a sit-to-stand position (assess rectus muscles).

Pregnant Client with a Herniated Disc

Subjective: This 38-year-old multiparous woman was in her 7th month of pregnancy when she developed sudden excruiating unrelenting back pain a 10 on a 0-10 scale 75% of the day. She was able to have some relief when sidelying.She was unable to care for her two other children and was at home resting as much as possible. She did have a history of back pain in her other two pregnancies.

Objective: Client had positive nerve root irritation on straight leg raising at 40° bilateral-ly. Patient was unable to complete the full exam due to severe pain on ROM testing in all directions. Slight decrease to reflex testing at the ankles at 1+ bilaterally.

Assessment: Client with extreme pain who is unable to complete ADL activities or care take of her children. Although the full exam could not be completed as there would be too great a potential of causing more back pain, a likely assessment is that she has a herniated disc at the L5-S2 level. Other diagnostic tests could not be done because of a contraindication in pregnancy.

Treatment:

1. Frequent rest periods in side-lying positions with support at the waist, under the abdomen, and between the thighs

2. Cold compresses applied to the low back, 10 minutes at a time, frequently throughout the day with 1 hour between applications

3. Massage of the low back area in side-lying position

4. Exercises, including:
   a. Hands and knees position with head up, maintaining a slight, extended position in the back
   b. Hands and knees position, performing contralateral arm and leg lifts
   c. Standing position with hands on hips, slight lumbar extension
   d. Supine position, leg slides maintaining pelvic tilt and lowering legs with control
   e. Standing position, contracting abdominal muscles

5. Body mechanics and back care- avoiding bending or lifting; avoiding sitting as much as possible; taking meals standing up; coughing or sneezing in extension with both hands supporting the small of the back; avoiding constipation

6. Posture- maintaining correct posture through strengthening of the upper back, stretching tight muscles, and exercising with the wall exercise

7. Use of mid- and low back supports (see Figures 7-6, 7-20, and 7-21)

8. Consult with physician to arrange for home care and childcare for her other children

9. Consult with her obstetrician to discuss how best to position her for labor and what options she will have.

Pregnant Client with Low Back Strain

Subjective: This 41-year-old primigravida client was seen one week following her MVA when she was rear ended while at a stop light. She was two months pregnant. She did have her seat belt on and felt a slight strain over her left clavicle from the strain of the belt. She is complaining of pain in her low back from mid day on.

Objective: Client has decreased spinal range on forward bending with pain and severe spasms in both paravertebral muscle groups in the lumbar area. She stands with an increased curve in the lumbar spine and is holding her hand in the small of her back.

Assessment: Client has a low back strain following her MVA.

Plan and treatment consists of:

1. Rest in a side-lying supportive position with pillow between knees, under abdomen, and towel roll at waist

2. Heat applied for short periods in the side-lying position with strap above and below the abdomen to hold it in place

3. Massage of entire back in sidelying position

4. Myofascial release techniques

5. Mobilization and muscle energy balancing techniques

6. Exercises
   a. Alternate knee-to-chest movement, maintaining pelvic tilt, slightly abducting hip to avoid hitting abdomen

b. Pelvic tilt, both knees to chest
c. Hands and knees position, performing cat exercise
d. Modified buddha position
e. Contralateral arm and leg lifts
f. Ipsilateral arm and leg lifts
g. Sitting side bends
h. Knee rock: on back, knees bent, drop knees easily side-to-side, head turns in opposite direction
7. Posture correction, strengthening upper back, stretching tight muscles; wall exercise (see this chapter-Posture)
8. Lumbo sacral support (see Figures 7-20 and 7-21)
9. Home exercise program

SELF-ASSESSMENT REVIEW

1. When evaluating an obstetric client, two positions that should be avoided are _____ and _____.
2. List three reasons why posture changes occur during pregnancy.
3. The difference between adaptive shortening and stretch weakness is _____.
4. List three reasons why muscle testing positions may have to be changed for the obstetric client _____, _____, and _____.
5. The posterior innominate position will require stretching of the _____.
6. List four activities patients with SI joint problems should avoid:
7. List three or more treatment suggestions for low back pain in the obstetric client:
8. The symphysis pubis may be injured or ruptured during _____.
9. A presenting sign of possible piriformis muscle tightness is an _____ position of the leg.
10. During childbirth, the coccyx may become _____.
11. The tempormandibular joint may be painful after delivery because _____.
12. Primary treatment of carpal tunnel syndrome is _____.
13. Tendon and muscle injuries may be treated in pregnancy by _____, _____, and _____.

Answers

1. Prone lying, supine lying for longer than 3 minutes. 2. Added uterine and breast weight anteriorly, change in center of gravity. 3. Adaptive shortening occurs when a muscle is held in a shortened position without appreciable lengthening during relaxation and is associated with muscle strength; stretch weakness defines muscles that remain in a lengthened position and is weak to MMT. 4. No abdominal compression, avoid a supine position longer than 3 minutes, and side lying should be maintained with trunk and abdomen support. 5. Iliopsoas. 6. Walking on uneven terrain, frog kick in swimming, widely abducted legs in sexual positions, taking more than one stair at a time. 7. Heat, exercise, lumbar support, posture correction. 8. Childbirth. 9. Externally rotated. 10. Subluxed and extended. 11. Mother's head may be thrusted in extension. 12. Splinting of the wrist in neutral. 13. Heat, friction massage, and a tendon injury program.

REFERENCES

1. Perinatal Exercise Guidelines. *Bull Sect Obstet Gynecol.* APTA; 1986.

2. Griffin JE, Karselis TC. *Physical Agents for Physical Therapists.* Springfield, Ill: Charles C Thomas; 1982.

3. Fries EC, Hellebrandt FA. The influence of pregnancy on the location of the center of gravity: Postural stability and body alignment. *Am J Obstet Gynecol.* 1943;46:374.

4. Hassid P. *Textbook for Childbirth Educators.* New York, NY: Harper & Row; 1978.

5. Kendall FP, McCreary EK. *Muscle Testing and Function.* 3rd ed. 1983; Baltimore, Md: Williams & Wilkins.

6. Grieve E. Lumbo-pelvic rhythm and mechanical dysfunction of the sacroiliac joint. *Physiotherapy.* 1981; 67(6): 171-173.

7. Golighty R. Pelvic arthropathy in pregnancy and the puerperium. *Physiotherapy.* 1982;58(7):216-220.

8. Grieve GP. The sacroiliac joint. *Physiotherapy.* 1976;52(12):384-387.

9. Kim LYS. Pelvic torsion a common cause of low back pain. *Ortho Rev.* 1984;13(4):61-66.

10. Cyriax J, Cyriax P. *Illustrated Manual of Orthopedic Medicine.* London, England: Butterworth's; 1983.

11. Hoppenfeld S. *Physical Examination of the Spine and Extremities.* New York, NY: Appleton Century-Crofts; 1976.

12. Saunders HD. *Evaluation, Treatment, and Prevention of Musculoskeletal Disorders.* Minneapolis, Minn: Viking Press; 1985.

13. Erhard R. Bowling R. The recognition and management of the pelvic component of low back and sciatic pain. *Bull Sect Orthoped of APTA.* 2(3):4-15,1977.

14. Fast A. Low back disorders. *Arch Phys Med Rehab.* 69:880-891,1988.

15. Wilson JR, Carrington ER. *Obstetrics and Gynecology.* St. Louis, Mo: CV Mosby; 1983.

16. Retzloff EW, Berry AH, Haight AS, et al. Piriformis. *JAOA.* 1974; 73(6):799-807.

17. Travell JCG, Simons D. *Myofascial Pain and Dysfunction.* Baltimore, Md: Williams & Wilkins; 1983.

18. Iglarsh ZA. *Telephone Interview with R Gourley.* March 1989.

19. Howell JW, Roseman GF. The evaluation and treatment of carpal tunnel syndrome in pregnancy. *Bull Sect Obstet Gynecol of APTA.* 1987;11(2):10-11.

20. Curwin S, Sandish W. *Tendinitis: Its Etiology and Treatment.* Lexington, Mass: DC Heath & Co; 1984.

Chapter

8

Care of the Fetus:
Preconception to Birth

The physical therapist practicing in the field of obstetrics will undoubtedly have a patient who asks, "Will this treatment harm my baby?" While the number of studies about safety and modality use is severely limited, other basic physical therapy treatments, such as instruction in corrective exercises or in body mechanics, are considered safe. However, to answer some questions clients and medical personnel may have about positioning and general maternal health, knowledge of fetal safety, anatomy, and development is vital. Likewise, it is important here to introduce the idea that those in the OB/GYN health care team are becoming increasingly liable for advising couples to seek genetic counseling prior to conception and during pregnancy. Therefore, the physical therapist must be at least familiar with as many as possible of the issues surrounding women's health care today.

PRECONCEPTION CONCERNS AND GENETIC COUNSELING

A special word should be included about the period surrounding conception. Although the effects of teratogenic substances has been recognized for quite a while, especially since the thalidomide tragedy of the 1950s, recent studies suggest that there may be a link between the pre-pregnancy nutritional status of the mother and the eventual health of the fetus.[1] One study conducted with mothers who took vitamins before conception suggested reduced incidence of myelomeningocele in their infants, as opposed to a group of mothers who received no preconception supplementation.[1] Although this study has not been replicated to date, the idea of encouraging prospective mothers to improve their diets before conception cannot be refuted. Other recent studies suggest that smoking can alter sperm count and integrity. Additional maternal nutrition studies suggest that preconceptional lifestyle may strongly influence fetal health, especially if substance abuse is a factor.

A brief review of genetics may be useful for physical therapists dealing with pregnant women or those planning a pregnancy. Human chromosomes number 46; 2 sex chromosomes and 44 autosomes. The female chromosomes include XX sex chromosomes; the male chromosomes, XY. Although the autosomes are paired and numbered by morphologic traits, they are arranged in an arbitrary manner called the karyotype. In the female embryo, one of the two X chromosomes (one paternal and one maternal) randomly becomes inactive, condenses, and is known as the Barr body or sex chromatin. It is the active maternal or paternal X that determines the autosomal trait seen clinically.[2]

Genetic screenings typically focus on three general categories: single gene disorders (autosomal dominant, autosomal recessive, or X-linked), chromosomal anomalies (cytogenetics), and multifactorial disorders related to both hereditary and environmental factors.[3] Examples of each category are described in Table 8-1. Prior to conception, then, a number of these disorders can be screened for, and the occurrence of risk calculated, based on familial traits and history. A diagram, called a family pedigree, can map family members and generations affected by multiple or single traits. This information can also help determine homozygosity or heterozygosity of defects. Once a woman is pregnant, the same type of map can be drawn; however, additional tests will help diagnose the possibility that such a disorder exists in this particular fetus.

Prenatal tests are usually conducted via samples of amniotic fluid. Amniocytes are then cultured and "examined cytogenetically, assayed biochemically (for inborn errors of metabolism) or analyzed for DNA changes."[4] Other methods for prenatal diagnosis include alpha-fetoprotein analysis, chorionic villus or fetal tissue biopsy, ultrasound, contrast radiography, and fetoscopy. While a certain amount of risk is associated with each of these procedures, and there may be a considerable wait for results from such tests, women at risk for producing a child with genetic abnormalities may consider the risk worth the answer.

TERATOGENS AND ENVIRONMENTAL HAZARDS

In the 1950s, the consequences of administration of the drug thalidomide to pregnant females in their third to fifth week of gestation proved convincingly, that the pregnant female who was exposed to or who ingested certain substances might be risking the health of her baby. Thalidomide is a tranquilizing agent or hypnotic drug and was then used to calm the anxious expectant mother. Yet the stress increased considerably when an infant with phocomelia (absence of the proximal part of a limb) was born. The relative rarity of this anomaly enabled epidemiologists to track the teratogen to thalidomide administered early in the pregnancy. This unfortunate incident, however, stands as a hallmark of expanding obstetric and epidemiologic awareness, especially concerning agents that affect the fetus. Correspondingly, the nonsteroidal estrogen, diethylstilbestrol (DES) was used, supposedly to decrease the incidence of miscarriage. This drug was administered from 1940 to 1971 until researchers linked it epidemiologically to congenital anatomic and reproductive anomalies in the offspring of women receiving DES.

A variety of factors can result in abnormal fetal development. Teratology is the study of those factors—called teratogens—substances that cause congenital abnormalities. Congenital abnormalities can include anything from gross structural defects down to cellular defects. Anomalies may be transmitted genetically, environmentally, or spontaneously. Examples of specific anomalies of each category are listed in Table 8-2. What is important to remember when answering patients' questions about potential birth defects is that not every mother who has a maternal infection will deliver an abnormal infant. In fact, only a very small percentage of children will have birth defects. Neither will every woman who has had a child born with birth defects deliver another the same. In some cases, however, such as genetically based anomalies, some disorders are more likely to occur in any offspring. Mothers with children who have genetic disorders should be referred to a genetic counselor to determine the risk of producing similar offspring.

Table 8-1

Overview of Genetic Screening Categories

Single-gene disorder
    Autosomal recessive (homozygous alleles)
        Sickle-cell anemia
        Cystic fibrosis
        Phenylketonuria
        Albinism
        Tay-Sachs disease
        Werdnig-Hoffman disease
    Autosomal dominant (heterozygous alleles)
        Huntington's disease
        Myotonic dystrophy
        Osteogenesis imperfecta, types I and IV
    X-linked (mutant gene on X chromosome)
        Dominant
            Vitamin-D resistant rickets
        Recessive
            Becker's muscular dystrophy
            Duchenne's muscular dystrophy
            Hemophilia A and B
Chromosomal anomalies
    Numerical
        Trisomy (21 = Down syndrome)
        Turner's syndrome (monosomy 45,X)
        Triple X syndrome (47,XXX)
        Klinefelter's syndrome (47,XXY)
    Structural
        Isochromosomes
        Ring chromosomes
        Duplications, Inversions, Deletions, Translocations
        Fragile X
        Inactive X
Multifactorial
    Cardiac defects
    Legg-Calves-Perthes disease
    Scoliosis
    Cleft palate
    Spina bifida
    Dislocated hip

It is important, too, for practitioners to keep aware of research in this field. Recent studies have implicated video display terminals on computers, smoking, alcohol, social drug abuse, and chemicals used in the workplace or at home, as potential teratogens. For instance, pregnant women were warned to avoid changing cat litter boxes because of the risk of toxoplasmosis carried in cat feces. In other research, initial suspicions of harm induced by caffeine consumption during pregnancy could not be conclusively proven, at least in regard to certain birth deformities, although there is data for both sides of the issue.[5] Therefore, the well-informed practitioner needs to keep updated to help clients answer questions about nutrition and environmental hazards. The physical therapist may also receive questions about the safety of analgesics, over the counter medications, and anesthetics used for labor and delivery, and even about the safety of certain fetal diagnostic procedures (amniocente-

Table 8-2

Modes of Transmission and Examples of Congenital Anomalies

Mode of Transmission	Trait	Cause
Genetic	Sickle-cell anemia Color blindness Huntington's chorea Chromosomal aberrations (Turner's syndrome, Klinefelter's syndrome, Down syndrome) Tay-Sachs disease	Aberrations of genes or chromosomes; hereditary
Environmental	Depends on gestational age at time of exposure	Radiation, maternal infection, maternal nutritional deficiency, chemicals, maternal-fetal blood difference
Spontaneous	Depends on gene affected	Possible genetic strain weakness

Table 8-3

Confirmed Teratogens

Substance	Possible Fetal Effect
Alcohol	Microcephaly, growth and developmental retardation (fetal alcohol syndrome)
Birth control pills	Bony and respiratory tract anomalies
Vaccines	Infection in fetus
Phenobarbital	Limb or heart defects, mental retardation
Cancer drugs	Assorted malformations
Cocaine	Assorted malformations
Diethylstilbestrol (DES)	Reproductive tract anomalies, cancer
Antibiotics	Assorted malformations
Thalidomide	Fetal death, assorted malformations

sis and diagnostic ultrasound). Tables 8-3 and 8-4 list a small sample of proven and suspected teratogenic substances; however, these lists are by no means exhaustive.

Clients should be advised to consult their physicians or caregivers if any doubt exists as to the safety of a substance. It is also wise to refer these clients to their caregiver even if a substance used is a confirmed teratogen. For some unexplained reason, teratogenic substances do not always induce birth defects. The substances identified as teratogens are associated with a significant increase in congenital anomalies. But that does not mean that an identified substance will always cause a defect. Legalistically, the practitioner is better off referring questions about general physical and mental health during pregnancy to a specialist in that field.

Table 8-4

Suspected Teratogens

Substance	Possible Fetal Effect
Smoking and passive smoking	Decreased birth weight
Nutritional deficiencies	Inadequate growth
Aspirin	Jeopardized homeostasis
Prolonged hyperthermia induced by hot tubs and saunas	Neural defects
Nasal decongestants	Anomalies
Allergy medications	Anomalies

CONCEPTION

Once sperm is introduced into the vagina, the journey becomes even more perilous. The acidic environment of the vagina could spell disaster for the alkaline sperm if not for their ability to mobilize rapidly to the cervical region. The semen forms a gel to protect itself, although the sperm are believed to be immobilized within 2 hours after ejaculation if left in the vagina. The gel is converted by prostatic enzymes to a liquid after about 20 to 30 minutes. Only the sperm enter the uterus, and uterine contractions propel the sperm into the fallopian tube within 5 minutes of insemination. Apparently only 200 of the 200 to 300 million sperm even get close to the egg; the others are either left in the vagina and digested by enzymes, or phagocytosized along the way.

Once the sperm move close to the egg, they undergo a process of capacitation, by which they prepare to penetrate the ovum. The head of the sperm changes to allow specific enzymes to egress for fusion with the egg membrane. Capacitation also causes altered receptor mobility and loss of seminal plasma antigens, as well as increased motility. These factors increase the chances of the sperm to penetrate the ovum and are required for in vitro fertilization to occur.

The ova and follicular cells rest on the surface of the ovary until muscular movements cause the cilia of the fimbriae to pick up an egg. To and fro propulsion through the fallopian tube causes the egg to reach the ampulla of the tube after about 30 hours. Any contact by the sperm with the egg occurs in the ampulla. It is believed fertilization occurs through random contact rather than by any mechanism that would attract the sperm to the egg. In the sperm head, the enzyme-containing acrosome undergoes a reaction that results in a fusing of the plasma membrane and the outer acrosomal membrane. As the sperm penetrates the egg, the zone pellucida surrounding the egg from ovulation to implantation appears to prevent additional fertilizations by prohibiting other sperm from entering. This is accomplished by enzymes that harden the extracellular layer and inactivate receptors for sperm.

How then does twinning occur? About once in every 80 births, a dizygotic or monozygotic twinning results either from the discharge of two ova or from the splitting of a single, fertilized ovum. In the case of two ova being released either from two or one ovarian follicle, twins are dizygotic or fraternal. These twins are like any other siblings. It is unclear whether the release of more than one ovum is directed by hereditary factors. The occurrence of monozygotic twinning, however, is believed to be hereditary, as two embryos arise from one fertilized egg. These twins are identical and of the same sex. Multiple births derive from the same circumstances.[6]

Once the male and female pronuclei migrate after the fusion of the sperm and egg membranes, the first cell division occurs. Two to three days after the embryo starts to develop and enters the uterus, implantation in the uterine endometrium begins. The cells of each surface mesh and the embryo becomes firmly situated.[4]

FETAL GROWTH

"How could one single cell, until then stored quietly in the body, suddenly give rise to a new human being with every feature that human beings have in common but still not exactly like any other living individual?" Prior to ovulation, the ovum, or primary oocyte, completes its first meiotic division (becomes haploid with 22 autosomes + 1 sex chromosome); the result is a secondary oocyte and a first polar body (one of the meiotic divisions that receives less cytoplasm than the other, and is therefore, nonviable as an oocyte). The first polar body eventually disappears, while the secondary oocyte begins a second meiotic division. If fertilized, a second polar body is discarded, and the fertilized ovum (now a diploid of male and female cells) is what remains.[7] During the first week after conception, that single fertilized cell (zygote) travels down the tube as it undergoes multiple mitotic divisions, still within the zygote. The zygote becomes a morula after several mitotic divisions (cleavage), then a trophoblast, and finally a blastocyst, as fluid accumulates, and fluid and cellular matter polarize. About 5 to 9 days after ovulation, the blastocyst burrows into the endometrium (implantation) and draws nourishment from the endometrial blood vessels as the placenta develops around it.

The location of the implantation is of great clinical importance. Most commonly, implantation occurs on the upper, posterior wall of the endometrium of the uterine body. Implantation involves cellular breakdown in the endometrium, closed over by a blood-clotting mechanism. This implantation bleeding may be mistaken clinically or by a woman as the start of a menses. If the blastocyst implants at sites other than the upper one third of the uterus, completion of pregnancy to term may be jeopardized. "In order of frequency they (abnormal implantations) occur as follows: (1) region of the internal os of the cervix, (2) ampulla of the uterine tube, (3) isthmus of the uterine tube, (4) angle of the uterine cavity, (5) infundibulum of the uterine tube, (6) ovary, (7) interstitial portion of the uterine tube, (8) peritoneum of the broad ligament, mesentery of the intestine or rectouterine pouch, and (9) pregnancy in a rudimentary uterine horn."[1] Outside the uterus, implantations are considered ectopic and can rarely reach full term within the abdominal cavity.

From here, the blastocyst differentiates into ectoderm, mesoderm, and endoderm to give rise to the brain, spinal cord, nerves, and skin; skeleton, urogenital system, heart, blood vessels, and muscles; and digestive system, liver, and pancreas, respectively. Rather than reiterate the contents of an embryology text, the information that is more useful for the practicing physical therapist regarding the development of the blastocyst focuses on the anatomy and function of the fetal membranes, the umbilical cord, the placenta, and the fetus, itself.

The fetal membranes include the yolk sac, allantois, amnion, and chorion. The yolk sac and allantois play a role in the development of the placental circulation and umbilical vessels. The amnion is the wall of the amniotic cavity, which holds the amniotic fluid. This fluid is produced by the amnion cells until the fetal kidneys start to function. The fluid is circulated, and the amount increases until the 5th month. Until then, there has been an increase up to about one quart; the volume reduces in the seventh month to allow growth of the fetus. It has been estimated that about one third of this fluid of water, protein, glucose, and inorganic salts is replaced every hour. Within the amniotic fluid, the embryo or fetus floats, is protected from injury, and temperature is regulated. The chorion helps in the establishment of fetal circulation as the decidua (lining of the uterus) in three different layers, fuses into one. The decidua meets the chorion to fill the uterus, except at the cervix where glands secrete mucus to form a mucus plug. This plug forms early to seal off the uterus from outside contaminants until labor begins.

Fusion of the amnion and the chorion creates the umbilical cord. Where this cord meets the ventral wall of the embryo is the umbilicus. Inside the cord is Wharton's jelly, a light blue-green substance, plus the yolk sac, a vitelline duct, allantois, and umbilical vessels. Two umbilical veins bring oxygenated blood from the chorion to the fetus, and two umbilical arteries return the deoxygenated blood from the fetus to the chorion. The umbilical cord is about 3/4 inch in diameter, and about 20 to 24 inches long at term. It is estimated that blood travels through the cord at a rate of 4 miles/hour and completes the trip from placenta, through the baby, and back in 30 seconds. This dynamic force makes the cord stiff and unlikely to knot as the baby moves within the womb.

The placenta is formed by fetal chorion and maternal decidua. The placenta is divided into sections called cotyledons and remains attached to the expanding uterus while thickening and increasing in area. At term, the placenta is flat, discoid, about 8 inches in diameter, about 1 inch thick, and weighs about 1 pound. The fetus is joined to the placenta via the umbilical cord. The placenta is capable of holding about 175 ml of maternal blood, flowing at a rate of 500 ml/minute. Uterine contractions force blood into uterine veins. Placental functions include respiration, nutrition, excretion, protection, and endocrine.[1] The placenta allows oxygen to reach the fetus and carbon dioxide to be carried away. Water, salts, carbohydrates, fats, proteins, and vitamins pass to the fetus, while excreted products pass to the mother to metabolize. The placenta can also protect the fetus from certain bacterial infections, plus it produces progesterone, estrogen, and gonadotropin. The placenta, however, cannot protect the fetus from everything, particularly from certain harmful substances ingested by the mother.

"The nutrient supply to a fetus is dependent on placental transport."[8] The ability to transport nutrients increases as pregnancy progresses, especially closer to term as the baby puts on weight. "Morphometric studies in human placentas have shown that the placental thickness decreases, and the surface area continues to increase exponentially until term." The conclusion drawn from these observations is that placental growth meets fetal nutritional requirements. It is believed that most of the protein transfer occurs after 30 weeks gestation; hence, fetal growth can be considered dependent not only on those substances ingested by the mother, but on the size and transport capacity of the placenta.

"The placental transport of nutrients to the umbilical circulation depends on the permeability of the placenta to each nutrient, the maternal-to-fetal concentration gradient for each nutrient, net placental nutrient consumption, and the magnitude and pattern of uterine, placental, and umbilical blood flows."[8] The placenta transports carbohydrates via diffusion, amino acids via active transport, and fats via a number of ways; the mechanism for fetal uptake of lipids is unclear. In fact, the mechanism for transport for most substances of high molecular weight is not totally understood. This applies to maternal antibodies as well as lipids. Vitamins B. C, D and dissolved substances such as sodium, chloride, and potassium transport easily; unfortunately, so do many drugs, some of which are teratogenic.

FETAL DEVELOPMENT

The birth of a normal, fully formed child is nothing short of a miracle when one considers the intricate balance of events that must occur to form all bodily systems accurately. "The normal development of the embryo is an integrated process in which the various organizing influences exert their inductive effects in a coordinated manner, in the correct sequence, at the correct time and place, and in the correct direction."[6] The sequence of systemic developmental events is important, not only to help researchers identify possible teratogenic substances if an anomaly should occur, but to determine clinically the health of the developing fetus. With the advent of diagnostic ultrasound and magnetic resonance imaging, fetal development has become more of an exact science. These events of human development are summarized in Tables 8-5 and 8-6 and in Figure 8-1. In addition to the events summarized in the tables, continued research has yielded interesting information about the fetus. Ultrasound imaging of the fetus has shown that "atropine, cigarette smoking, and frightening the mother produced a fetal tachycardia within 2 to 4 minutes."[2] Also, ductus arteriosus and secundum atrial defects are normally present in utero, and cannot be diagnosed until birth. Experiments have not linked fetal cardiac arrhythmia to congenital heart disease.[5] Craniocaudal development has been confirmed by several investigators. "Fetal movements (at 12 weeks) were characterized as (1) active movements of all body components, (2) sporadic kicking, and (3) strong, pulsed trunk movements that resemble the hiccups of a more mature fetus... Upper limb movements predominate at 26 weeks. The most powerful movements occurring at this gestational age include foot withdrawal and the lateral trunk incurvation reflex... by 28 weeks, bursts of activity involving the trunk and limbs occur, followed by a resting phase in which, although the fetus may perceive external stimulation, he is unable to react. One month later, spontaneous movements are more powerful and frequent...."[2] Although maternal counting of movements has not proven accurate because of the tendency to count fetal breathing movements, Braxton Hicks contractions, and the mother's own movements, observations by mothers of decreased fetal movement prior to fetal death have been documented in high and low risk mothers.[2]

Unlike fetal body movements, which typically occur as a burst of activity followed by as much as 2 hours of rest, fetal breathing movements normally occur at a rate of 40 to 70/minute.[5] These breathing movements tend to increase after meals and in rate, depth, incidence, and level of organization as pregnancy progresses.[5]

Testing of sensory stimulation in utero may prove to be valuable for diagnosis; such tests include using auditory stimuli instead of a contraction stress test to determine fetal status. Early research suggested that background noises of the maternal digestive and circulatory systems may calm the infant, but so far these sounds have not achieved the same effect when applied after birth.[5]

FETAL PHYSIOLOGY

During pregnancy, the uterine blood flow increases as uterine size increases with fetal growth. However, the increase of blood flow in proportion to the growth of the fetus is lacking; therefore, more oxygen is extracted per volume of uterine blood toward the end of pregnancy. The uterine arteries ultimately supply the placenta, which functions similarly to a lung for the fetus. The placental villi act in the exchange of oxygen and nutrition to the fetal

Table 8-5

Fetal Growth and Developmental Highlights

Week of Gestation	Event	Fetal size
0-1	Implantation	1-36 cells
1-2	Embryo takes shape Entoderm, mesoderm, ectoderm differentiate	
2-3	Body forms, heart beats Brain forms two lobes	1/10 inch
3-4 (1st month)	Head, trunk, arm buds	1/4 inch
4- 5	Arm buds with hand plates; ears and jaws form; yolk sac useless	
5-6	Ears form	1/2 inch
6-7	Resembles adult with eyes, ears, nose, lips, tongue, teeth buds, fingers, thumbs, knees, ankles, toes; fetal movements; brain directs other organs; stomach digests; liver makes blood cells; kidney extracts uric acid from blood; first bone cells replace	1 inch; 1/30 oz
(2nd month)	Cartilage skeleton Embryo becomes fetus	
9-10	Total body movements; threefold increase in nerve-muscle connections	2 inches
12 (3rd month)	Swallows amniotic fluid, fingernails form; eyelids seal; bony ribs and verte-brae form; palate fuses; excretes urine	
12-16 (4th month)		6-8 inches; 6 oz
16-20 (5th month)	Grows hair; skeleton hardens; settles into favorite lie	10 inches; 1 pound
20-24 (6th month)	Permanent teeth buds; eyes open; grip is strong; vernix and lanugo (hair) on body	13 inches; 1 3/4 pounds
24-28 (7th month)	Deposits adipose tissue under skin	15 inches; 2-3 pounds
28-38 (8th, 9th months)	Gains weight and length	20 inches 6-10 pounds

Table 8-6

Fetal Development by System

System	Time	Event
Cardiovascular	Day 22	Primitive tube forms
	4th week	Cardiac activity; cardiac loop
	4-7 weeks	Four chambers form
	7-8 weeks	Heart rate increases from week 4 until now when it decreases due to improved contractility
Respiratory	34 weeks	Primordium forms trachea and lung buds
	10 weeks	Left bronchus divides in two, right into three
	11 weeks	Fetal breathing movement
	4th month	24 bronchial divisions
	13-25 weeks	Canalization
	24 weeks	Alveoli form (this process continues until 8 years)
Nervous		
Vision	5 weeks	Optic cup, lens vesicle
	24 months	Retina differentiates
	5 months	Rods and cones form
	10-26 weeks	Eyelids fuse
	30 weeks	Eye responds to light
Taste	7 weeks	Taste buds
	12 weeks	Mature taste buds; swallows
	28 weeks	Taste established
Hearing	18 days	Ear develops
	6 weeks	Cochlea appears
	10 weeks	Cochlea has 2 1/2 turns; Scala vestibuli and tympani
	5 months	Cochlea complete
	6 months	Inner ear functions
	7 months	Eardrum forms
	26-29 weeks	Response to external sounds
Touch	7 weeks	Reflex response to touch
	8 weeks	Receptors to face
	10 weeks	Pressure receptors in fingers; light touch in hands
	11 weeks	Upper and lower extremities respond
	15-17 weeks	Abdomen/buttocks respond
	7 months	Meissner's corpuscles in hand (light touch)
	2nd/3rd trimester	Reflex grasp strengthens
Musculoskeletal	3 weeks	Nerve cells present
	5 weeks	Myotomes give rise to spinal muscles and three muscle layers on thorax/abdomen
	5-8 weeks	Forelimb and hind limb buds grow and angle to form elbows and knees
	6-8 weeks	Spinal reflex arc
	7.5 weeks	First reflex activity (neck contralateral flexion to perioral stimulation)
	8.5 weeks	Thorax/lumbar flexion
	9.5 weeks	Pelvic rotation; mouth opening
	10.5 weeks	Swallowing motions; sucking movements
	11 weeks	Hip movements
	12 weeks	Ankle movements; three motor patterns

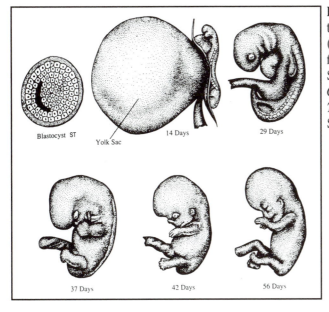

Figure 8-1. Development of the embryo and fetus (Reprinted with permission from O'Connor LJ, Gourley Stephenson RJ. *Obstetrics and Gynecologic Care in Physical Therapy.* Thorofare, NJ: SLACK Incorporated; 1990.)

blood, and carbon dioxide and fetal wastes to the maternal blood. Fetal circulation differs from that of the newborn and of the adult (Figure 8-2). Briefly the difference lies in extra flow from the placenta entering the fetal heart via the ductus venosus to the inferior vena cava. Additional fetal blood shunted to the liver from the umbilical vein flows to the inferior vena cava via hepatic veins, and blood from the gut reaches the ductus venosus from the portal vein. The inferior vena cava opens near the foramen ovate, causing blood to flow through the foramen ovate to the left atrium, while blood entering via the superior vena cava passes into the right-sided chambers. Blood in the left chambers pass into the aorta and then to the head, neck, and upper extremities. This blood appears to be better oxygenated than the blood that passes to the caudal regions via the pulmonary trunk. Little blood flows into the lungs because of the resistance, flowing instead to the patent ductus arteriosus and the descending thoracic and abdominal aortae to the lower extremities. These openings in the ductus arteriosus and in the foramen ovate cause the left and right sides of the fetal heart to pump in parallel rather than in series, as in the adult. Fetal blood then travels to the placenta through the umbilical arteries, and circulation repeats.

At birth, blood flowing through the umbilical cord will continue to diminish over several minutes, although it is believed that most of it reaches the infant within a minute after delivery.[1] Part of the reduction in flow is due to swelling of the Wharton's jelly inside the cord, which compresses the two arteries and one vein.[9] As the placental circulation stops, peripheral resistance rises until the aortic pressure exceeds that in the pulmonary artery. The infant becomes asphyxic, gasps, and these responses added to negative intrapleural pressure cause the lungs to inflate. This first breath apparently draws in additional placental blood. When the lungs expand, pulmonary blood flow can increase, pressure in the left atrium rises and shuts the foramen ovate by pressing on the valve. The ductus arteriosus also shuts after a few minutes, possibly because of a rise in arterial oxygen pressure. The complete mechanisms for these closures are unknown, but may be linked to vasoreactive factors.[7] Experimentation with prostaglandins suggests they may play a role in the adjustment of fetal circulation to birth. In any event, peripheral circulation may take longer to establish, and the hands and feet of the newborn may be cold for the first few hours.

Figure 8-2. Maternal-fetal circulation. (Reprinted with permission from O'Connor LJ, Gourley Stephenson RJ. *Obstetrics and Gynecologic Care in Physical Therapy.* Thorofare, NJ: SLACK Incorporated; 1990.)

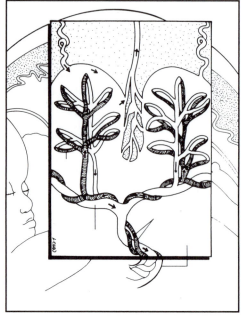

After the cord is cut and ligated, the placenta remains inside the uterus for a short time, then peels off the uterine wall and is delivered, designating the third stage of labor. This peeling tends to leave a wound on the uterine wall which bleeds for a few weeks after the birth.

FETAL AND NEONATAL ASSESSMENT

The status of the mother is relatively easy to assess compared to the status of the fetus. Several methods have been devised in recent years to help obstetric attendants learn more than the information gained by fetal heart monitoring and feel more confident that the fetus is healthy during pregnancy and during labor. Tests for early pregnancy include amniocentesis, chorionic villus sampling, and maternal serum alpha-fetoprotein. Other tests for later pregnancy include electronic fetal monitoring, ultrasonography, magnetic resonance imaging, antepartum fetal heart rate testing (nonstress test and the contraction stress test), and fetal movement charting. A biophysical profile (a composite score of fetal breathing movements, gross body movements, muscle tone, amniotic fluid volume, and the nonstress test) also may be conducted (Table 8-7).

Amniocentesis can be used for a variety of analyses. This sampling of amniotic fluid drawn by needle from the area around the baby can be done early to detect genetic disorders, or later in pregnancy to assess fetal lung maturity. Fetal lung maturity is assessed by several other tests, but the most widely used one determines the ratio of lecithin and sphingomyelin (L/S ratio). These substances are phospholipid components of surfactant, which increases alveolar surface tension. A ratio above 2:1 is considered a normal proportion. Amniotic fluid can also be examined for signs of maternal or fetal infection. There is a certain risk of maternal infection and fetal demise from the procedure.

Chromosomal analysis can also be done by chorionic villus sampling of about 30 mg of chorionic tissue drawn by suction catheter through the vagina and directed by ultrasound. Again, a risk is associated with the procedure.

Table 8-7

Fetal Assessment Methods & Tests

Amniocentesis
Chorionic villus sampling
Maternal serum alpha-fetoprotein
Electronic fetal monitoring
Ultrasonography
Magnetic resonance imaging
Antepartum fetal heart rate testing
    Nonstress test
    Contraction stress test
    Oxytocin challenge test
Fetal breathing movements
Biophysical profile
Hepatitis B virus
Herpes simplex virus
Congenital toxoplasmosis

Sampling of maternal serum alpha-fetoprotein is a screening for neural tube defects and has been recently used with encouraging results to detect Down syndrome.[10] Concentrations of this alpha-globulin synthesized in the fetal yolk sac, liver, and gastrointestinal tract are much higher in fetal serum than in amniotic fluid, and higher in amniotic fluid than in maternal serum; however, the ease of sampling maternal serum makes this test more practical.

Another test that used to be performed routinely with maternal blood typing is for Rh incompatibility. An Rh-negative mother may become sensitized if the fetus is Rh-positive. Rh immune globulin can be administered several times during pregnancy and immediately after delivery.

Electronic fetal monitoring has become a legalistic necessity during labor and delivery in the minds of many obstetric physicians and nurses. The readout from the electronic monitor assures the physician that fetal heart rate is within normal limits (120 to 160 bpm) over time and that the uterus is contracting efficiently. Two tracings record fetal heart rate variations and pressure of uterine contractions (mm Hg) The fetal heart is monitored through a sound transducer placed externally or internally and contractions, via a pressure transducer. The internal electrode is attached through ruptured membranes to the fetal scalp. If monitored externally, there are two belts that must be worn (Figure 8-3). If the woman changes position the reading may be disturbed. Many women find these belts uncomfortable, but a great number of physicians and hospitals require continuous monitoring for medicolegal records. Women who do not want these procedures should be advised to shop around for a physician and hospital that will meet their needs.

Diagnostic ultrasound, to be differentiated from therapeutic ultrasound and surgical ultrasound, is used to determine gestational age and to detect fetal anomalies, intrauterine growth retardation, fetal position, multifetal pregnancy, uterine size, and placental location. There are three basic systems of diagnostic ultrasound, usually in the range of 3.5 to 5 MHz, static B scan, real-time imaging, and the Doppler. The static B scan is a pulse-echo method, real-time is a rapid-pulse scan, and the Doppler is a continuous transmission of ultrasound waves. The echoes received from the sound waves that bounce off the fetal heart are then converted to audible range. With ultrasound, the higher the frequency is, the less the depth

Figure 8-3. Electronic fetal monitor: external and internal(in circle) electrode placements. (Reprinted with permission from O'Connor LJ, Gourley Stephenson RJ. *Obstetrics and Gynecologic Care in Physical Therapy.* Thorofare, NJ: SLACK Incorporated; 1990.)

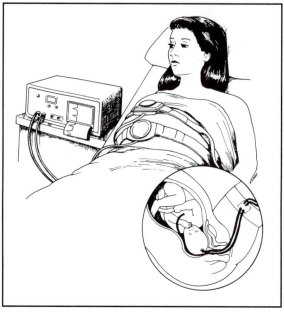

of penetration will be. Therefore, the intensity must be increased to maintain the desired depth of penetration with good resolution.[11,12]

Unfortunately, the effects of higher intensity ultrasound on fetal tissue are not well documented. The American College of Obstetricians and Gynecologists has developed guidelines for use of diagnostic ultrasound, but the guidelines are broad and include almost any use except as a routine screening tool.[13] The International Childbirth Education Association published a position paper on this topic to encourage use "only in the presence of medically valid criteria," and discouraged use "in the absence of a high-risk indication."[14] It may be many years before the long-term impact of routine use of diagnostic ultrasound is known. Until then, women should question routine screening with ultrasound. Obstetricians and nurses can listen to fetal heart tones without a Doppler device. This does not imply, however, that if a woman is at high-risk, or there is a question of fetal safety, she should refuse. What it seems to boil down to is trust and respect between physician and client. If a woman feels comfortable and confident of the physician's abilities, she should also be able to ask questions and have them answered in a logical way. Physicians need to provide facts when asked if a procedure is necessary and whether it is safe for the fetus, and women need to demand these facts before making an informed decision.

Magnetic resonance imaging has been used for better resolution of hydrocephalus and other fetal anomalies. It is also believed to be useful for measuring the bony pelvis. Few studies have been done to determine safety and cost-effectiveness.

The stress tests do as their name suggests, place stress on the fetus. Even the nonstress test places stress if the fetus is unhealthy. These tests are done, if indicated, during the last trimester. In the nonstress test, patients are placed in a semi-Fowler position, while maternal blood pressure and pulse and fetal activity and heart rate are assessed in serial readings for 20 to 40 minutes. The test may be reactive or nonreactive; the reactive test results in two to three or more fetal heart rate accelerations in this period. An acceleration is 15 beats/minute above baseline for 15 seconds or longer. The contraction stress test repeats the nonstress test plus stimulates uterine contraction, either by the mother stimulating her nipples or by infusing oxytocin (the substance that should be naturally produced by nipple stimulation and causes uterine contractions; if oxytocin is used the test is referred to as the oxytocin challenge test).[15] Again fetal heart rate is the criteria for a positive, suspicious, or negative test, but late decelerations are the key. The test is positive if there are repetitive late decelerations coincident with uterine contractions, suspicious if late decelerations are noted but not persistent, and negative if none occur with uterine contractions. A contraction stress test, though, may also be reactive or nonreactive should accelerations occur as well. The predictive value of these tests is debatable in terms of fetal outcome. The worst scenario is a nonreactive positive contraction stress test, suggesting that elective delivery may be needed to save the fetus.[16] The mother must plan to rest in a lateral recumbent position for at least an hour to chart fetal movements. This test depends heavily on the mother's perceptions of fetal movement as she charts gross motions. Four or more fetal movements in an hour are considered normal, although a healthy fetus may move far more often.

The factors associated with the biophysical profile have been explained, except for the amniotic fluid measurement and fetal tone assessment. The examiner looks for pockets of amniotic fluid, greater than 1 cm in size, surrounding the fetus. One or more pockets of this size are normal. The assessment of fetal tone examines active flexion and extension of the limbs or trunk. Each of the five factors of the profile can earn 2 points if normal; if the patient achieves 8 to 10 points, the fetus is considered healthy. A score of 2 or less suggests consideration of elective delivery. Additional tests are constantly being developed. Recent research has introduced pre-natal screenings for hepatitis B virus, herpes simplex virus, and congenital toxoplasmosis.

Immediately at birth, the newborn receives its first medical examination. Several scales have been developed to assess the status of the newborn, but perhaps the best known is the Apgar scale, named after pediatrician Virginia Apgar. This scale assesses the infant's color, respirations, reflex responses, heart rate, and muscle tone. Each category is scored by someone present at the delivery who assigns 0 to 2 points for the five areas at 1 and 5 minutes after birth. Thus, a perfect score is 10, but scores between 7 and 10 at 1 and 5 minutes are considered high. This scale has been in use since the 1950s, and studies have confirmed its reliability and value in predicting neonatal mortality. The most useful aspects of this scale are the categories for heart rate and respirations. Heart rate should be over 100 beats/minute, and respirations should be deep and even, usually with crying as well. It is becoming increasingly obvious, however, that the Apgar scale is indeed merely a screening. Additional problems can arise after 5 minutes, and therefore a more careful examination is necessary. In addition to tests for neurologic integrity, the neonate may be subject to state-imposed tests for phenylketonuria, a Vitamin K shot to insure clotting, or ophthalmic treatments within 2 hours of birth to prevent venereal disease.

Most infants delivered in a hospital or clinic will have a thorough examination by a pediatrician or family physician before discharge. This examination includes careful scrutiny of skin, bony development, weight and weight gain, muscle tone, behavior, and neurologic maturation. The Apgar scale is not the assessment of choice to detect subtle differences or systemic dysfunctions that show up later in the infant's life, including the potential effects of anesthesia used during labor or delivery. This observation has been apparent for many years, however, and numerous scales have been developed to assess the infant's health. Perhaps one of the best known scales is the Brazelton Neonatal Behavioral Assessment Scale, developed by T. Berry Brazelton, M.D. a pediatrician and author of several books on infant care. Like Brazelton's scale, other similar screenings and evaluation tools focus on the neonate's neurologic status, including motor and sensory components, behavior, and reflex activity. Within the physical therapy realm, pioneers like the Bobath's, Rood, Knott, and

Fiorentino have offered techniques for assessment and treatment of infants with neuromuscular dysfunction that are based on these neurologic screenings. The reader is referred to pediatric literature for specific testing items.

SELF-ASSESSMENT REVIEW

1. It is of great clinical importance that the placenta implant in the _____ of the uterus.

2. The placenta serves as a means of _____ for nutrients needed by the fetus.

3. Drugs cannot pass through the placenta to the fetus, true or false?

4. An example of a suspected teratogen is _____.

5. An example of a confirmed teratogen is _____.

6. Pregnant women should be concerned about working with chemicals and computers, true or false?

7. Commercial formulas are the same composition as human breast milk, true or false?

8. Newborns need a precise combination of nutrients such as _____, _____, and _____ to thrive and grow.

9. The _____ scale is a screening immediately after birth to assess the health of the newborn.

10. More detailed tests of newborn health include tests of _____.

Answers

1. Upper third. 2. Transportation. 3. False. 4. Smoking (or others in text). 5. Cocaine (or others in text). 6. True. 7. False. 8. Carbohydrates, proteins, fats. 9. Apgar. 10. The neonate's neurologic status, including motor and sensory components, behavior, and reflex activity.

REFERENCES

1. Snell RS. *Clinical Embryology for Medical Students*. Boston, Mass: Little, Brown & Co; 1972.

2. Hill LM, Breckle R. Wolfgram KR. An ultrasonic view of the developing fetus. *Obstet Gynecol Surv*. 1983;38:375-398.

3. Rayburn WF, Lavin JP. *Obstetrics for the House Officer*. Baltimore, Md: Williams & Wilkins; 1988.

4. Nilsson L. *A Child is Born*. New York, NY: Dell Publishing; 1965.

5. Rosenberg L, Mitchell AA, Shapiro S, Slone D. Selected birth defects in relation to caffeine containing beverages. *JAMA*. 1982;247:1429-32.

6. Warwick R. Williams PL. *Gray's Anatomy*. 35th ed. Philadelphia, Pa: WB Saunders; 1973.

7. Ganong WF. *Review of Medical Physiology*. 11th ed. Los Altos: Lange Medical Publications; 1983.

8. Kennaugh JM, Hay WW. Nutrition of the fetus and newborn. *West J Med*. 1987;147:435-448.

9. Flanagan GL. *The First Nine Months of Life*. New York, NY: Simon & Schuster; 1962.

10. DiMaio MS, Baumgarten A, Greenstein RM, Saal HM, Mahoney MJ. Screening for fetal Down syndrome in pregnancy by measuring maternal serum alpha-fetoprotein levels. *N Engl J Med*. 1987;317:342-6.

11. O'Brien WD. Ultrasonic bioeffects: A view of experimental studies. *Birth*. 1984;11:149-57.

12. Petitti DB. Effects of inutero ultrasound exposure in humans. *Birth*. 1984;11:159-63.

13. American College of Obstetricians and Gynecologists. Diagnostic ultrasound in obstetrics and gynecology. ACOG *Technical Bulletin*. 1981;63:Oct.

14. International Childbirth Education Association. ICEA position paper: Diagnostic ultrasound in obstetrics. *ICEA News*. 1983;22.

15. Beckman CRB, et al. *Obstetrics and Gynecology*. 2nd ed. Baltimore, Md: Williams & Wilkins; 1994.

16. DeVoe LD. Clinical features of the reactive positive contraction stress test. *Obstet Gynecol*. 1984;63(4):523-7.

9

Physical Therapy
Care During Labor

There is increasing appreciation of the role of the physical therapist in the care of the laboring woman. Pain relief measures that can be provided by the therapist include instruction in positioning, childbirth education (see Chapter 4 Early Pregnancy Classes and Chapter 10 Childbirth Preparation Classes), and the use of transcutaneous electrical nerve stimulation (TENS).

LATE PREGNANCY: PRODROME TO LABOR

In the last trimester, the fetus takes up most of the room inside the uterus, and the uterus takes up most of the room inside the abdominal cavity. The mother may find it difficult to breathe deeply or catch her breath after exertion. That is, until the last few weeks of the pregnancy (Figure 9-1). Towards the end of term, the baby may approach the bony pelvis, and the mother may feel as though she can take a deep breath again. This event is termed "lightening," and may be accompanied by additional maternal symptoms such as increased pelvic pressure and need to urinate, constipation from pressure on the intestines, vulvar or rectal varicosities, and edema in the lower extremities related to pressure on blood vessels. Throughout the pregnancy, and especially starting around the seventh month of gestation, uterine contractions may be felt by the expectant mother. These contractions are thought to be similar to warm-up exercises as the uterus prepares for a long, continuous workout. Sometimes called Braxton Hicks contractions (named after their founders), they may be strong enough in the latter months to cause some cervical effacement or dilation.

The part of the fetus that lies closest to the cervix is the presenting part; this is most commonly the head, but may be the feet, knees, buttocks, and occasionally an arm. Any position, or lie, of the fetus other than head first is considered breech presentation and is a potential complication for delivery and the progress of labor. The obstetric caregiver can tell by physical examination, and by listening to the fetal heartbeat, the position of the fetus. This position may change frequently during pregnancy, but less often as term approaches. Babies have been known to change from breech to cephalic presentation (head down) in the beginning of labor, but usually once labor starts the position is fixed. As the fetus draws closer to the bony pelvis it is considered to be floating (freely moving), dipping (presenting part passes into the inlet), or engaged (the presenting part at its widest diameter passes through the pelvic inlet). In the primigravida, or a woman in her first pregnancy (as opposed

Figure 9-1. Full-term pregnancy. (Reprinted with permission from O'Connor LJ, Gourley Stephenson RJ. *Obstetric and Gynecologic Care in Physical Therapy.* Thorofare, NJ: SLACK Incorporated; 1990.)

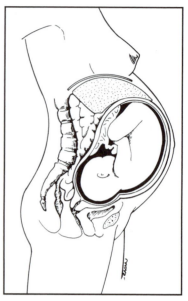

to multigravida), engagement often occurs 2 to 3 weeks before labor. In the multigravida(a woman who has been pregnant more than once), engagement may not occur until labor starts, or may even occur during labor. In either case, engagement is often associated with cervical effacement. The neck of the uterus thins, shortens, and softens and becomes quite stretchy during labor. In the multipara (a woman who has delivered two or more viable children), the uterus is often thinner and softer; therefore, engagement may not seem to occur as suddenly as it might in the primipara (a woman who has delivered one child after 20 weeks of gestation). Also, near the onset of labor, women may lose a few pounds, feel renewed energy and have an intense need to finalize preparations for the newborn. This intense need is known as nesting.

NORMAL LABOR

The onset of labor happens primarily in three ways: rupture of the amniotic sac, bloody show, or contractions that become stronger and rhythmic. False labor episodes occur often, usually mimicking true labor with contractions that get stronger, longer, and closer together. While these contractions may be exciting, and seem like the real thing, it is this false labor that may stop if the woman changes activities (goes for a walk or takes a rest) or, more commonly, after she arrives at the hospital. The contractions of real labor, though, do not disappear with activity.

Bloody show is the passing of the mucus plug that formed early in the pregnancy to seal off the uterus from the external world. As the cervix thins and softens, the plug simply dislodges. When it dislodges, it tends to break free from the uterine wall, and in so doing breaks some of the small blood vessels. As a sign of impending labor though, it is unreliable since it may pass whenever the cervix starts to dilate and soften. Many women never see the bloody show; it may pass unnoticed while using the bathroom.

Rupture of the membranes, however, is a more reliable indicator of impending labor. In fact, if the membranes rupture, the woman will either start labor on her own or it may be started for her via intravenous oxytocin drip anywhere from 8 to 48 hours afterwards. Many labors, however, continue with the membranes intact until the end of the first stage. It is believed that the fluid in the amniotic sac provides a cushion between the fetal head and the cervix, thereby reducing stress on the fetus.

After the membranes rupture, the inside is exposed to the outside, infection is a possibility, and contractions seem to increase in frequency and intensity, because of the firmer pressure exerted on the cervix by the presenting part. The mother may experience either a sudden gush of fluid or a trickle, depending on where the membranes rupture. If the tear is high towards the fundus, there will probably be a trickle with each contraction. If the tear is low, fluid will gush forth, mostly during one or two contractions; however, there is still plenty of fluid left around the baby, and the membranes continue to produce fluid during labor. Women can be advised to investigate the fluid for odor, color, and ability to stop the flow if they are unsure whether the fluid is amniotic or urine.

Some physicians start infusing oxytocin (usually a synthetic - pitocin) after 8 hours with no regular contractions, while some will wait longer and allow the woman to monitor her temperature at home for signs of infection. Pitocin drip or "pit" causes contractions in uterine muscle. For some reason, these artificially-induced contractions seem stronger to women who have had previous labor contractions. The woman must also labor with an intravenous line in place, which is uncomfortable for many. The idea behind using pitocin is to stimulate the uterus to start contracting on its own. When contractions start on their own, the pitocin is stopped.

Although some people describe their 24-hour labor or their 10-hour labor, it is always difficult to compare the two experiences, since the perception of when labor starts can vary greatly. For instance, one woman may consider labor started at the first contraction; another may consider labor started when contractions became regular; and another when the membranes ruptured. Studies of length of labor suggest an average first labor of 12 to 14 hours and subsequent labors of 6 to 8 hours. Since these are average figures, however, labor may be longer or shorter; but usually after 24 hours of labor, the health care provider considers intervention by forceps or by cesarean section. The decision to intervene depends on the fetal and maternal health during labor and on the policies of the physician or obstetric department.

Labor is simply the process by which the uterus expels the fetus. What triggers labor to start is unknown: theories range from a preset lifetime of the placenta to some type of stretch initiated response as the fetal size increases. This latter theory does little to support premature birth. It is known that oxytocin is secreted around the time of labor onset and that oxytocin causes uterine contraction. What is even more interesting is that oxytocin is purely specific to uterine contraction. Oxytocin is also secreted in response to nipple stimulation, particularly during lactation; and in fact, this response has been tried as a method to stimulate post-mature labor, with limited success. It is believed this response is nature's way of returning the uterus to prepregnant size as the mother nurses the infant.

The muscle fibers of the uterus run longitudinally, transversely, and in a figure-eight pattern. Therefore, muscle contraction causes a downward force and an upward pull starting from the fundus and moving caudally to the cervix area. The contractions tend to become stronger, longer, and closer together if labor progresses normally and efficiently. Contractions may start approximately 20 minutes apart and gradually occur less than 1 minute apart, or in an erratic fashion close to delivery. These contractions may also start out fairly mild and build in intensity; although when a beginning labor contraction is considered mild, it is definitely a relative term. To the woman having her first labor, the early contractions may seem very strong-that is, until she experiences those of later labor.

Figure 9-2. Effacement and dilation. (Reprinted with permission from O'Connor LJ, Gourley Stephenson RJ. *Obstetric and Gynecologic Care in Physical Therapy.* Thorofare, NJ: SLACK Incorporated; 1990.)

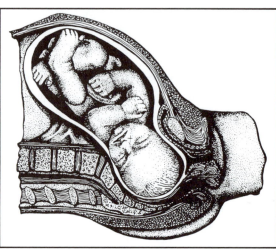

Figure 9-3. Station. (Reprinted with permission from O'Connor LJ, Gourley Stephenson RJ. *Obstetric and Gynecologic Care in Physical Therapy.* Thorofare, NJ: SLACK Incorporated; 1990.)

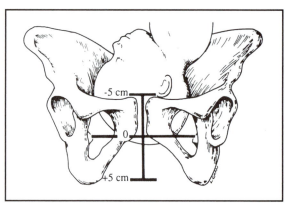

In any event, the sum force of these contractions is to thin out or efface the cervix, measured as a percentage of complete effacement of 100% (about 0.25 mm thick), and to dilate or open the cervix completely from 0 cm to 10 cm (diameter of the cervical os) for passage of the fetus. Effacement and dilation are measured manually. The cervix also tends to soften as labor starts or during the weeks prior to onset (Figure 9-2).

As the contractions occur and the cervix effaces and dilates, the fetus is being assisted down into the birth canal. The descent of the fetal presenting part is measured by station (centimeters above or below the ischial spines; -5 is 5 cm above the ischial spines, +5 is 5 cm below or caudal to the ischial spines- Figure 9-3). When the fetus passes through the cervix, passes through the vagina, and the largest diameter of the fetal head is seen at the vaginal opening in the perineum, the fetus is considered to be "crowning." Prior to crowning, however, the mechanism of labor may be described as follows: in the cephalic presentation, engagement is followed by an attitude of flexion of the fetal neck, then the neck rotates (internal rotation) with the occiput anterior (baby's face to the mother's spine) to fit through the pelvis, followed by neck extension as the head passes under the pubic arch and continues to the outside. After this event, delivery is hopefully imminent, barring any complications in extracting the rest of the body. Once the head is born, the head again rotates (external rotation) to realign with the shoulders, the upper shoulder maneuvers under the pubic bone, then the lower shoulder, and the rest of the body slides out. This is the moment of birth, and technically, labor has ended.

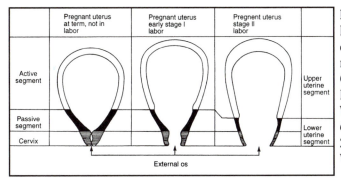

Figure 9-4. First stage of labor; cervix starting to dilate. (Reprinted with permission from Beckman CRB, Ling FW, Barzansky BM, Bates GW, Herbert WNP, Laube DW, Smith RP. *Obstetrics and Gynecology.* 2nd ed. Baltimore, Md: Williams & Wilkins; 1994.)

The easiest way to understand human labor is to divide it into stages and phases. Four stages divide labor into the period of thinning and dilating of the uterine cervix as the baby descends (Stage I-see Figure 9-4), delivery of the infant (Stage II), delivery of the placenta (Stage III), and post-partum (Stage IV). Stage I is actually what is commonly known as labor and is further divided into three phases: early labor or latent phase, active labor or active phase, and late labor or transition. The basic characteristics of the first stage and its phases, as well as relief measures, are described in Table 9-1. These characteristics have been placed in a chart form that has been used as a patient handout for couples attending childbirth education classes. Stages II, III, and IV will be discussed in other chapters.

The early or latent phase of labor is usually the longest because contractions are milder and stay at the peak for a shorter time than later contractions. Again, it is difficult to judge exactly how long this phase will be, but on average, it lasts from a few up to 10 or more hours. During this time, the mother is excited and probably initially unsure whether this is true labor or not. The hallmark of this phase is effacement of the cervix and dilation to 3 cm.

Between 4 cm and 7 cm dilation is the active phase of first stage labor. This is typically a busy time for the mother, and not only because the contractions are getting longer, stronger, and closer together. If she is having a hospital birth, it will most likely also be the time that contractions are about 5 minutes apart, regular, and of a stronger intensity than in early labor. It is at this time that physicians usually suggest the woman be admitted to the hospital. Women that attend childbirth education classes learn how to relax, breathe, and deal with the pain associated with labor contractions during admission procedures. This time can be particularly stressful to some women and couples.

Late labor, or transition, is marked by 7 cm to 10 cm dilation, frequent, lengthy, intense contractions, and possibly by symptoms of nausea, vomiting, trembling legs, and feelings of discouragement. This is generally the most difficult phase of labor, but also the shortest. At 10 cm dilation, the woman in the hospital is allowed to push, whether or not she experiences any urge to do so. This magic number, estimated by manual measurement, is the signal that the cervix is completely open and ready for passage of the fetus. The transition phase may take about an hour or so, and pushing may take an hour or longer, if left alone. Once the fetal presenting part (hopefully the head) passes through the cervix, it enters the birth canal. The vagina is capable of instant expansion to accommodate the fetus as it rotates under the pubic bone and down to the perineum. As the widest part of the fetal head passes through the vaginal opening, crowning has occurred, and delivery is imminent.

Preparation for labor and delivery in the hospital, depending on the policies of the hospital and the policies of the physician, can include enemas, pubic hair shaving, hooking up of an electronic fetal monitor, and many questions. Enemas to cleanse the lower bowel and

Table 9-1

Phases of First Stage Human Labor

Phase	Characteristics	What to do	How to help
Effacement 0-3 to 4cm dilation, 20~5 min apart	Cervix softens, thins, begins to dilate; mild contractions begin; length of phase varies; may see show or fluid leakage; may have backache, nausea	Relaxation; continue light activity at home; deep breathe when no longer can walk, talk; rest; urinate often	Assist in relaxation with touch, imagery; watch for signs of tension; time contractions; observe type of contractions; apply back pressure; prepare for hospital
Active 4-7cm dilation, 60 see long, 5~1 min apart	Cervix opens; baby comes down; contractions increase; 2-9 hours; may feel pressure in low back, groin, and perineum	May feel busy or discouraged; concentrate on breathing; change positions; urinate often; conserve energy; use effleurage	Encourage relaxation; relieve tension; help with positioning; breathe with her; watch for hyperventilation; apply counterpressure; give ice chips; praise her; ask about progress
Late (Transition) 7-l0cm dilation, 60-90 sec long, erratic	Cervix is open; baby enters birth canal (20-60 min); may feel irritable, out of control, hot, dizzy, tingly; may have rectal or perineal pressure, hiccups, nausea, shaky legs, desire to push	Relax body, perineum; remember baby is coming; rest between contractions; change positions; relax; maintain breathing	Help with relaxation and position; time contractions; help her breathe at the start of each contraction; breathe with her; watch for hyperventilation; praise her; apply counterpressure; remind about baby coming

pubic hair shaving to reduce the risk of infection from bacteria used to be standard procedures. Research has suggested that no greater risk exists without pubic hair shaving and that bowel evacuation is solely to encourage uninhibited pushing by the mother. For these reasons, many physicians no longer insist on these procedures. Other options for labor and delivery exist aside from the traditional hospital birth. Women need to look for hospitals that will let them walk and move around during labor, assume different positions for labor or delivery than standard lithotomy, and receive minimal intervention from nursing staff if that is their choice. Women should also be advised to explore a variety of childbirth education classes that exist to help women reduce anxiety and pain of labor. Each class may utilize different methods to cope with labor. All are based on relaxation and some type of breathing techniques, as well as education about the birthing process. Even if women are introspective and tuned in to the changes in their body during labor, childbirth education classes are probably a good idea to learn varied pain relief methods, to share feelings with other pregnant couples, and to understand what will happen before, during, and after labor.

One of the most important aspects of care is providing the woman with a support partner during labor—it may be the father, a friend, a health professional, or another family member. The support for the woman in labor is so important that studies have shown reduction in length of labor, reduction in pain analgesia, and in some a reduction in operative deliveries. Studies have also recorded improved mental state in the post-partum woman with greater self-esteem, more women breastfeeding, and women have more positive responses to their babies in those who had support of a doula (a trained lay person).[1] Similarly a large California-based health-maintenance organization showed reduced epidural use and a more positive birth experience in those women who were provided a doula versus those who were not. There was no difference in rates of operative deliveries, need for oxytocin, breastfeeding, nor self-esteem in this study.[2]

COMPLICATED LABOR

Although it may seem that the phases of labor are fairly well delineated and that the normal labor will run a predictable course, there is no such thing as a classic textbook case when it comes to labor. The figures we hear about as being average are just that, average. Researchers do know, however, that in normal labor the contractions tend to get stronger, longer, and closer together; the cervix effaces and dilates at a certain rate; and the fetus moves down against the cervix as labor progresses. Occasionally, though, contractions do not cause cervical dilation, the fetus does not descend, or other delays in progress occur. These situations present complications in labor and are generally called dystocia.

Premature labor contractions can result in the birth of a premature infant (weight less than 5 pounds 8 ounces) and can be caused by several factors. Among these are premature rupture of membranes, incompetent cervix, trauma, placenta previa, abruptio placentae, or illness. A recent study suggests premature contractions might be linked to maternal standing with little movement.[3]

There is no known cause for premature rupture of the membranes. It occurs in 10% to 12% of women, resulting in a premature infant 20% of the time.[4] In some cases, premature rupture of the membranes is associated with cervical incompetency. But other times, the cervix is unfavorable or unripe (less than 80% effaced and 2 cm dilated).

An incompetent cervix is a weak cervix that may shorten, efface, and dilate during pregnancy. If the woman makes it to labor, progress is often rapid as well. This weakness has been treated a variety of ways: either by cerclage, which involves placing a suture around the cervix; by placing the patient on bed rest; or by using tocolytic therapy if premature contractions occur. Tocolytic therapy employs medications such as ritodrine or terbutaline that inhibit uterine contractions. The drug may be infused and then administered orally in a maintenance dosage. Physical therapists have become more involved with this clientele by providing instruction in bed exercises and transfer methods to reduce intraabdominal pressure and pressure on the cervix (see Chapter 6).

On the opposite end of the spectrum is the post-date pregnancy, over 42 weeks' gestation. Studies suggest a greater risk of fetal mortality and morbidity from post-date pregnancies than in those delivered at term, probably related to the decay of the placental function.[5] Stress testing and induction of labor have not been associated with reduced mortality, but maternal breast stimulation to induce uterine contractions has shown some success. Another method currently being researched to induce labor is the use of prostaglandins administered vaginally.[6]

Abnormal placement of the placenta is a potentially serious complication causing significant fetal mortality.[7] Placenta previa is an implantation of the placenta low in the uterus that remains low or even covering the cervical os at term. This happens only 2% to 3% of the time.[8] Cesarean section is usually recommended unless the placenta is only marginally covering the os and there is little danger of the placenta preceding the delivery of the infant. If the placenta or the umbilical cord precedes the infant, blood supply and, therefore, oxygen supply is jeopardized.

Occasionally the umbilical cord will prolapse through the vagina if membranes are ruptured. This presents a hazardous situation as the infant may compress the cord against the sides of the birth canal as it descends.

Abruptio placentae is a premature peeling away of the placenta from the uterine wall. Again, this is a dangerous situation that may require cesarean section.

Aside from these less common complications of labor are episodes of malpresentation, malposition, uterine dysfunction, pelvic contraction, and passage of meconium. Malpresentation refers to any part, other than the fetal head, that is presenting to the cervix, and therefore will be born first. This presenting part can be a breech (buttocks, knees, or feet first), shoulder, face, or brow of the fetus. Any of these presentations complicate the progress of labor. Researchers have conducted studies that suggest that the mother who assumes a lateral position on the same side as the fetal spine may correct an occipito-posterior position and thereby reduce the need for cesearean delivery.[9]

Breech presentations prior to labor are fairly common, but remain that way for delivery only 3% to 4% of the time. When the fetus is breech, the mother may feel kicking against the rectum and fetal movement more in the lower abdomen. Because of the uneven pressure from the presenting part, as opposed to the pressure when the head is down, it has been theorized that the cervix dilates more slowly and labor and descent take longer. However, research does not bear out this theory.[4] The major problem with a breech presentation is that the largest and least moldable part, the head, must be born last. If the pelvic outlet will not accommodate the head, or if the cervix is not dilated completely and the body slips through, the fetus may be jeopardized. For this reason, many physicians elect to deliver breech babies by cesarean section, especially if the baby appears to be large. Specific types of breech deliveries are discussed in a later chapter. Basic breech presentations may be complete (knees and hips flexed), frank (hips flexed, knees extended; the most common type), footling (hips and at least one knee extended with the foot coming first) or kneeling (one or two hips extended, knees flexed and coming first) (see Figure 10-6).

Fetal heart tones will be heard at different locations depending on the presentation and position. Position refers to the orientation of the presenting part and is designated by stating where a certain point on that part is located in relation to the front, back, or sides of the mother's pelvis. That certain part is called a denominator and is the occiput for the cephalic presentation, sacrum for breech presentations, and scapula for shoulder presentations. The most common is the left occiput anterior, abbreviated LOA. For brow presentations, the chart may note Fr for forehead; for face presentations, an M for mentum or chin.

Another way fetal position is described is by lie, that is the orientation of the longitudinal axis of the fetus to that of the mother while standing. Lie may be longitudinal (cephalic or buttocks), transverse, or oblique. Transverse lie that persists is almost always an indication for delivery by cesarean.[4]

The uterus is subject to a variety of dysfunctions, prolapse, anatomic anomalies, sacculation (the presence or formation of sacs), torsion, poor quality contractions, or failure of the cervix to dilate. Cervical dystocia may arise from anatomic anomaly, scarring, or carcinoma. Contractions may intensify until the cervix ruptures or detaches. However, if parts of the uterus do not work in synergy, contraction strength diminishes, and labor is slower. The uterus can also develop an inefficient type of tetany that produces few, if any, productive contractions. Incoordinate uterine action occurs most frequently in primigravidas.

A contracted pelvis, at the inlet, midpelvis, or outlet, can also jeopardize labor progress because of bony impedance to the fetus. A past history of pelvic fracture mandates careful examination of the pelvic capacity, hopefully prior to pregnancy. There is also a variety of pelvic deformities linked to spinal deformity and to leg length discrepancy from childhood.

MATERNAL POSITION AND STATE

Contrary to the "flat on the back" position assumed by many laboring women for many years, it is believed that the instinct to remain upright and moving can help labor progress. In fact, studies of the effects of maternal position during labor show that fetal oxygen saturation may decrease more when mother is in the supine position than when she is in the left lateral position.[10] Likewise, if mother has had an epidural for pain relief, the supine position may reduce cardiac output more than if mother remains in lateral position.[11] When a woman is ambulatory, it is believed that she utilizes the forces of gravity to assist fetal descent. Research does exist to support the theory that ambulation shortens the length of labor,[12] and reduces the risk of operative delivery,[13] yet other studies have found no harm or benefit from ambulation during labor.[14] Sitting versus laying down in labor also tends to increase the pelvic outlet.[15] Therefore, even if a woman must be strapped to an electronic fetal monitor or intravenous line, she should try to stay upright and change positions fairly often.

Another misconception about labor is the idea that a full bladder impedes the progress of labor. A study on this topic found no effect of a full bladder on uterine activity and labor duration.[16] However, she will be more comfortable with her bladder empty during labor. It is also believed that labor may be complicated in the very young and very old. A study of nulliparas under 15 years of age compared to nulliparous women aged 20 to 29 years showed no difference in cervical dilatation at admission, need for labor induction, use of epidurals, frequency of preterm birth or birth weight. Length of active phase of labor and cesarean delivery were reduced in the adolescent group.[17] However, the rate of cesarean delivery was higher in older women having their first baby.[18]

PAIN MECHANISMS AND RELIEF

Although labor pains were for many years a woman's cross to bear, the acceptance of anesthesia for obstetric practice changed that way of thinking. And with Queen Victoria's approval of and insistence upon using chloroform for her own birthing process, physicians thereby gained approval for its use with the common folk. The pains of labor vary from woman to woman. One woman can have little pain; in fact, it is not uncommon to hear stories about someone who unknowingly delivers a child. These stories may be farfetched, because there are legitimate physical causes of pain in addition to any psychological overlay. "Labor pain is not of a single intensity but of varying intensities and is usually greatest only for a few seconds at the peak of contractions. Labor pain is not the lancing pain of injury, but rather an aching, cramping pain that can be associated with positive functioning, great pressure, or the accomplishing of an important task."[19]

The pain of labor is not easily forgotten, but in many ways the pain of labor is welcome; each pain of the uncomplicated labor signals that the infant is closer to being born. It is also a relief to many to have the pregnancy draw to an end, because the baby becomes heavy and weari-

Table 9-2

Causes of Pain in First Stage Labor

I. Physiological Causes
  Anoxic uterus due to inadequate relaxation of muscle between contractions of late labor

II. Physical Causes
  A. From stretching as fetus descends:
    1. Cervix
    2. Fallopian tubes
    3. Ovaries
    4. Peritoneum
    5. Uterine ligaments
    6. Pelvic floor muscles
    7. Perineum
  B. From pressure (exerted by the fetus and uterine contractions):
    1. Nerve ganglia near cervix
    2. Nerve ganglia near vagina
    3. Urethra
    4. Bladder
    5. Rectum
    6. Nerve Pathways
      Sympathetic sensory: Uterine contractions and cervical dilation - sympathetic-uterosacral ligaments- uterine, pelvic, hypogastric, aortic plexuses- dorsal roots T11, T12 - spinal cord.
      Sympathetic motor: Uterus- aortic, hypogastric, pelvic, and uterine plexuses to ventral rami of T10-T12.
      Pudendal: Anterior S2-4; passes near ischial spine and to urogenital diaphragm; breaks into inferior hemorrhoidal to lower rectum and rectal area, dorsal clitoris to clitoral area, perineal to vulva, skin, fascia, and deep perineal muscles.
      Posterior femoral cutaneous: may pass impulses to S2-4
      Ilioinguinal: may pass impulses to L1.

some to some women in the last month, in particular. Women may also find they have to get up at night to urinate because of pressure from the fetus on the bladder. Although this may be good practice for those night feedings after the baby is born, the broken sleep tends to wear on many women and bearing the pregnancy becomes tiresome. Once labor does start, there are real causes of pain (Table 9-2). As the fetus descends and the uterus contracts, there is increased pressure on organs, tissues, and nerves and increased pull on ligaments, tissues, and muscles. Women may also experience pain in the lower abdomen or in the back related to posterior position of the fetus, inefficiency of uterine contractions, or a cervix resistant to dilation. The uterus that contracts uncoordinatedly or spasms may cause additional pain as well.

What happens to the patient with back pain during pregnancy when she goes into labor? Anecdotal evidence suggests that back pain does not interfere with labor or delivery. In fact, women with back pain during the entire pregnancy may have no back pain during labor, and conversely, women who had no significant back pain during pregnancy may have severe back pain during labor. However, the back pain experienced only during labor, referred to as "back labor," arises from pressure on lumbar and sacral nerves from the fetal head as it works its way into the pelvis and birth canal. In a retrospective study of 170 women with 400 pregnancies and deliveries, 42.5% of the pregnancies were complicated by back pain. Of these pregnancies, 72% also reported back labor.[20] Successful vaginal deliveries have occurred even in women with herniated discs.

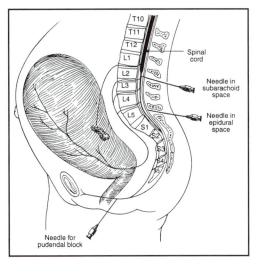

Figure 9-5. Anesthetic blocks. (Reprinted with permission from Beckman CRB, Ling FW, Barzansky BM, Bates GW, Herbert WNP, Laube DW, Smith RP. *Obstetrics and Gynecology.* 2nd ed. Baltimore, Md: Williams & Wilkins; 1994.)

Since the Victorian era, relief of labor pain has shown little progress, although measures have been developed to lessen that pain in varying degrees. Three general categories of pain relief exist: medications/anesthesia, prenatal childbirth education, and more recently, TENS. The practicing physical therapist may receive questions about the types of drugs used for labor pain. Basically, these drugs fall into categories of analgesia or anesthesia and are used specifically for either first stage or second stage. Analgesic agents are used to raise pain thresholds or induce sleepiness and are administered either orally or by injection. Anesthetic agents block nerves and are administered by infusion or inhalation (Figure 9-5). The phase of first stage, during which pain relief is needed, may also determine the type of medication selected by the physician or anesthesiologist. The dosage required, length of action by the particular drug, or maternal and fetal side effects warrant careful selection (Table 9-3).

In some cases, analgesia or anesthesia may be titrated or administered more than once during a labor. In other cases, analgesia may be given later to be followed by an anesthetic for stronger contractions in active labor. It is wise to remember that, while some drugs cause less pain and have been proven entirely safe for the fetus, all drugs are believed to cross the placenta. Drug companies perform tests under specific conditions of dosage, time during labor, and health of the mother and baby. In cases that do not follow these specific criteria, outcome is undetermined. This does not mean that the physical therapist then warns mothers not to use drugs for labor pain relief. The role of the physical therapist is to educate expectant parents (without bias if the parents decide to use medications) about the risks and benefits of therapeutic drug use and to encourage discussion of their concerns with their birth attendant. Parents should be told the effects of medications and anesthetics used by their birth attendant and whether there have been any long-term deficits associated with administration of that drug during labor. Patient-controlled epidural analgesia in labor has been in use for about a decade, but researchers have been attempting to provide optimal pain relief with minimal side effects. Recent combination of spinal-epidural analgesia may be effective.[21] In a retrospective study of over 6,000 combined spinal and epidural blocks in which over 4,000 were used for labor pain relief, patients who received systemic narcotics less than 6 hours before the blocks were more likely to require intravenous treatment for low oxygen saturations, dysphagia, or pruritius. The authors of this study believe that this form of labor analgesia is safe

Table 9-3

First Stage Medications

Type	Action	Example	How Administered, Time to Work, How Long Lasts	Side Effects Mother	Baby
Narcotics	Pain relief	Demerol	IM, 5-20 min, 1-4 hrs	Nausea Respiration decrease, contractions decrease	Respiration decrease
Tranquilizer	Relaxant	Vistaril	IM, 15-20 min, 3-4 hrs	BP decrease, lethargy, sleepiness	Respiration decrease
Barbiturate	Relaxant	Seconal	PO, 20-30 min, 3-4 hrs	Hangover, lethargy, moodiness, anxiety, effects long-lasting	Respiration decrease

and effective, but that mothers should be monitored with continuous pulse oximetry.[22] Epidural analgesia has also been implicated in delay of labor necessitating obstetrical intervention. However, a study by the National Institute of Child Health and Development determined that epidural analgesia with low-dose bupivacaine may increase the need for oxytocin administration, but not cesarean delivery.[23] There is some evidence to suggest that drugs used during labor may have effects on children,[24] reaching into their school-age years or longer. The decision, then, belongs to the parents to make after they have collected enough information to feel comfortable about using therapeutic drugs during labor without regrets (Tables 9-4 and 9-5).

Many women who go through labor and birth are disappointed; many are not. Those who are, often say, "Next time it'll be different." This usually means they will obtain a different birth attendant, hospital or setting, or avoid medications. Another factor to consider is that one medication often leads to another and may result in complicating labor. For instance, some drugs slow labor contractions, and because regional anesthesia can also affect motor control, forceps may be required if the mother is unable to push the baby out during delivery. One other point worth mentioning is that the contractions of late labor are generally the most painful, and last the least amount of time. Often, strong encouragement and support from a spouse or loved one can help the woman bear the last few contractions before the cervix is fully dilated. Because the contractions of the second stage involve active pushing, the excitement increases, and the pain may seem to decrease. Prior studies showed that women with first labors and deliveries had more pain than women with subsequent labors and deliveries. However, in a recent study of labor pain in women with a minimum of five previous deliveries compared to those delivering their first child, all women had intense pain during labor.[25] In addition, the women who had given birth before did not receive epidurals, compared to 40% of the first time women. The women with several prior births believed their pain relief was inadequate, particularly at the end of labor, during delivery, and in the days following delivery.

Despite all the pain, few women who want children avoid subsequent pregnancies because of the labor of the first. The birth of a healthy child, for most women, is worth any amount

Table 9-4

First Stage Anesthetics: Regional

Type	Site	Area Numbed	Time to Work, How Long Lasts	Side Effects Mother	Baby
Epidural	Lumbar epidural space	Below navel	10-20 min, 60-90 min	BP decreased Possible, numbing on 1 side, forceps use	HR decreased O2 decreased
Caudal	Sacral below cord	Pelvic area	10-20 min, 60-90 min	Pushing urge decreased forceps use	HR decreased
Spinal	Spinal fluid	Below injection site	Immediate, 60-90 min	BP decreased Headache, forceps use	O2 decreased

Table 9-5

First Stage Anesthetics: Local

Type	Site	Area Numbed	Time to Work, How Long Lasts	Side Effects Mother	Baby
Paracervical	Cervix	Cervix	5-20 min, 1 hr	Weak/numb LEs	HR flux

of pain. Every woman's labor is different, and only she knows the amount of pain she experiences. An informed decision is the goal of education. If a woman decides emphatically that she does not want to take medications unless absolutely necessary, the only other option that is fairly well accepted by physicians, primarily because of consumer demand, is childbirth education. The most popular forms are psychoprophylaxis (ASPO/Lamaze) and variations of relaxation techniques combined with patterned breathing methods. Psychoprophylaxis is a technique adopted by Dr. Fernando Lamaze after he visited Russia, where this breathing and relaxation method was taught to laboring women. Lamaze introduced the idea of the monitrice, or labor attendant, to help women learn these methods. In the 1950s, the method worked its way to the United States, primarily with the assistance of a book, titled *Thank You, Dr. Lamaze*, and promotion by Elisabeth Bing, PT, who was instrumental in the development of the early childbirth organization and pro-consumer movement. This technique uses physical and psychological relaxation as a foundation, to which deep, shallow, and paced breathing techniques are added as the pains increase in intensity and frequency. Instructors of other methods utilize relaxation and deep breathing methods more than some Lamaze instructors (see chapter on delivery for childbirth preparation classes). Basic philosophies are similar, and classes are eagerly sought by many women. Reasons for the popularity of childbirth education classes center mainly around the need for women to take an active rather than a passive role in the birth of their child. These methods also usually include instruction for the father at the same time, a trend set by Dr. Robert Bradley of the Bradley Method and the American Academy of Husband Coached Childbirth. However, even patterned breathing may take its toll on the laboring woman. A study of use of patterned breathing showed that women exhibited more fatigue during the latent phase of labor, whereas during the active phase, differences were less between groups of women. The researchers concluded that patterned breathing should be encouraged but may increase the mother's fatigue if started too early.[26]

The third alternative for the control of labor pain is TENS. Physical therapists should be aware that use of TENS during labor is not listed as an indication for TENS by the Food and Drug Administration, nor has TENS been proven safe or unsafe for the fetus. Research on the safety of TENS for use in labor and delivery is scant and inconclusive.[27-30] Recent studies continue to conflict, with review of trials conducted on 712 women concluding that "randomized controlled trials provide no compelling evidence for TENS having analgesic effect during labor," with "weak positive effects in ... analgesic sparing and... choosing TENS for future labors," perhaps "due to inadequate blinding causing overstimation of treatment effects."[29] Another recent study, however, found that about two-thirds of 104 women thought TENS was effective during labor and would use it again. This population also had a reduced duration of labor and reduced amount of analgesics used with no adverse effects on mothers or newborns.[30] Although some physicians will authorize use of the TENS unit for their patients, a legal challenge of the safety of this has not yet occurred. Because obstetrics is a high-risk profession, malpractice rates for obstetricians are exorbitant. Therefore, the physical therapist practicing obstetrics and using TENS during labor and delivery should be aware of the risks and clarify malpractice insurance coverage with his or her carrier.

The theory of pain relief by TENS in labor was developed out of the work by Melzack and Wall in their work on the gate theory of pain. Activation of pain reduction, they theorized, was due to the stimulation (stimulation is low-intensity, high-frequency at 100 to 200 Hz) of low-threshold nerve fibers, mechanoreceptors and A beta fibers by a TENS unit. Therefore, this stimulation reduces the excitability of A delta and C pain fibers. Consequently, this stimulation by TENS reduces the amount of pain messages passing up the spinal cord so the brain does not receive the client's own message of labor pain. Melzack and Wall also theorized that activation of A delta and C fibers enhanced the release of the body's own natural pain inhibitors, namely endorphins and encephalins. This activation occurs with low-frequency high-intensity stimulation of the TENS unit at 2-10 Hz.[31]

Protocol for the application of the TENS electrodes suggests placement of one pair of electrodes paravertebrally over the T10-T12 area during early labor and another pair over S2-S4 if there is additional back pain (Figure 9-6). Otherwise add the S2-4 electrodes for additional pain relief during delivery to correspond to the nerve pathways. Some experimentation has been done suprapubically, but this evidence is mostly anecdotal.[32] The physical therapist interested in conducting a TENS program for obstetric clients would be wise to collect as much documentation as possible to support research in this area (see Appendix).

SELF-ASSESSMENT REVIEW

1. Symptoms of pregnancy include _____, _____, and _____.
2. By the third or fourth month of pregnancy the uterus may move _____ into the _____ and relieve the pressure on the _____.
3. Toward the end of term, the fetus may approach the bony pelvis. This event is called _____ . Once in the pelvis, _____has occurred.
4. Warm-up or preparatory contractions of the uterus that begin about the seventh month

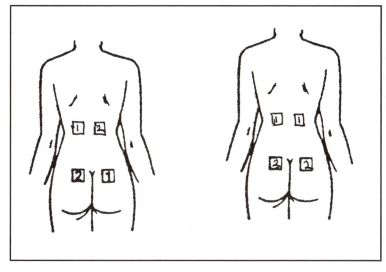

Figure 9-6. Placement of electrodes for labor (a or b) with a two channel set-up. (Adapted from Empi, Inc.. *Clinical Guidelines.* St. Paul, Minn: 1997; 30-32.)

of pregnancy are called _____.

5. The way the fetus is oriented in the abdomen is described by _____, _____, and _____.

6. Signs of true labor include _____, _____, and _____.

7. Labor may be described by stages and phases. Name and define the stages and phases.

8. Labor may be complicated by problems of _____, _____, or _____.

9. Three ways a woman may obtain relief from labor pain are _____, _____, and _____.

10. The physical therapist using TENS for obstetric clients should obtain physician's authorization, clarify insurance coverage, and _____.

Answers

1) Breast tenderness, weight gain, nausea, frequent urination. 2) Upward, abdomen, bladder. 3) Lightening, engagement. 4) Braxton Hicks contractions. 5) Lie, position, presentation, station. 6) Regular contractions, bloody show, rupture of membranes. 7) Stage I, labor or cervical effacement and dilation; Stage II, delivery of the fetus; Stage III, delivery of the placenta; Stage IV, post-partum; Phases- Early or latent (effacement and 0-3 cm dilation), Active (4-7 cm dilation), Late or transition (7-10 cm). 8) poor cervical dilation, poor fetal descent, placental anomalies. 9) Childbirth education, TENS, and medications/anesthetics. 10) Carefully document cases and submit for publication.

REFERENCES

1. Klaus MH, Kennell JH. The doula: An essential ingredient of childbirth rediscovered. *Acta Paediatr.* 1997;86:1034-6.

2. Gordon NP, Walton D, McAdam E, Derman J, Gallitero G, Garrett L. Effects of providing hospital-based doulas in health maintenance organization hospitals. *Obstet Gynecol.* 1999;93:422-6.

3. Schneider KTM, Huch A, Huch R. Premature contractions: Are they caused by maternal standing? *Acta Genet Med Gemellol.* 1985;34:175-7.

4. Oxorn H, Foote WR. *Human Labor & Birth.*3rd ed. New York, NY: Appleton-Century-Crofts; 1975.

5. Elliott JP, Flaherty JF. The use of breast stimulation to prevent post-date pregnancy. *Am J Obstet Gynecol.* 1984;149:628-32.

6. Jagani N, Schulman H, Fleischer A, Mitchell J, Blattner P. Role of prostaglandin-induced cervical changes in labor induction. *Obstet Gynecol.* 1984;63:225-9.

7. McShane PM, Heyl PS, Epstein MF. Maternal and perinatal morbidity resulting from placenta previa. *Obstet Gynecol.* 1985;65:176-82.

8. Rayburn WF, Lavin JP. *Obstetrics for the House Officer.* Baltimore, Md: Williams & Wilkins; 1988.

9. Ou X, Chen X, Su J. Correction of occipito-posterior position by maternal posture during the process of labor [in Chinese]. *Chung Hua Fu Chan Ko Tsa Chih.* 1997;32:329-32.

10. Carbonne B, Benachi A, Leveque ML, Cabrol D, Papiernik E. Maternal position during labor: Effects on fetal oxygen saturation measured by pulse oximetry. *Obstet Gynecol.* 1996;88:797-800.

11. Danilenko-Dixon DR, Tefft L, Cohen RA, Haydon B, Carpenter MW. Positional effects on maternal cardiac output during labor with epidural analgesia. *Am J Obstet Gynecol.* 1996;175:867-72.

12. Flynn AM, Kelly J, Hollins G, Lynch PF. Ambulation in labour. *Brit Med J.* 1978;2:591-3.

13. Albers LL, Anderson D, Cragin L, et al. The relationship of ambulation in labor to operative delivery. *J Nurse Midwifery.* 1997;42:4-8.

14. Bloom SL, McIntire DD, Kelly MA, et al. Lack of effect of walking on labor and delivery. *N Engl J Med.* 1998;339:76-9.

15. Noble E. Controversies in maternal effort during labor and delivery. *J Nurs-Midwifery.* 1981;26:13-22.

16. Kerr-Wilson RHJ, Parham GP, Orr JW. The effect of a full bladder on labor. *Obstet Gynecol.* 1983;62:319-23.

17. Lubarsky SL. Obstetric characteristics among nulliparas under age 15. *Obstet Gynecol.* 1994;84:365-8.

18. Ragosch V. Effect of maternal age on the course of labor-analysis of women over 40 years of age. *Z Geburtshilfe Neonatol.* 1997;201:86-90.

19. Shearer MH. Labor and delivery. In Cooper PJ. ed. *Better Homes and Gardens Woman's Health and Medical Guide.* Des Moines, Ill: Meredith Corp; 1981.

20. Diakow PR, Gadsby TA, Gadsby JB, Gleddie JG, Leprich DJ, Scales AM. Back pain during pregnancy and labor. *J Manipulative Physiol Ther.* 1991;14:116-18.

21. Paech M. New epidural techniques for labour analgesia: Patient-controlled epidural analgesia and combined spinal-epidural analgesia. *Baillieres Clin Obstet Gynaecol.* 1998;12:377-95.

22. Albright GA, Forster RM. The safety and efficacy of combined spinal and epidural analgesia/anesthesia (6,002 blocks) in a community hospital. *Reg Anesth Pain Med.* 1999;24:117-25.

23. Zhang J, Klebanoff MA, DerSimonian R. Epidural analgesia in association with duration of labor and mode of delivery: A quantitative review. *Am J Obstet Gynecol.* 1999;180:970-7.

24. Matheson I, Nylander G. Should pethidine still be administered to women in labor? *Tidsskr Nor Laegeforen.* 1999;119:234-6.

25. Ranta P, Jouppila P, Jouppila R. The intensity of labor pain in grand multiparas. *Acta Obstet Gynecol Scand.* 1996;75:250-4.

26. Pugh LC, Milliagn RA, Gray S, Strickland OL. First stage labor management: An examination of patterned breathing and fatigue. *Birth.* 25(4):241-245, 1998.

27. Section on Obstetrics and Gynecology, APTA. TENS special issue. *Bull Sect Obstet Gynecol.* APTA 1983;7(3).

28. Kaplan B, Rabinerson D, Lurie S, Bar J, Krieser UR, Neri A. Transcutaneous electrical nerve stimulation (TENS) for adjuvant pain-relief during labor and delivery. *Int J Gynaecol Obstet.* 1998;60:251-5.

29. Carroll D, Tramer M, McQuay H, Nye B, Moore A. Transcutaneous electrical nerve stimulation in labour pain: A systematic review. *Br J Obstet Gynaecol.* 1997;104:169-75.

30. Wattrisse G, Leroy B, Dufossez F, Bui Huu Tai R. Transcutaneous electric stimulation of the brain: A comparative study of the effects of its combination with peridural anesthesia using bupivacaine-fentanyl during obstetrical analgesia [in French]. *Cah Anesthesiol.* 1993;41:489-495.

31. Sapsford R, Bullock-Saxton J, Markwell S. *Women's Health: A Textbook for Physiotherapists.* London, England: WB Saunders Company; 1998.

32. Empi, Inc.. *Clinical Guidelines.* St.Paul, Minn: 1997; 30-32.

10

Physical Therapy
Care During Delivery

Multiple factors determine the duration of labor. These include parity, position and size of the fetus, pelvic shape, cervix malleability, medications or anesthesia, medical interventions, abdominal muscle contractions, contractions of the diaphragm, power of the uterine contractions, and the mother's ability to assist her body in labor and delivery. The physical therapist can assist the mother in delivery by; instruction in childbirth preparation classes, suggesting alternative positions, and application of TENS for pain relief.

SECOND STAGE OF LABOR

The stages of labor delineate phases the mother's body goes through during preparation to deliver, delivery of the infant, delivery of the placenta, and return of the uterus to its prepregnant size. The first stage, detailed in the last chapter, includes the time from the onset until the cervix is fully effaced and fully dilated to 10 cm. The second stage encompasses the time of full dilation to delivery of the infant, and usually requires about 20 contractions in the primigravida and 10 or less contractions with a multipara. The median duration of second stage is 50 minutes for primigravidas and 20 minutes for multiparas. Succeeding labors tend to be shorter until the fifth or sixth labor, after which labor tends to lengthen. The shorter labors are credited to a more lax cervix, which offers less resistance. There is, however, an increase in connective tissue in the myometrium after the fifth or sixth delivery that decreases the intensity of uterine contractions.[1]

Pauls, in her study of the relationship between selected variates and the duration of second stage labor (all women were primigravidas with vaginal deliveries and episiotomies), found that about one-quarter of the variation in duration related to infant weight (13%) and fetal station (9%).[2] The strength of the abdominal muscles has been thought of as an important variant in the duration of the second stage of labor; however, this study did not substantiate this hypothesis. Maternal positioning, a full bladder, and pelvic floor fatigue are but a few factors that may have an influence on the effectiveness of the abdominal muscles.

The second stage of labor is distinguished by involuntary contractions of the uterus coupled with voluntary pushing by the mother to assist in delivery of the infant (Figure 10-1). The fetal position changes in the birth canal so that it may accommodate the passageway. Pushing begins after the mother is fully 10 cm. dilated, as verified by the physician or midwife. Sometimes the mother will begin bearing down or grunting, signaling that she is expe-

Figure 10-1. Second stage of labor. The baby is turning and moving down. The membranes, still intact, are bulging in front of the baby's head. (Reprinted with permission from O'Connor LJ, Gourley Stephenson RJ. *Obstetric and Gynecologic Care in Physical Therapy.* Thorofare, NJ: SLACK Incorporated; 1990.)

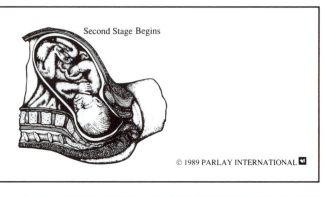

Second Stage Begins

© 1989 PARLAY INTERNATIONAL

Figure 10-2. Second stage continues. The baby's head crowns. Membranes have ruptured. (Reprinted with permission from O'Connor LJ, Gourley Stephenson RJ. *Obstetric and Gynecologic Care in Physical Therapy.* Thorofare, NJ: SLACK Incorporated; 1990.)

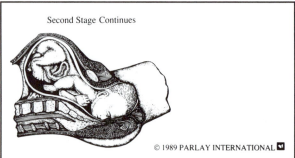

Second Stage Continues

© 1989 PARLAY INTERNATIONAL

riencing the pushing reflex. She should still be checked for full dilation to avoid possible bruising of the cervix.

The mother is encouraged to work with her uterine contractions, at the same time, relaxing the perineum and allowing the pelvic floor to stretch as comfortably as possible. Once given the go-ahead to push, she should wait until the urge to push is irresistible. She should then take a deep breath and bear down with a steady push, allowing air to escape so that she is not holding her breath against a closed glottis. In this way, she is not susceptible to large fluctuations in blood pressure and is able to maintain respiration while the rib cage, abdominal muscles, and diaphragm interact to supplement the uterine contractions. The mother will often moan and grunt as she releases air through the open glottis. These are natural sounds and should be encouraged to decrease the possibility of prolonged breath holding. When the mother needs to take another breath, she should take that next breath while still maintaining the pressure of the ribs and the abdominal muscles, allowing the diaphragm to ascend slowly. This controlled breathing will decrease the natural backward movement of the infant in the birth canal. Once the baby has crowned, (Figure 10-2) it may be necessary for the mother to pant, maintaining the baby on the perineum, allowing for the muscles of the pelvic floor to stretch slowly. She will feel an intense burning and stretching, followed by a naturally induced numbness that results when the tissues are fully stretched and blood circulation is depressed. This numbness is referred to as "nature's anesthesia."

An episiotomy may be done when the perineum bulges and the fetal scalp is visible. An episiotomy is an incision of the perineum performed to enlarge the vaginal opening. This is a common but controversial, obstetric procedure. The two types, midline and mediolateral, are usually performed to prevent extensive lacerations, (Figure 10-3) fetal head trauma, and post-partum pelvic relaxation from stretching of the endopelvic fascias. Although pain and edema result from an episiotomy, Niswander believes that episiotomies are simpler to repair

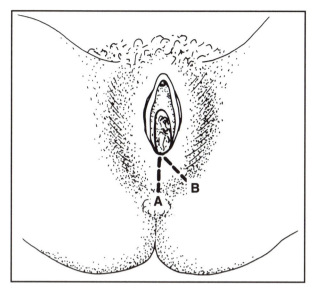

Figure 10-3. Episiotomies: A) midline episiotomy, B) mediolateral episiotomy. (Reprinted with permission from O'Connor LJ, Gourley Stephenson RJ. *Obstetric and Gynecologic Care in Physical Therapy.* Thorofare, NJ: SLACK Incorporated; 1990.)

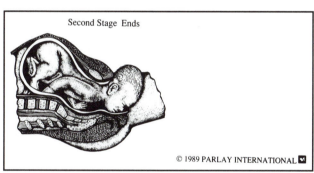

Figure 10-4. Second stage ends as the baby's head emerges from the vaginal opening and lifts upward. (Reprinted with permission from O'Connor LJ, Gourley Stephenson RJ. *Obstetric and Gynecologic Care in Physical Therapy.* Thorofare, NJ: SLACK Incorporated; 1990.)

than lacerations.[3] This, of course, depends on the laceration, but an episiotomy may indeed be larger than a small tear. Perineal massage may help increase the flexibility of the perineum during this crowning phase (when the largest diameter of the presenting part passes through the vaginal opening). Midwives have long advocated perineal massage during pregnancy, labor, and delivery as a way of increasing circulation and increasing flexibility of the perineum. As Niswander states, "Most deliveries can be performed without one (an episiotomy), and the proposed benefits (of an episiotomy)have never been proven."[3]

A slow, controlled delivery often results in minimal trauma to the pelvic floor and birth canal (Figure 10-4). The mother will be instructed to push the baby out easily, allowing the uterus to readapt to the pressure changes once the baby's head is born (Figure 10-5). The shoulders are delivered one at a time, and the mother's bearing down efforts should be controlled for slow, easy delivery. The fetal position changes in the birth canal to accommodate the passageway.

Molding of the infant's head occurs as it passes down the birth canal. The head is usually the widest part of the infant, and this molding, obvious at birth, helps to decrease the overall width of the cranium; molding is possible because the cranial sutures overlap slightly. The cranial bones reapproximate within a few days after birth. The infant's head rotates from a transverse orientation to an anterior alignment (usually occiput anterior, ie, the presenting fetal occiput faces the anterior of the mother, or baby's face to the mother's spine).

Figure 10-5. The baby's head turns as it is being born, and the shoulders rotate. (Reprinted with permission from O'Connor LJ, Gourley Stephenson RJ. *Obstetric and Gynecologic Care in Physical Therapy.* Thorofare, NJ: SLACK Incorporated; 1990.)

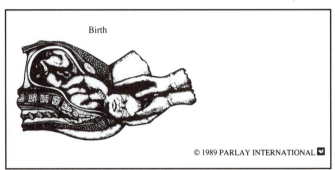

Birth

© 1989 PARLAY INTERNATIONAL

The vagina expands as the infant's neck extends while passing under the symphysis pubis, which acts as a fulcrum point, and the head emerges (see Figure 10-4). Between the time that the head is delivered and when the shoulders press on the perineum, the mother may not have an urge to push. The uterus takes a few moments to accommodate to the decreased volume. Yet, the muscle fibers and fundus of the uterus can retract and reduce the size of the uterine cavity within 30 seconds.[4]

Mucus, maternal blood, and amniotic fluid may be seen in the infant's nose or mouth. The midwife or physician will check for loops of the umbilical cord around the neck, slip them off, and aspirate the mucus from the infant's nose and mouth. The infant's head then rotates back toward the original position it had assumed (transverse orientation), and the uppermost anterior shoulder is delivered first. The posterior shoulder, which has been in the hollow of the sacrum, is then delivered (see Figure 10-5). The rest of the body follows easily. The exact and documented time of birth occurs when all of the infant is outside of the mother's body. This may be before the infant breathes or cries and usually before the cord is cut.

The cord will pulsate for about 2 minutes after delivery, during which time a significant amount of blood will be transferred, depending on the position in which the baby is held. If held at or below the vagina, the placental transfusion may be as much as 100 ml; if held above the mother's uterus, the amount of blood will be much less. The cord should generally be clamped between 20 to 40 seconds post-delivery. However, if the mother received general anesthesia the cord should be cut promptly, or if there is maternal-fetal blood group incompatibility, severe fetal asphyxia, or obvious cardiovascular anomalies requiring resuscitation.

THIRD STAGE OF LABOR

The third stage of labor is the delivery of the placenta. Although this occurs in a short period of time, there are many hazards for the mother. Post-partum hemorrhage is the leading cause of maternal death, and manipulations required to decrease blood loss increase the possibility of infection, which can result in illness or death. The placenta will usually separate from the uterine wall spontaneously, 5 to 10 minutes after delivery of the infant, when the sudden reduction in the size of the uterine cavity results in a reduction of the placental site. The placenta, which is non-contractile, cannot change its surface area and, at this time, becomes separated from the uterine wall. If the placenta has not separated after 10 minutes, the attendant will manually remove it with adequate anesthesia administered to the mother. The placenta is examined for possible abnormalities that might suggest congenital anomalies of the newborn. After separation, gentle, firm fundal massage and gentle traction on the cord will assist in delivery of the placenta. Pressure on the abdomen prevents uterine inversion.

If an episiotomy was done, local anesthesia is administered to the perineum for the repair after delivery of the placenta. External fundal massage is continued in recovery to help decrease blood loss by encouraging contraction of the uterus. Early suckling of the infant on the mother's breast is encouraged as soon as possible as this stimulates release of oxytocin and thereby increases uterine contractions. Additional oxytocin may be given to augment uterine contractions which will decrease uterine size and decrease blood loss. Oxytocin is often given to women who are susceptible to post-partum hemorrhage (eg, previous twins, over 35, grand multiparity [a woman who has given birth seven or more times], hydramnios, prolonged labor, general anesthesia, and post-partum hemorrhage after a previous delivery). Recovery care should continue for at least 1 hour; with 15-minute observations of pulse, blood pressure, consistency and height of the fundus, and amount of uterine bleeding (slight, moderate, heavy).

ALTERNATIVE BIRTH

The expectant couple has many options to consider when designing the birth of their baby. They can choose location, who will be present, and often the type of pain management they wish to use if labor is uncomplicated. They may even consider alternative delivery methods or positions.

Options for location include birthing rooms, birthing centers, home births, hospital delivery rooms, or hospital birthing rooms. Hospital birthing rooms are comfortably designed for labor and delivery. Some feature rocking chairs, decorated bathrooms, and special beds to give the appearance of home. The bed may be sectioned, so that the lower half can be removed and stirrups added, if needed, for delivery. Most complications, however, would necessitate a move to the delivery room. Birthing centers are usually located within 10 minutes of a nearby hospital. Here a family-centered approach to delivery may take place, where mothers may labor with assistance from family and midwives. If a labor or birth is complicated, the mother can be transferred quickly to the local hospital. Birthing centers and even some hospitals now offer programs to prepare siblings to view the birth. These classes generally present discussions of mother's limitations; terms such as uterus and placenta, labor and delivery; and adjusting to the new family. The sibling is usually forewarned about the possibility of seeing blood and hearing the different sounds of childbirth. Many sessions also include discussion of potential feelings of being left out, sibling rivalry, and jealousy.[5] How much the sibling or siblings are involved in the labor and delivery process depends on the parents. The presence of siblings at birth is a controversial topic because some believe that children will be frightened at birth and unable to understand its complexities. It appears, however, that with proper explanation and communication of the vast emotions and events in a birth, children are able to understand, give support, and bond with their new sibling.

An increase in home births has been noted since the 1970s. This trend has been examined to document consumer dissatisfaction with hospital childbirth and excessive use of technology. As of 1997 there were more than 40,000 out-of-hospital births in the United States annually, most of them being in birth centers, clinics, and in the home. Of this about 25,000 were home births, representing 0.6 % of all births.[6] The safety of the mother and child is the major concern in any out-of-hospital delivery. In a Michigan study,[7] it was found that better-educated women are more likely to make informed choices about their deliveries and take necessary preparations, and that women who choose to deliver at home tend to have higher birth weight babies, a factor that leads to a significant decrease in neonatal mortality. Nevertheless, guidelines are necessary for safe home births.

Burst suggests that five criteria must be met to insure safety in alternative out-of-hospital birth settings: attendance by a home-care professional; adherence to strict, stringent screening and transfer criteria; appropriate care at birth; immediate transport be available; and immediate availability of a consulting physician in a hospital.[8]

In the United States, physicians seem to favor mothers positioned on their backs for delivery. In this dorsal lithotomy position, with the mother's legs in stirrups, physicians have easy access to the perineum; unfortunately, prolonged pressure by the stirrups may cause nerve palsies or thrombosis in leg veins. In England, the left lateral side-lying position is preferred; this position physiologically avoids compression of the inferior vena cava by the gravid uterus. Asian women have long preferred giving birth in the squatting position. This position has the advantage of using gravity to assist the descent of the infant through the birth canal, plus eliminates compression on the inferior vena cava, and allows expansion of the pelvic opening.

Birthing chairs, adjustable recliners with an opening in the seat, were brought back into popularity in the late 1970s as an effective compromise between mothers and obstetricians. The chair may be raised and lowered so that the obstetrician or midwife has maximal ease in delivering the child; and because the mother is upright and assisted by gravity, there is no compression on the inferior vena cava, and perineal support is maintained. There appears to be no change in the length of second-stage labor or time spent in bearing down efforts while using a birthing chair.[9,10] There have been, however, some cases of vulvar edema resulting from the prolonged use of birthing chairs.[11]

PAIN MANAGEMENT FOR DELIVERY

The goal of pain management is to help the mother to easily and effectively work with her body to safely and comfortably deliver her infant. Methods include psychoprophylaxis, TENS, analgesics, and narcotics. The mother works with the contractions, bearing down without holding her breath. Forced muscular efforts while breath holding, known as the Valsalva maneuver, may cause large fluctuations in circulation and respiration, and are discouraged. Pushing with a partially closed glottis will lead to the production of a guttural sound or moan. Moaning as an auditory focus, helps the woman in labor, relieve tension and is instinctive.[12] When the presenting part stretches the pelvic floor (as long as there is no anesthesia given), the brain receptors are stimulated to release oxytocin and, thereby, further stimulate contractions.

During delivery, the mother and her partner who have attended childbirth classes will find they use what they have learned. These classes prepare them both for the physical and psychological aspects of childbirth. Not all women have the benefit of partners or classes, however, in those cases the midwife, physician, or other attending staff may act as a support person. In delivery, the support person can provide the mother with feedback about the intensity of her pushing efforts, progress on how she is doing, and general encouragement. Because fetal monitors can sometimes detect the beginning of a contraction before the mother can, this technology, if necessary, can be used by the support person, as well, to help the mother prepare for the next contraction. Whether an electronic monitor is used or not, the mother must be encouraged overall to listen, trust, and work with her own body. Her job is to assist the uterine forces by contracting her abdominal muscles, while at the same time relaxing and opening the pelvic floor to allow passage of the infant. Pain during delivery will be increased by fear of the unknown, previous unpleasant experiences, anxiety, insecurity, and anger. The mother may reduce her pain and discomfort, through education, and, as a result, gain confidence, better understand the birth process and need for outside support, learn relaxation, breathing exercises, and distraction techniques, plus develop realistic expectations.

In addition to standard childbirth pain relief methods, some women can use hypnosis for pain relief. They initiate the hypnotic trance once in labor, and continue it throughout delivery. Hypnosis probably works as a pain reliever through suggestion, conditioned reflex, education, and motivation.

TENS applied on the site of pain or paravertebrally over the related nerve roots, will decrease the perception of pain. Two sets of paired electrodes generally provide the greatest relief. The first set placed over the T10-T11 nerve roots, which supply nerves for the uterus during the first stage of delivery and the second two electrodes placed over the S2-S4 nerve roots, which will diminish the pain experienced in back labor and during delivery. See discussion on the mechanism of pain relief with TENS in Chapter 9 (see Figure 9-6).

If there is evidence of fetal distress, expulsive efforts need to be assisted at the time of delivery, and the need for pain relief is immediate. A mixture of 50% nitrous oxide and 50% oxygen may inhaled during contractions. If there is a need for Cesarean section, however, choices include general anesthesia, subarachnoid block, and epidural analgesia.

General anesthesia is chosen when there is a contraindication for conduction anesthesia, or there is a need for rapid delivery. It is believed that uterine relaxation is maximal with general anesthesia, but it has the disadvantage that the mother needs to be intubated to prevent aspiration of vomitus. Antacid may be given to counteract the effects of aspirations, should they occur, and an injection of thiopental 4 mg/kg may be used with an injection of a muscle relaxant (eg, succinylcholine 1 to 1.5 mg/kg) to facilitate incubation. Muscle relaxants have a low transmissibility across the placenta due to their low lipid solubility, high water solubility, and high ionization. Anesthesia is maintained with inhalation of enflurane, halothane, isoflurane, or similar agents.

Subarachnoid blockage is used for Cesarean section when there is no critical fetal distress or urgency. Spinal anesthesia has the advantage that the mother is awake, and her reflexes are intact; therefore, aspiration pneumonia is less of a problem. There is a lower risk of cardiovascular or central nervous system toxicity, as well. This regional anesthetic is given in one dose, injected into the subarachnoid space to achieve a dermatomal block up to T5. This produces anesthesia for all the pelvic organs and nerves supplying the pelvis and abdomen. The injection may consist of 5% lidocaine, 1% tetracaine, or 0.75% bupivacaine, and a 7.5% dextrose mixture. The main disadvantage is that spinal anesthesia may cause maternal hypotension. To counteract this problem, the uterus is displaced to the left so that good venous return to the heart may be maintained. Epinephrine can be administered in 10 mg increments to maintain blood pressure between 90% and 100% of its original level. Blood pressure is continuously monitored, and oxygen can be given by mouth, if necessary.

Epidural analgesia for Cesarean section can be dangerous because of the increased possibility of cardiovascular and central nervous system toxicity. It is superior to spinal anesthesia, because encroachment on respiratory function is less. With continual, carefully titrated dosage, the block can be maintained for postoperative analgesia as well. Generally, epidural success rate for Cesarean section is lower than with the spinal and is more complicated, but it is valuable in conditions where sudden and marked fluctuations in blood pressure impose a great risk.[3]

POSITIONS FOR DELIVERY

The physical therapist is uniquely qualified to assist women to labor and deliver in positions that prevent hip and spinal pain while prevent paresthesias that can result from pressures placed on the nerves of the lower extremities.

Women choose positions to deliver in that may be the same or different that what they labored in (see Chapter 9). At times her position may need to be changed because of difficulty of delivering a child's impacted shoulder. Flexion of the mother's leg, the MacRobert's maneuver, has the effect of straightening her sacrum relative to the lumbar spine. This may free the impacted shoulder and prevent a potential brachial plexus injury. During delivery, when the mother has had anesthesia, she will be unable to control or sense pressure on her legs. Placing her legs in a supported hip and knee flexion position without pressure on the skin will reduce the likelihood of peripheral neuropathies.

Alternative positions for delivery include birthing chairs, special split beds that allow for the variability from being upright to supine lying, and squatting bars. The squatting position allows the pelvis to be free of pressure while assisting with the gravitational forces. As the woman holds, the squatting bars provide for stability and balance when the contractions are intense.

COMPLICATED DELIVERIES

Complicated deliveries often follow dysfunctional labor, precipitous labor, or dystocia secondary to pelvic and fetal factors. Danforth describes the four "Ps" that are concerned with influencing the success and failure of delivery: the *powers*, which represent the expulsive forces of the contracting uterus; the *pelvic* architecture and its boundaries; the *passenger* (the fetus) as it passes through the pelvis and birth canal; and the *psyche* of the mother, which has an important impact on the force and duration of labor and delivery.[1]

Precipitous labor and delivery occur in 10% of all deliveries.[4] This indicates completion of the first and second stages of labor in less than 1 hour. It occurs more in multiparas than in primigravidas. The infant is sometimes injured during this rapid, uncontrolled labor because of the force on the presenting part. The baby should be delivered in as safe a place as possible, and no anesthesia should be given to delay delivery. The diagnosis is often made by serial pelvic exams that reveal a rapid cervical dilation accompanied by severe, violent contractions. There is no known etiology for precipitous labor. Patients who have had one precipitous labor are prone to subsequent ones, however. The infant needs to be evaluated, post-delivery, for possible fetal intracranial bleeding and depression.

A breech presentation is one in which any part other than the fetal head is the presenting part. The fetal sacrum becomes the designated reference point. There is a 4% incidence of breech presentation. Breech births are defined by the posture of the lower extremities of the infant: frank breech, complete breech, footling breech. A frank breech (Figure 10-6a) refers to hips that are flexed and legs extended so that the feet are at the level of the chin. In a complete breech (Figure 10-6b), the infant's legs are fully crossed at the level of the buttocks, so that it is sitting in a tailor fashion. A footling (single or double) or incomplete breech (Figure 10-6c) means that one or both of the feet and legs are extended through the birth canal.

Breech presentations that can be delivered vaginally should meet the following criteria: fetal weight is between 2500 to 3500 gm,[13] the pelvis must be able to accommodate the fetus

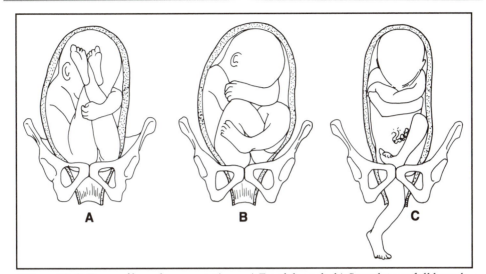

Figure 10-6. Types of breech presentations: a) Frank breech, b) Complete or full breech, c) Singe footing breech. (Reprinted with permission from O'Connor LJ, Gourley Stephenson RJ. *Obstetric and Gynecologic Care in Physical Therapy.* Thorofare, NJ: SLACK Incorporated; 1990.)

without hyperextending the fetal neck during vaginal breech delivery (the risk of spinal cord transection is 25%); labor progression must be normal (labor longer than 18 hours will often proceed to a Cesarean section); fetal heart rate patterns must be normal and fetal monitoring continuous; mother's pre-pregnancy weight must be less than 180 pounds (with increased maternal size, there is an increase in perinatal morbidity due to inability to estimate fetal weights); and a complete or footling breech presentation associated with a high risk of prolapsed cord requires the cervix to be completely dilated to avoid entrapping the fetal head.

The mortality of vaginal breech deliveries is 5.5 times that of infants presenting head first. The major causes of perinatal deaths in breech births are cord prolapse, other cord complications, tentorial tears, and cerebral hemorrhage of the after-coming head. The molding of the infant's head, which usually takes several hours, must occur in moments. As a result, sudden stresses that may be highly damaging are placed on the infant's cranium. This is especially true in a pre-term infant whose head is larger than the presenting part, and the cervix and lower uterine segment are dilated only enough for the passage of the presenting part. Other injuries include damage to the spinal cord, liver, adrenal glands, or spleen (from abdominal manipulations), and delayed responses to injury that can include cerebral palsy, learning disorders, and cerebral dysfunction.

If a vaginal delivery is selected, the infant is allowed to deliver to its umbilicus, usually with a wide episiotomy. The umbilical cord is pulled down to prevent any tension. The infant's thighs are flexed and abducted to deliver the feet and legs, then traction is applied to the infant's body with a downward rotation of the chest, away from the shoulder to be delivered. The fetus's arm is flexed across its chest and splinted; then, with traction and 180-degree rotation, the posterior shoulder is advanced to the anterior position and that shoulder and arm are delivered. The head is often delivered by forceps with gentle flexion and suprapubic pressure, which will assist in maintaining the infant's head in flexion during the descent.

Shoulder dystocia is a serious obstetric problem that occurs when the infant's shoulders are too large for the pelvic inlet. Diagnosis is made after the head is delivered and downward pressure exerted on the head meets with obstruction from the pubic bone. The incidence of shoulder dystocia is 1.5 in 1000 deliveries; and in babies over 4000 gm, 17 in 1000 deliveries.[2] An ultrasound evaluation of the bisacromial-to-head/diameter ratio has been suggested as a screening for shoulder dystocia. Infants with an estimated weight of more than 4500 gm should be delivered by Cesarean section. Management includes a large episiotomy and fundal pressure and attempts to dislodge the anterior shoulder while exerting modest pressure on the fetal head. Stretching of the fetal neck can result in brachial plexus injuries. Flexion of the mother's leg (MacRobert's maneuver) has the effect of straightening her sacrum relative to the lumbar spine, which may free the impacted shoulder. Other maneuvers involve delivery of the infant's posterior shoulder first or purposely fracturing the infant's clavicle, a difficult procedure to perform.

Forceps

Two types of obstetric forceps are used today; classic forceps with cephalic curves or pelvic curves, and specially-designed forceps for specific problems, such as breech birth or unusual head presentations. In the past, forceps were applied to the pelvis without regard to the position of the fetal head. This application is rarely used today (unless under most extraordinary circumstances), because it places forces on the head that the fetus cannot tolerate. Generally, in modern obstetrics, if the forceps cannot be applied properly to the fetal head, a Cesarean section is indicated. Conversely, in a cephalic application, the forceps are placed along the occipitomental diameter of the head (occiput to chin). Forceps may also be used for the after-coming head as in a breech presentation.

Low forceps or outlet forceps are used to supply the final force needed to deliver the infant's head through the vaginal opening. If the infant's head does not emerge after it has descended to the pelvic floor, forceps can be indicated, especially if there is prolonged pressure on the fetal head. The following four criteria must be met before forceps are to be used: the scalp must be, or has been, visible at the introitus without separating the labia, the skull must have reached the pelvic floor, the sagittal suture must be in the sagittal plane of the pelvis, and the membranes must be ruptured. Anesthesia and an episiotomy are part of this procedure.[1] Because of the controversy over when low forceps can be used safely, a standardized description of use has not been developed.

The American College of Obstetricians and Gynecologists defines other forceps operations. Mid-forceps is the application of forceps to the fetal head after it is engaged.[1] Danforth suggests that definition be expanded to include that mid-forceps delivery be limited to use when the fetal head lies at a station between 0 and + 3.[3] Mid-forceps delivery has changed greatly in the last 19 years. Reviews of mid-forceps delivery have revealed a high incidence of neonatal death and increased frequency of long-term intellectual deficits among the survivors. A high-forceps operation was previously used to apply forceps before the fetal head was engaged in the pelvis. This type of procedure deferred to Cesarean section and is now obsolete.

Vacuum extraction has been found, in some cases, to be less traumatic than forceps to the infant and the birth canal. The extractor consists of a cup, a rubber hose, and a pump. The cup is inserted into the vagina without an episiotomy and secured to the occiput of the infant. The air is pumped out so the cap forms a partial vacuum to the fetal occiput. Traction is then applied to the hose sufficient to pull the head through the birth canal. The vacuum extractor has been found to be easier to use in multiparas and in patients with a transverse arrest than in primigravidas or in those with an occiput posterior presentation.[3] Although this device shows a great deal of promise, it has shown an alarming association with shoulder dystocia and hematoma.

Attempts were made in the 17th and 18th centuries to save the mothers; all but a few died from hemorrhage or infection. In the mid-1800s, Edoardo Porro discovered that by doing the Cesarean hysterectomy, he was able to circumvent the problem of uterine hemorrhage and save the mother as well as the child.

Cesarean

Cesarean section, or laparotrachelotomy, refers to delivery of fetuses 500 gm or more by abdominal surgery requiring an incision through the uterine wall. Cesarean sections are one of the earliest operations known and have been traced to Rome during the reign of Numa Pompilius 715-672 BC. He decreed that any woman who died late in pregnancy was to have the child removed from her womb. This law continued under Caesar, when it acquired the name lex caesarea. Another explanation for its name, is from the Latin words, caedare (to cut), and caesareus (abdominal birth).

Prior to 1960, Cesareans were performed only when a mother was dying, to deliver a viable infant, or to save the mother's life when labor was obstructed. Between 1960 and 1965, the reported Cesarean rate was 5% of all deliveries made. Today, hospitals and clinics report a range of deliveries by Cesarean section from 12% to 25%.[1,3] Expectedly, perinatal mortality has decreased with the rise in Cesarean sections; however, there is a three to four times greater risk of maternal mortality with a Cesarean than with a vaginal birth (8 to 10 deaths per 10,000 with Cesarean delivery versus 2.7 deaths per 10,000 deliveries with vaginal deliveries).[3]

The four general indications for Cesarean section are: When delivery of the infant is necessary but cannot be induced; when labor is unsafe for the infant or mother; when fetal and maternal dystocia contraindicate a vaginal delivery; and when an emergency situation demands immediate delivery, and a vaginal delivery is not possible. Specifically, indications for a Cesarean include failure to progress, pelvic disproportion, malpresentation, fetal distress, pregnancy-induced hypertension, mothers with placenta previa or abruptio placenta, prolapse of the umbilical cord, diabetes mellitus, herpes progenitalis, severe Rh incompatibility, failed forceps delivery, failed induction of labor, and sometimes repeat Cesarean section.[3]

There are two major techniques for performing a Cesarean section. In cases of prematurity, before the lower uterine segments have formed sufficiently, in placenta previa, and when the infant is lying in a transverse position, the incision is made longitudinally in the anterior wall of the uterus. Often, these incisions extend into the fundal area, constituting a classical type of Cesarean section (Figure 10-7A).

In this classical incision, the Cesarean operation proceeds rapidly with the layers of the abdomen opened and the abdominal wall retracted, bladder reflected, vessels clamped, and pads put in place to decrease the amount of amniotic fluid entering the peritoneum. The underlying veins in the broad and cardinal ligaments are avoided, because the incision is made laterally without entering the broad ligament. Fingers are insinuated between the uterine wall and the fetal head. The most preferred incision in the United States is the low-segment approach (Figure 10-7B), because it is associated with a lower immediate and later morbidity. The incision is made in the peritoneum overlying the lower uterine segment. The bladder is dissected away from the lower segment, and the deeper incision is made to the uterus transversely in the non-contractile portion. With pressure on the fundus, the fetal head pushes up through the incision, and the nose and mouth are then suctioned. The shoulders are delivered one at a time after this.

After the fetus is extracted, it is placed head down to facilitate drainage from the mouth and nose and decrease the chance of aspiration. The cord is clamped and cut. The placenta

Figure 10-7. Cesarean sections: A) Classic incision, B) Transverse incision made in the lower portion of the uterus with the bladder displaced downward. (Reprinted with permission from O'Connor LJ, Gourley Stephenson RJ. *Obstetric and Gynecologic Care in Physical Therapy.* Thorofare, NJ: SLACK Incorporated; 1990.)

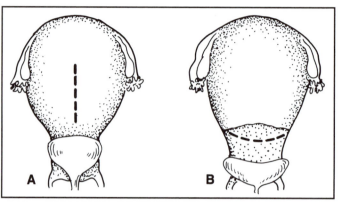

is removed and layers of the uterus and abdominal wall are approximated and sutured in layers. Oxytocin is given to augment the uterine contractions. Care is given to the mother's legs to decrease the risk of developing thrombophlebitis and thromboembolism. Spontaneous movements of the legs and early ambulation are strongly suggested.

Vaginal Births After Cesarean

Despite the famous dictum of 1916 made by Edward Cragin, M.D., to the Eastern Medical Society of New York, "Once a Cesarean section, always a Cesarean section," women who have had Cesarean births now demand a chance to deliver vaginally. In response to this demand, the New York State Health Department has started a statewide program to reduce the rate of Cesarean sections. In 1988, Cesareans accounted for 20% of all New York births. State medical experts, however, believe that many of those were unnecessary, and they have set up an independent team to review each Cesarean procedure.[14] The national health objective for the year 2000 is to have an overall Cesarean section rate of 15%, a primary section rate of 12%, and a vaginal birth after Cesarean section (VABC) rate of 35%.[15] The rate for 1995, was 21% for overall rate, 15% for primary Cesarean section, and VABC rate of 28%.[15]

The major concern for vaginal birth after Cesarean (VBAC), is the increased possibility of uterine rupture (ie, the uterine surgical scar will be unable to withstand the forceful labor contractions). Rupture of the uterus is very serious but occurs only once in every 1500 to 2000 deliveries, or in 1% of births, most often as the result of a rupture of a scar from previous Cesarean sections or from direct trauma.

In women with a classic Cesarean section incision (see Figure 10-7a), there is a substantially increased chance of uterine rupture over those with a low transverse scar. If rupture occurs, it is more likely to be a complete rupture and result in perinatal death. However studies show that the infant does well if delivered within 17 minutes of a uterine rupture.[16] Flamm further suggests crash Cesarean drills to respond to these emergency situations. There has been no objective evidence to support the thought that multiple Cesarean sections predispose women to increased uterine rupture in subsequent pregnancies. An extensive review of the literature from 1950 to 1980 showed some surprising results about vaginal deliveries in patients with prior Cesareans. It was found that with a properly conducted vaginal delivery after Cesarean, there was a 0.7% incidence of uterine rupture, a 0.93% incidence of perinatal mortality, and no maternal deaths associated with uterine rupture. In 1974, however, 99% of those patients who had a previous Cesarean section were delivered by repeat

Cesareans in American hospitals. Although controversy continues about the safety of vaginally delivering breech presentations and twins after previous Cesarean sections, a review by Lairn shows that many breeches and twins have been delivered successfully in women with prior Cesareans.[17]

Traumas causing rupture include excessive oxytocin in patients with obstructed labor and those from surgical delivery, such as version, breech extraction, and manual removal of the placenta.[4] Symptoms include sudden abdominal pain followed by blood loss. Treatment consists of surgery, Cesarean section, blood transfusion, and possibly a hysterectomy if there is extensive rupture.

Rarely, in labor, the anterior lip of the uterus may be pinched as the head descends between the pubic bone, often following cephalopelvic disproportion. The uterus may become edematous and rupture at the lower segment and may tear the entire cervix (annular amputation). The entrapped lip may be freed by the physician or midwife by disengaging the head and pushing the anterior lip upwards with the fingers. Injuries to the lower segment of the uterus can result from cephalopelvic disproportion or malposition. Because the presenting part cannot descend through the pelvis, muscle fibers in the upper segment continually contract and retract. The lower segment is then thin and stretched to the point of separation.

There are apparently no ill effects, but physicians' opinions are divided as to whether to artificially rupture amniotic membranes or not. If ruptured, internal fetal monitors may be used early. The use of anesthesia for VBAC is also debated. Some believe that with anesthesia, the mother's inability to perceive pain, especially in uterine rupture, would be masked. Lavin, however, emphasized the unreliability of abdominal pain as a symptom of uterine rupture, and this pain may actually be secondary to peritoneal adhesions, round ligament tension, hypersensitive bladder, or scarring of the abdominal wall.[17]

The duration for labor in VBAC was found to conform to the norms for delivery of patients without a history of Cesarean section, and there is no evidence to support the routine use of forceps. In a study that measured the effect of a previous Cesarean, in women who had both one vaginal and one Cesarean delivery (in either order), those whose most recent delivery was vaginal had a lower rate of Cesarean and an shorter duration of labor than those who most recent delivery was Cesarean.[18] Post-partum exam is encouraged to assess scar integrity, but the medical need for this test is uncertain. Most agree that the following criteria must be met to be a candidate for VBAC: no indication for Cesarean section in the current pregnancy; previous low transverse incision, documented in hospital records; mother is admitted to hospital when labor begins; mother is blood-typed and cross-matched; mother is carefully monitored, and the obstetrician is present during labor; the facility and personnel must be ready to perform an immediate Cesarean; and the mother must be counseled about risks and benefits, and informed consent must be obtained.[17,19]

Because over 90% of all Cesareans in the United States today are performed with a low transverse incision,[20] chances are increasing that women will not have a repeat Cesarean section simply because they needed one in the past. Favorable outcomes for vaginal births following Cesarean sections are high if the woman's physician has a 20% or less Cesarean rate, is younger than 54 and if their at risk population is less that 5%.[21] The benefits of such a trend will be increased participation by the parents in delivery, less recovery time, more comfort, and reduced medical and financial costs to the family and insurance carrier.[18]

Multifetal Birth

Most mothers with twin gestations will go into labor by 37 to 38 weeks and those with triplets and quadruplets at 35 and 34 weeks, respectively. Consequently, more than 50% of all twins will be delivered at 37 weeks and will weigh less than 2500 gm. Presentation is very important in the delivery of twins, because statistics show that the first twin will present head down in 80% of all cases, but the second in only 50%. Other combinations (first twin to second twin) occur with varying frequencies: cephalic-cephalic, 39%; cephalic breech, 37%; breech-breech, 10%; cephalic-transverse, 8%; breech-transverse, 5%; and transverse-transverse, 1%.

Another potential combination (also a complication) is fetal interlocking, which occurs in 1 of every 817 twin deliveries. This usually occurs at or below the pelvic inlet, and usually the first twin is breech. The neck of the first baby is elongated and locked above the head of the second. Other entanglements, termed collisions, occur above the pelvic brim. When both heads try to descend at the same time, neither is able to enter the pelvis. Usually, Cesarean section is indicated for a collision situation or where twins are conjoined.

When a vaginal delivery is desired with twins, the physician or midwife must be skilled in podalic version. Podalic version describes the external or internal manual manipulation of the fetal position while in utero. Forty percent of second twins require a manipulative delivery. It is suggested that a Cesarean section be done when one twin is of low birth weight or when either infant is in a malposition. Low birth weight, prematurity, and intrauterine growth retardation put the malpositioned fetus at a higher risk for head entrapment and complications of a traumatic delivery.

With twins, the cervix only needs to dilate once, but the uterus must contract for both deliveries. The first twin is delivered as any infant previously described. There is some discussion, however, regarding how long to wait before delivery of the second infant. Classic obstetric instruction suggests a wait of 5 to 20 minutes after the first twin,[1] unless there is bleeding or fetal distress. Noble states that a midwifery text from the last century describes a 4-hour wait before intervention. She further points out that until recently, 30 minutes were generally allowed to elapse between births, so that the uterus could adjust and prepare for the next delivery.[22]

However, the membranes of the second twin usually rupture (depending on the sac configuration) within 5 minutes after delivery of the first twin, and longer waits for the delivery may result in placental insufficiency, premature separation, cervical retraction, and cord accidents.[6] The second twin will most likely change position after delivery of the first and be delivered either head first, breech, or by Cesarean. If the second is in an undesirable position and cannot be helped by internal or external inversion or is distressed, Cesarean section is performed in about 40% of the cases. Occasionally, low forceps may be needed to facilitate delivery.

After either spontaneous or manual delivery of the placenta, it is inspected to determine zygosity and any vascular communications between the twins. Oxytocin is given to augment uterine contractions. Because the uterus is arranged in layers, contraction of the layers cuts off any bleeding vessels and prevents hemorrhage from the placental site. The uterus is manually explored for rupture which may have occurred during the manipulative maneuver. A fundal massage is also given to stimulate uterine contractions. Early suckling of the twins at the mother's breast will stimulate uterine contraction.

REPAIR OF THE PERINEUM

The birth canal, cervix, vagina, and perineum should be inspected for lacerations after delivery. Some damage to the soft tissue structures (of the birth canal and surrounding organs) usually occurs after every delivery, especially in primigravidas, because the firm tissues are more resistant to the delivery of the infant. Perineal lacerations are categorized into four types, depending on their depth: *first-degree* laceration extends through the skin and superficial structures above the muscles; *second-degree* lacerations are tears that extend through the muscles of the perineum; *third-degree* laceration tears into the sphincter; and *fourth-degree* laceration includes a tear in the anterior wall of the rectum, as well.

These injuries occur if the vaginal opening is stretched too quickly or over-distended during delivery, usually by the infant's head. If the perineum is torn, the lower vagina is also injured, and tears that involve the medial surfaces of the labia minora bleed profusely because of the many veins in this area. Any tears in the perineum are repaired immediately, the layers of tissue approximated by absorbable sutures. Special care is given to the repair of third- and fourth-degree lacerations. Local anesthesia is administered to the perineal wall before intestinal sutures are placed. Frequent ice packs on the perineum after stitching will reduce swelling and increase the mother's comfort. It is suggested that the stools be kept soft for several days so that the sutures are not overstressed during elimination.

Vaginal lacerations may result at the level of the ischial spines or in the vault of the vagina. Vaginal tears are usually circular and result from using forceps in a rotational manner. These lacerations may bleed profusely and are repaired with catgut sutures. Careful investigation is warranted to insure that all tears are inspected and repaired. Injuries to the anterior vaginal wall may be accompanied by injuries to the bladder neck and urethral wall, if they are compressed against the posterior surface of the pubic bones or pushed ahead of the infant's presenting part.

If the pelvis is small, the delivery precipitous, or the infant unusually large, more damage than usual will occur. As the uterus contracts. the soft tissue structures are pushed ahead and will eventually stretch and become injured. Injury to the bladder may also occur if it is distended or if the presenting part is high. The mother should be catheterized if she cannot void.

If posterior lacerations are not repaired to give support to the rectal walls, the levator bundles will retract laterally and destroy the perineal body, thereby eliminating the normal support of the lower vagina. When standing, the weight of the abdomen will then increase the descent of the rectal wall; it will increase with each rectal movement and result in a rectocele (rectum protrudes into the vagina and forms a large pouch). After menopause, with the withdrawal of estrogen hormones, a preexisting rectocele will increase rapidly.

An episiotomy decreases the resistance of the muscles and fascia posteriorly, and endopelvic fascia may be injured even if the skin and vaginal wall appeared uninjured. As the head descends through the vaginal canal, the levator bundles are separated, and the levator fascia is stretched. Often, the fascial layers will tear, allowing the levator to separate and laterally retract. This is especially true if the labor is forceful and the structures are torn apart rather than stretched slowly. If the mother has a narrow pubic arch, the infant's head cannot fit closely beneath the symphysis, and it will be forced backward toward the posterior pelvis putting added strain on the soft tissues. Wilson advocates episiotomy to avoid posterior wall injury, the use of regional or local anesthesia before episiotomy, and that episiotomy be done before the tissues have been injured. He argues that episiotomy performed on an overstretched, blanched perineum offers no protection to the deep fascia and muscles, also stretched to the maximum.

INJURIES INVOLVING UTERINE SUPPORT

The cardinal ligaments rarely become torn during labor and delivery, but they may be stretched a great deal if labor is delayed by cephalopelvic disproportion, or if delivery is forced before full cervical dilation. If the supporting ligaments are stretched or injured during labor and the vaginal wall is compromised, the uterus can invert and distend towards the introitus. In a first-degree prolapse, the cervix lies between the ischial spines and the vaginal opening. In a second-degree prolapse, the cervix protrudes through the vaginal opening. The cervix in the third-degree position is completely prolapsed, and the vaginal canal is inverted. The advanced stages of uterine-prolapse seem to occur in post-menopausal women with atrophied tissues, causing diminished uterine support. Treatment consists of surgical repair through the vagina to reposition a cystocele, rectocele, and the uterus. After delivery, a cystocele may develop where the bladder protrudes downward into the vaginal canal as a result of the supporting structures in the vesicovaginal septum losing their integrity. The weak anterior vaginal wall will descend due to the force of gravity and weight of the abdominal contents when standing. Added stresses from straining, lifting, and coughing, along with the added weight of the bladder, will stress the septum until the bladder bulges into the vagina. Cystoceles that produce a bulge in the vagina and cause difficulty voiding are often repaired surgically through the vaginal levator sling.

Some women develop a mild incontinence after the delivery of a child, often the result of injury during childbirth to the urethrovesical junction and urethra. Anatomically, the posterior urethrovesical angle changes, and the relationship of the urethra to the pubis changes (see Chapter 3). The amount of incontinence depends on how much damage was done and the amount of recovery that has taken place post-injury. Multiparous women may experience stress incontinence during menstruation, and in cases of extreme dysfunction, the incontinence may continue throughout the entire month. Treatment of incontinence is included in Chapter 3.

Retrodisplacement of the Uterus

Retrodisplacement, wherein the uterus rests posteriorly, may result from congenital anomaly, from adhesions from pelvic inflammatory disease or endometriosis, or may develop after childbirth when supporting structures are injured. If the retrodisplaced uterus is enlarged, there may be low back pain, pelvic pressure, dyspareunia, and interference with rectal evacuation. Treatment may include a pessary to hold the uterus in place, which remains in place for 2 to 3 months.

INJURY TO THE PELVIC JOINTS

The symphysis pubis tends to separate to some extent during delivery. If, however, there is a great deal of force used, or if the baby is unusually large, the symphysis pubis may be injured. If so, the mother will experience severe pain in the symphysis pubis and possibly the sacroiliac joint on weightbearing. The pubic bones will appear abnormally separated and the symphyseal area may be extremely tender. Ultrasound is used to confirm a symphysis pubis separation. Increased mobility is noted and the bone ends may shift several centimeters when the woman shifts weight from one foot to the other. Urine may be bloody from injury to the bladder neck and urethra. Treatment includes instruction in comfort positions and mobility instruction, plus immobilization of the pelvic girdle by a snug low fitting support. The mother is also advised to avoid widely abducted legs, walking on uneven terrain, large strides, and exaggerated pelvic movements. Heat and activities to decrease pain and increase healing are recommended.

Occasionally, the coccyx can become dislocated or even fractured during delivery. The mother will most likely complain of localized pain in the coccyx area and, possibly, radiation down both legs. With digital manipulation through the rectum, the dislocated coccyx can be felt overlying the sacrum and may be reduced. Ice or heat, and perhaps a donut pillow or TENS, plus instruction in comfort positions may help relieve pain. Refer to Chapter 7 for treatment suggestions.

GENITAL FISTULAS

Genital fistulas, requiring surgical repair, are abnormal openings between two internal organs. Fistulas of the vesicovaginal, vesicocervical, or vesicouterine (opening between the bladder and the genital tract), rectovaginal fissure (opening between the rectum and the vagina), or ureterovaginal (opening between the ureter and vagina), can be caused by injuries during labor and delivery, surgical trauma, or radiation. Vesicovaginal, rectovaginal, or ureterovaginal fistulas can result from intrapartum injury or from later avascular necrosis in response to the crushing of pelvic organs between the presenting fetal part and the bony pelvis. Diagnoses are confirmed by clinical exam and by cystoscopy and pyelography.

CHILDBIRTH PREPARATION CLASSES

Physical therapists can help mothers prepare for delivery by instructing childbirth preparation classes. Classes in psychoprophylaxis describe physical and psychological preparation for labor and delivery. These classes are designed to be held as close to the mother's due date when motivation peaks. The repeated practice of the techniques learned in this class will encourage a conditioned response by the mother and her partner when they need it during labor and delivery. Women are again encouraged to bring their partner or other support person. Labor and delivery is a time when support is most definitely needed. A class is usually 1 1/2 to 3 hours each time, with a break in the middle. Fees for the classes will vary, depending on how the teacher will be reimbursed. A hospital or physician may pay the instructor directly and charges to the client included in the hospital's or doctor's fees. If the instructor is in private practice, fees will probably need to be calculated to cover the length of class, rental of equipment (films, projectors), and space; or the fee charged to students may be a reflection of the resources and customs of the community. Some childbirth classes may be covered by the couples' insurance. Class size should probably be limited to 8 couples.

Publicizing the classes is often another job of the instructor; if she is in private practice or works for a sponsoring agency, articles written periodically in a local newspaper may help remind the community of available classes. Calling local hospitals and physicians is a must to exchange information between instructor and referral sources. Some hospitals and doctors ask that the instructor show them some of the class handouts and information used. Prepared packs given to these potential referral sources will supplement the initial contact. Offering to stock the hospital or doctor's office with brochures allows them to give out some information about the instructor and classes (objective, content, and logistics). Some instructors keep a running calendar at the doctor's office to post when the next class will start. When starting up a new class, it may be helpful to advertise and show a childbirth film free to the public.

Table 10-1

Suggested Outline for 7-Class Series in Childbirth Preparation

Class 1	Content
	Introduce self. Give background information. Have students introduce them selves. Discuss course content and goals, overview of class. Introduce psychoprophylaxis and its relevance to pain, labor, and delivery. Discuss fetal and maternal development. Introduce relaxation. Give overview of labor and delivery, showing charts. Teach pregnancy stretches.
Class 2	Answer questions. Practice relaxation. Show exercises for pelvic floor and abdominal muscles. Discuss body mechanics and positions of comfort. Discuss labor and coaching role. Start basic breathing techniques.
Class 3	Answer questions. Review breathing techniques. Practice breathing techniques. Practice relaxation. Discuss transition and review labor. Discuss variations of normal labor. Review pregnancy stretches.
Class 4	Answer questions. Practice relaxation exercise. Teach expulsion. Discuss second stage of labor. Discuss coach's role. Discuss what to bring to the hospital.
Class 5	Answer questions. Review labor, including hospital procedures. Show film on labor and delivery. Discuss appearance of the newborn. Discuss post-partum period expectations, emotional and physical changes.
Class 6	Answer questions. Review all breathing exercises. Review all relaxation exercises. Show film of post-partum period, adjusting to the newborn. Instruct in post-partum exercises and supplement with handouts.
Class 7	Visit the hospital. View labor and delivery rooms, birthing rooms, and birthing chair, if provided.

A hospital tour should be arranged or encouraged for the class members. Communication is enhanced for the participants if there are realistic expectations between hospital, doctor, and childbirth educator. At the final class, a course evaluation and scheduled post-partum meeting with all the babies will encourage further group contact and support.

A suggested outline of a 7-class series in childbirth preparation is included and a list of items for couples to bring to the hospital are provided for ideas (Tables 10-1 and 10-2).

No matter what type of childbirth education is offered, relaxation exercises are the stepping stones to controlled breathing and to a prepared response to the pain of labor (Figure 10-8). To achieve a conditioned response, relaxation and breathing start automatically in response to a uterine contraction; however, participants must practice relaxation and breathing exercises daily.

There are two basic breathing techniques taught in preparation for labor and delivery: rhythmic, deep breathing, which is about 8 breaths per minute or 2 per 15-second period, and shallow chest breathing, which is 30 to 40 breaths per minute.[1] The mother uses rhythmic or slow breathing when she can no longer walk or talk through a contraction. She signals the beginning of a contraction with a cleansing breath. She focuses on one spot to enhance concentration, rhythmically and gently inhales through the nose, and exhales through the mouth. After the contraction is over, she gives another cleansing breath (Figure 10-9A). Coaches are encouraged to breathe along with mother during practice and in late labor.

Shallow chest breathing is used when the rhythmic chest breathing is no longer adequate to cope with the contractions. This technique begins with a cleansing breath, the mother

Table 10-2

What to Bring to the Hospital

For the Labor Bag: A watch with a second hand, lip balm, ice pack, socks, money for phone calls, phone list, powder for abdominal stroking, pen and paper, food for partner, cards, books, magazines, focal point, camera/flash and film, lollipops to decrease nausea, labor guide, tennis ball for counterpressure in case of back labor, paper bag for hyperventilation.

For the Mother: Slippers, two to three nursing nightgowns, bathrobe or bed jacket, bras, underpants, sanitary pads, toilet articles, address book and birth announcements, reading material, writing material, loose fitting going home outfit (probably one worn at ~5 months of pregnancy).

For Baby: Pacifier, undershirt (newborn size), diapers, pins, plastic pants, going home outfit, blanket, sweater, hat, and car seat.

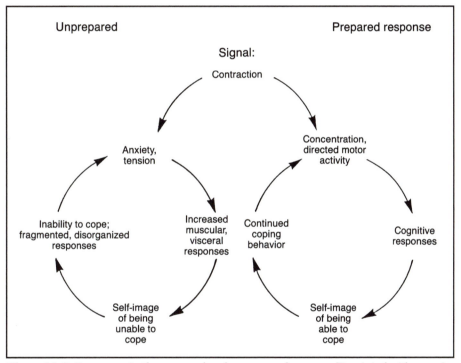

Figure 10-8. Responses in the prepared and unprepared woman. (Reprinted with permission from O'Connor LJ, Gourley Stephenson RJ. *Obstetric and Gynecologic Care in Physical Therapy.* Thorofare, NJ: SLACK Incorporated; 1990.)

focuses, and continues with 30 to 40 breaths per minute. It should be practiced for at least 1 minute and should end with a cleansing breath. These breaths are shallow, brief, held high in the chest, and are very light. There is little chest exertion noted (Figure 10-9B).

Based on these two breathing methods, other breathing patterns and activities are adapted to suit the needs of the laboring woman. For example:

1) Add abdominal stroking to rhythmic chest breathing to increase concentration and sensory input.

Figure 10-9. Breathing for labor and delivery. (Reprinted with permission from O'Connor LJ, Gourley Stephenson RJ. *Obstetric and Gynecologic Care in Physical Therapy.* Thorofare, NJ: SLACK Incorporated; 1990.)

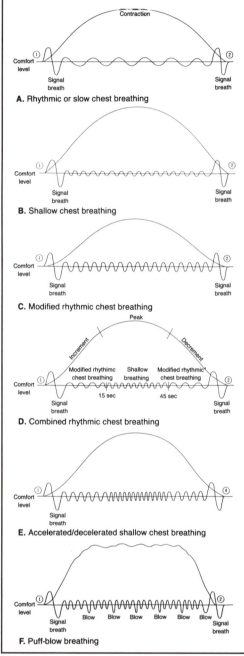

2) Modify rhythmic chest breathing by incorporating variations, such as inhaling for a count of 1, exhaling for a count of 2 to 3 (Figure 10-9C)

3) In active labor, perform combined rhythmic breathing by starting with a cleansing breath, continuing with modified rhythmic chest breathing, but, during the peak of contraction, use shallow chest breathing, and end with a cleansing breath (see Figure 10-9D).

4) Use accelerated/decelerated shallow chest breathing when labor has been prolonged or during difficult labor. It is more complicated and requires more concentration. After a

cleansing breath, start with shallow breathing, 1 every 2 seconds; after 15 seconds, increase to the rate of 1 per second, then at 45 seconds decrease to 1 every 2 seconds, alternating with shallow chest breathing (Figure 10-9E).

5) Use puff-blow for transition. After a cleansing breath, take a series of three shallow breaths (inhale and exhale) and a blow. By counting these breaths, more concentration is required, which helps pass the transition contractions that may last 90 seconds or more. The coach can also have the mother vary the puff-blow techniques to encourage distraction, (eg, 3 breaths to 1 blow, 2 breaths to 1 blow, 3 breaths to 1 blow again, and 1 breath to 1 blow-Figure 10-9F). Add abdominal stroking for greater comfort in transition.

6) Use rapid repeated blows when feeling a premature urge to push (not pictured).

Hyperventilation may result from repeated blowing, prolonged exhalations or breathing at a rapid rate. As the CO_2 blood level drops, respiratory alkalosis may occur, and vasoconstriction may cause dizziness or tingling around the mouth and fingers. If the alkalosis state is continued, spasms of the wrist and feet may occur. To relieve symptoms, exhaled CO_2 can be reinhaled by placing a paper bag over the mouth or cupping hands over the nose and mouth. To avoid recurrence, instruct the woman to slow down and pay more attention to relaxation.

Preparing a couple for pushing involves using relaxation as well as muscle contraction simultaneously. To practice the technique, mothers should first empty their bladders. Women are then instructed to assume a comfortable position. The most common are sitting or semi-reclining, described as follows:

Position: Sit with feet touching the floor and hands grasping the thighs, or recline to about 40 degrees from sitting (three to four pillows behind) with knees pulled up, hands under thighs.

Breathing: Take a deep breath in to lower the diaphragm, lean forward, if sitting; if reclined, pull thighs to chest. Relax jaw and perineum. Direct the push low down in front, increasing the pressure in the abdomen as you bear down, letting breath out. Refuel with 1 to 2 slow deep breaths at the end of the contraction.

Women who have been experiencing many Braxton Hicks contractions or who have had previous miscarriages should practice only the positions and breathing, and not the actual pushing. Some instructors, in fact, do not allow any women in late pregnancy to practice pushing in class or at home for fear of causing premature labor.

Discussion about drug analgesia and anesthesia should be presented in an overview fashion, so that the couple can make informed choices. It should not be the role of the teacher to discuss every type of analgesia or anesthesia available. The mother is given guidelines so that she will know when to ask for medication. If she is unable to cope with contractions at 4 cm of dilation, she may need intervention because of the many hours left until delivery. She may request medication at 8 cm dilation, but with strong support from her doctor, midwife, and coach, she may be able to get through without medications. The idea of a psychoprophylaxis class is to teach the mothers how to better cope with pain through the many techniques she has learned. These techniques should greatly reduce her need for medication,[23] a factor which can only help both mother and infant.

Mothers and their partners should be introduced to the possibility of a Cesarean section, because these surgeries account for one out of every four births. In a class of eight couples, then, two may have a Cesarean section. The reasons Cesarean sections are performed should be the focus of the instruction. A few reasons for Cesarean birth are cephalopelvic disproportion, placenta previa, abruptio placentae, malposition, malpresentation, fetal distress, toxemia, premature rupture of the membranes without labor, and prolapsed cord. Participants should be encouraged to talk about their fears, and realize that having a section is, indeed, having a baby. Medications, incisions, and post-partum care after Cesarean can also be covered in the class. If the mother is to have a general anesthesia, or if the father is not there, a picture taken at the time of delivery may make the transition from pregnancy to parenting easier.[23] A film about Cesarean delivery can be shown to reduce anxiety and fear (see resource section in Appendix).

Many emotional and physical changes occur during post-partum. Initially, even if the mother is exhausted, she may feel an emotional high. Soon after, however, she may be more concerned about her body image and about how she has managed her labor. These feelings may have an effect on her nurturing abilities. She may feel that she did not live up to her own expectations, and as a result, may have less confidence in herself. The dramatic physical and hormonal fluctuations after birth will have an influence on the mother's well-being as well. Her family, partner's love and support, rest, and exercise will help speed her recovery.

Understanding these changes will enable partners to be supportive, even if the mother has days of emotional stability and strong, uncharacteristic dependency needs. Special time should be set aside for partners to spend together, perhaps necessitating child care arrangements. Even a walk around the block together may become a scheduling hassle. New parents need this time to sort out their new roles and priorities and to maintain mutual support for each other. In childbirth preparation classes, these emotional needs can be brought to the attention of the father. He should be encouraged to schedule time with the mother and to share child care responsibilities so mother can feel she has some time alone as well. Group support can be very important to both the new mother and father. A class roster with home phone numbers can be useful to the class. The instructor may also want to make a follow-up call to each family, post-delivery, before the class gets together after everyone has delivered. Extended families and friends can also be solicited to help with household tasks, so mother can rest and attend to child care.

Self-Assessment Review

1. Cephalopelvic disproportion refers to _____.

2. A third-degree laceration of the perineum is a tear _____.

3 A cystocele is _____.

4. _____, _____, and _____ may influence the duration of the second stage of labor.

5. Stress incontinence often results from injury during birth to the _____ and _____.

6. Breech birth refers to a presenting part _____.

7. Shoulder dystocia occurs when _____.

8. VBAC means _____.

9. Ten indications for Cesarean are: _____, _____, _____, _____, _____, _____, _____, _____, _____, and _____.

10. Usually, mothers with twins will go into labor by _____.

11. The third stage of labor is _____.

12. The two basic types of breathing for labor and delivery are: _____ and _____.

Answers

1. Disproportionate ratio between the child's head and the mother's pelvis; the head is not able to pass through the pelvis. 2. Into the anal sphincter. 3. Bulging of the bladder into the vagina after damage to the supporting structures of the bladder. 4. Maternal position, full bladder, pelvic floor fatigue. 5. Urethrovesical junction and urethra. 6. Other than the head. 7. The infant's head is delivered, but the shoulders are too wide for the pelvic inlet. 8. Vaginal birth after Cesarean. 9. Failure to progress, pelvic disproportion, malpresentation, fetal distress, pregnancy-induced hypertension, placenta previa, prolapse of the umbilical cord, herpes progenitalis, sometimes repeat Cesarean section and severe Rh incompatibility. 10. 37 to 38 weeks. 11. Delivery of the placenta. 12. Shallow chest breathing and rhythmic chest breathing.

REFERENCES

1. Danforth DV, Scott JR, eds. *Obstetrics and Gynecology*. 5th ed. Philadelphia, Pa: JB Lippincott; 1986.

2. Pauls J. The relationship between selected variates and the duration of second stage labor. *J Obstet Gynecol PT*. 1986;10(4):6-9.

3. Niswander KR, ed. *Manual of Obstetrics Diagnosis and Therapy*. 3rd ed. Boston, Mass: Little, Brown & Co; 1987.

4. Wilson JR, Carrington ER, Ledger WJ. *Obstetrics and Gynecology*. St. Louis, Mo: CV Mosby; 1983.

5. Malecki MP. *Mom and Dad and I are Having a Baby*. Seattle, Wash: Pennypress; 1982.

6. Murphy PA, Fullerton J. Outcomes of intended home births in nurse-midwifery practice: A prospective descriptive study. *Obstet Gynecol*. 1998;92:461-470.

7. Simmons R, Bernstein S. Out-of-hospital births in Michigan 1972-79. *Public Health Reg*. 1983;98:161-170.

8. Burst H. Issues and concerns of healthy pregnant women. *Public Health Reg (Suppl)*. 1987;102:57-61.

9. Stewart P. Hillan E, Calder A. A randomized trial to evaluate the use of a birth chair for delivery. *Lancet*. 1983;1:1296-1298.

10. Liddell HS, Fisher PR. The birthing chair in the second stage of labour. *Aust NZ J Obstet Gynecol*. 1985;25(1):65-68.

11. Goodlin RC, Frederick IB. Post-partum vulvar edema associated with the birthing chair. *Am J Obstet Gynecol*. 1983;146(3):334.

12. Rehn M. The moaning method. *CBE Reporter*. 1996;8(8).

13. Queenan JT, Hobbins JC. eds. *Protocols for High-Risk Pregnancies*. 2nd ed. Oradell, NJ: Medical Economics Books; 1987.

14. Effort launched by New York to reduce Cesarean sections. *PT Bull*. Feb 22, 1989;7.

15. Miller ES, Partezanna J, Montgomery RL. Vaginal birth after Cesarean: A 5-year experience in a family practice residency program. *J Am Board Fam Pract*. 1995; 8:357-360.

16. Flamm BL. Point/counterpoint: I. Vaginal birth after Cesarean: Where have we been and where are we going? *Ob Gyn Survey*. 1998;53(11):661-662.

17. Lairn JP, Stephens RJ, Miodovnik M, Barden TP. Vaginal delivery in patients with a prior Cesarean section. *Obstet Gynecol*. 1982;59(135):135-148.

18. Caughey AB, Shipp TD, Repke JT, Zelop C, Cohen A, Lieherman E. Trial of labor after Cesarean delivery: The effect of previous vaginal delivery. *Am J Obstet Gynecol*. 1998;179:938-941.

19. Keolkirk K. *Vaginal Birth after Cesarean*. Seattle, Wash: Pennypress; 1981.

20. Eglinton GS, Phelan JP, Weh S, Diac FP, Wallace Tm, Paul RH. Outcome of a trial of labor after prior Cesarean delivery. *J Reprod Med*. 1984;29(1):3-8.

21. Goldman G, Pineault R, Potvin L, Blais R, Bilodeau H. Factors influencing the practice of vaginal birth after Cesarean section. *Am J Public Health*. 1993;83:1104-1108.

22. Noble E. *Having Twins*. Boston, Mass: Houghton-Mifflin; 1980.

23. Noble E. Rationale for prenatal and post-partum exercise. In: Simkin P, Reinke C, eds. *Kaleidoscope of Childbearing Preparation, Birth, and Nurturing*. Seattle, Wash: Pennypress; 1978.

Chapter 11

Physical Therapy and Post-Partum Care

The puerperium period follows the delivery of the placenta and ends about 6 to 8 weeks later, although some references suggest that the post-partum period ends with the resumption of the menstrual cycle. In nursing mothers, the puerperium is not as clearly defined because lactation delays ovulation for weeks or months. Many dramatic changes occur during this time as the uterus shrinks, the birth canal and perineum repair, and the endocrine system rebalances.

ANATOMICAL AND PHYSIOLOGICAL CHANGES POST-PARTUM

The Uterus

At delivery, the uterus weighs about 1000 gm and measures 14 cm long, 12 cm wide, and 10 cm thick, about the same size at 16 weeks of pregnancy. Within a week, it weighs 500 gm and decreases in size so that it again lies within the true pelvis. This decrease is attributed to the decrease in both the amount of cytoplasm and size of the individual cells.[1] Uterine contractions increase in intensity after delivery, probably because of the decreased uterine volume within the surrounding, contracting myometrium. After the first 1 to 2 hours, these contractions are diminished and become uncoordinated. However, when oxytocin is released in response to the baby's suckling, the uterine contractions (after pains) can once again become smooth, intense, and coordinated and continue through the beginning of the puerperium. These pains can become quite severe in the multipara.

Exfoliation occurs at the placental site of attachment. The shedding of the endometrial tissue prevents scar formation. The outer-most layer of decidua becomes necrotic after the first few days. Consequently, the sloughed tissue of serum and leukocytes makes up the vaginal discharge. Within the third week post-partum, the cells of the endometrial glands (in the remaining decidua) grow across the bare surface and complete regeneration of the area.

Lochia is the name given to the vaginal discharge after delivery. It undergoes many changes during the next 4 to 6 weeks. In the first 6 to 8 days, it is called lochia rubra because of its bright red color and consists of decidua, blood, and trophoblastic material. For the next several days it becomes more serous and darker and is termed lochia serosa; it is made up of sloughed tissue, leukocytes, old blood, and serum. During the following 2 weeks, the lochia becomes whitish-yellow, and is composed of decidua, leukocytes, epithelial cells, serum, bacteria, and mucus. This latter form of lochia is called lochia alba because of its whitish color.

It is important to remind the mother that the uterus may be sensitive after delivery and after fundal massage. In the days that follow delivery, the bleeding will be heavy and gradually diminish, but if a mother physically overexerts herself, she may have a period of red flow, and she should slow down.

The cervix constricts and returns to its pre-pregnancy shape in about 2 weeks post-delivery. The cervix undergoes dramatic remodeling from a maximally effaced and dilated condition at delivery to its normally closed position. The vagina resumes its non-pregnant size by 6 to 8 weeks.

The Perineum

The introitus is red and swollen, especially locally around an episiotomy or lacerations. The perineum will also feel sore from stretching, even if an episiotomy was not done. The mother may find some comfort from applying ice packs to the perineum to decrease pain and swelling. Early pelvic floor exercises should help decrease discomfort while urinating. These exercises can be started immediately upon delivery and should be done every hour after that. This will promote an increase in circulation, which will decrease stiffness and edema. Sitz baths and careful cleaning, perhaps with a water-filled squeeze bottle, are recommended to help promote healing, avoid infection and irritation to the healing sutures of an episiotomy.

Urinary Tract

There is often trauma to the urethra and bladder after the birth of the baby through the vaginal canal. The bladder wall may be swollen and hyperemic, and there may be slight bleeding in the muscle. The bladder may also be insensitive to the intravesical pressures that stimulate urination. This insensitivity will be even more marked if anesthesia has been used in labor. As a result, the mother may have some loss in sensitivity to pressure build-up in the bladder. She should be reminded to frequently empty the bladder, especially during the first week post-partum, when there is considerable natural diuresis. By doing this, she avoids overdistention and to helps the bladder return to normal function. Some women need a catheter.

Due to diaphoresis during the first week post-delivery, urinary output will greatly exceed intake. The glomerular filtration rate remains elevated to handle the increased urine flow, often reaching 3 liters per 24 hours.[1] Physiologic proteinuria may appear during the first week and less often, glycosuria, but these usually resolve within a few days. The ureters and renal pelves return to their normal prepregnant size within 6 weeks.

Gastrointestinal Tract

There is a minor slowing of intestinal motility, in an unmedicated birth, which may be intensified if the mother received anesthesia. Early ambulation, a diet rich in fiber and a mild laxative will assist in normal motility. If there has been a third- or fourth-degree laceration into the rectal sphincter, laxatives are often prescribed to eliminate straining the rectal wall during bowel movements. In addition, mothers often experience hemorrhoids following delivery due to the increased pressure on the rectal veins from pushing. Sitz baths, laxatives, commercial preparations, and pelvic floor and abdominal exercises tend to stimulate healing and decrease swelling of mild hemorrhoids.

Circulation

An initial heat loss in the post-partum mother results from delivery of the infant, placenta and loss of amniotic fluid, possibly resulting in shaking and chills. Cardiac output after the first minute post-partum may increase approximately 40% to 50% above prelabor values, but should return to non-pregnant values by 2 to 3 weeks post-partum. These changes are due to fluctuations in stroke volume. There is little change in blood pressure, however. With the decreased size of the uterus and descent of the diaphragm, normal cardiac access is restored, and an electrocardiogram at this time will show normalized features.[1] Blood volume changes will depend on the amount of blood lost during delivery and the amount of extravascular water excreted. In the first 72 hours, there is a greater decrease in plasma volume than in cellular components. Consequently, there is a slight increase in the hematocrit level as compared to immediate post-partum levels. Volume changes and reduced pressures often result in the resolution of lower extremity or vulvar varicosities after delivery.

Musculoskeletal

Post-partum abdominal muscle tone is very slack, and the muscles may not provide adequate support for the trunk, specifically for the low back. Hormonal influence continues to affect ligaments as well. Therefore, the back is at greater risk for injury due to this lack of support and lack of protective ligaments. The ligaments usually return to their shortened length during the post-partum weeks, but until that time, abdominal exercises should be performed in a stable position to avoid over stretching ligaments or exacerbating a rectus diastasis.[2]

Diastasis Recti Abdominus

To accommodate the expanding uterus, and because of the hormonal influences of pregnancy, the linea alba becomes stretched and softened. This places the abdominal muscles at a disadvantage, and often the rectus abdominis muscles will separate from the uniting linea alba. If not during pregnancy, a diastasis recti can instead develop during the second stage of labor, particularly if there is excessive breath holding during pushing. Consequently, the abdominal wall should be checked for diastasis recti post-partum.

Exam for Diastasis Recti
1. The woman lies flat on her back with her knees bent.
2. She raises her head and shoulders until her neck is about 8 inches, her chin should be tucked and her arms stretched out front.
3. The therapist should check the presence of a bulge in the central abdominal area, which is evident when the muscles have parted.
4. The numbers of the therapist's fingers inserted horizontally into the gap at the level of the umbilicus, 2 inches above and 2 inches below, defines the amount of separation between the taut rectus muscles.

Any separation of more than two fingers wide constitutes a restriction on any type of curl-up or leg lowering exercises without approximation of the rectus. Trunk rotational exercises should be avoided until there is no rectus separation. Unless there is significant diastasis recti, however, abdominal exercises with the pelvic floor contracted should be started within the first 24 hours to restore abdominal tone. A jack-knifed position (sitting straight up from a supine position) and double leg lifts should be avoided, because of the possibility of increasing a separation between the rectus abdominis muscles or injuring the low back.

Emotional Adjustments

On the third day post-partum, 70% to 80% of women will go through a transient depression, sometimes known as the "post-partum blues." Contributing to this emotional depression are the emerging physical body changes, endocrine upheaval, and readjustment of intracellular fluid level, coupled with adjustments to parenting responsibilities and the infant's demands. Usually this depression is gone within a few days, but rarely, serious psychiatric disorders do occur. If the mother's lingering depression interferes with her effectiveness and her ability to cope with day-to-day responsibilities, a psychiatrist's help must be obtained. Psychological problems of this nature may have a long-reaching history. True psychoses after delivery can occur when a constellation of psychotic factors has been set up prior to pregnancy; the stress of pregnancy and delivery become the precipitating and nonspecific factors.[1]

Lactation

During pregnancy, high levels of estrogen block the secretion of milk. This causes an adherence of prolactin to breast tissue which prevents a milk-producing effect on the epithelium.[1] After delivery, high levels of estrogen and progesterone, human placental lactogen (HPL), and insulin are decreased, and milk engorgement begins in 2 to 3 days. Sucking enhances milk production by signaling the brain to release prolactin and oxytocin. The prolactin stimulates the let-down reflex in the breast. It is believed that the tactile nerve endings in the areola send a stimulus to the hypothalamus, resulting in an increase in production and transport of oxytocin to the posterior pituitary, where it is released into the circulation.[1] Oxytocin signals the alveoli and ducts in the breast to contract and squeeze milk through the nipple. The level of prolactin is gradually decreased during the first weeks of pregnancy. By the fourth or fifth month, the prolactin level has returned to its non-pregnant value. The factors that maintain milk production after this point remain unclear.[1]

There are three types of human milk, the first being *colostrum*, a clear or yellowish fluid, containing more antibodies, serum chloride, potassium, protein, minerals, and fat soluble vitamins than mature milk. This milk will often leak out of the breast prenatally, but mothers should not encourage expression. It is believed that colostrum readies the infant's intestinal tract for later milk and helps to clean out the infant's digestive tract, by stimulating the elimination of the meconium that fills the gastrointestinal tract of the infant at birth. On the second or third day, the breasts become gorged with milk. Frequent feedings will decrease the distended breasts. *Transitional milk* comes next and lasts up to 2 weeks post-partum. It changes over a two week period to a higher fat and lactose content, thereby increasing its total caloric value. *Mature milk*, the last to come, 2 weeks post-delivery, decreases in fat content in the latter part of the first year, and works in concert with the additional nutrition the baby receives from other sources.

The composition of milk changes in response to the different stages of lactation, time of day, time within a feeding, and a mother's level of nutrition. Usually, the milk fat comes in the later part of a feeding. In addition, there is an additional rise in fat between the morning and mid-afternoon feedings.

A mother's nutrition, rest, and fluid intake are crucial to a good supply of milk. The nursing mother will need 500 calories more a day than what she was eating before she was pregnant, along with 20 gm more of protein for milk production. If the mother is not nursing, an injection of estrogen and testosterone is given to inhibit milk production. Supportive bras, cold applied to the breasts, aspirin, and a lowered fluid intake, will decrease the engorgement of the breasts.[3]

The breasts in a nursing mother will retain 2 or 3 pounds until weaning. Breasts may leak before and after delivery, and some women use nursing pads inside their bras. Mothers can often toughen their nipples during pregnancy, preparing them for nursing by frequently pinching, rolling, and gently rubbing them with a towel. Because the newborn will nurse on demand, the nipples are subjected to a great deal of manipulation and moisture, which encourages cracking and soreness. To prevent mastitis or cracked and sore nipples, the mother should allow nipples to dry between feedings, feed the baby frequently so that the breast does not become full, use good nursing positions, break suction correctly, avoid use of soap or oils on the nipples, get plenty of sleep, and maintain good nutrition.

If only one breast is sore, the baby should nurse on the unaffected side first. When both sides are sore, the milk should be (manually or with a pump) expressed until a letdown reflex occurs. This will make the milk more available for the infant and, thereby, decrease the intensity of the baby's initial suckling. Heat and breast massage can decrease sore breasts, as well. If the nipple does become sore or cracked, a breast shield or a 1- to 2-day rest from suckling on that side may help relieve symptoms. The affected breast will need to be pumped or milk expressed to maintain the milk production.

The mother should build up the sucking time gradually in each breast from 5 to 15 minutes. The feedings may stretch out to every 3 to 4 hours after the first few weeks. An experienced mother or nurse can offer assistance for the first-time mother when nursing is started. The nipple and areola should be held between the second and third fingers of one hand with the opposite hand held behind the baby's head to bring it to the nipple. This way, the nipple and areola can be placed well back into the baby's mouth so that it is sucking on the areola. If the baby needs some encouragement, stroking the cheek next to the nipple will elicit the rooting reflex, and the baby will turn to the nipple and suck. The baby will suck quite naturally; the letdown reflex may come slowly at first, but continued suckling will encourage it.

Sometimes the suction with which a baby holds on may be a problem. It will need to be broken so that the baby can be switched to the other side. A finger placed in the corner of the infant's mouth will relieve the suction. The baby needs to be burped before changing sides, and at the end of the feeding to expel swallowed air. The next feeding should start on the breast that was finished last. A safety pin attached to the bra, changed from side to side after each feeding will help the mother remember which side to start on.

Sometimes the baby will strongly prefer one breast over the other. This may mean that the baby has an inborn cerebral dominance, expressed as a preference for a certain head position that he was accustomed to in utero.[4] By changing from the standard cradling position, the mother can still have the child nurse from the non-preferred side. Other possible positions are mother and child side-lying, or the football hold, in which the baby is held on the forearm alongside the mother rather than across her (Figure 11-1). The mother should bring the baby up to her and avoid leaning to the baby when feeding, or upper back pain may result. A pillow placed under the child and behind the mother, so that she can maintain a supported position, will decrease back strain.

Comfortable clothing, such as tops that facilitate nursing and supportive nursing bras, are helpful. Sometimes mothers have difficulty allowing their milk to let down in public. Mothers can usually find a private place to nurse or can drape a cloth over the top of the baby's head and across her own shoulder to facilitate the letdown reflex by decreasing her own inhibition.

Figure 11-1. Breast-feeding positions. A) sitting with pillows under child, B) sidelying, C) football hold.

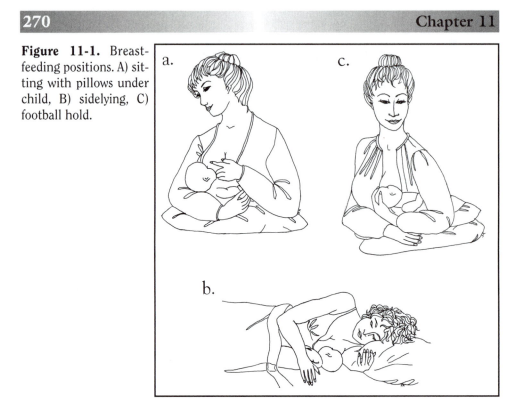

EXERCISE

Exercise in the post-partum period is key to rapid and maximum muscle function and restoration of the mother's health. A complete exercise program done at this time can often prevent problems in later life, such as: pelvic floor dysfunction, poor posture, decreased gastrointestinal motility, back and neck discomfort, poor abdominal strength, fatigue, difficulty nursing, and possibly a poor self-image. Post-partum, the body must adjust to sudden weight loss, change in center of gravity, and accompanying postural adjustments. Fundamentally, the pelvic floor and abdominal muscles deserve a great deal of attention, but the rest of the trunk is also undergoing changes related to postural readjustment. The low, mid, and upper back, buttock, and deep hip muscles should be exercised to facilitate their return to normal. Pelvic floor and abdominal exercises can begin as soon as the infant is delivered.

Mothers should receive clearance from a physician before beginning an exercise program, because there are conditions that may limit or contraindicate certain activities. These include myocardial disease, congestive heart failure, rheumatic heart disease (class II or above), recent pulmonary embolus, acute infectious disease, uterine hemorrhage, severe hypotensive disease, diabetes mellitus, radicular arm or leg signs, sacroiliac pain, excessive vaginal bleeding, and marked rectus diastasis.[4,5] Abdominal exercises should be prescribed after the abdominal wall has been fully evaluated for rectus diastasis A woman who has been on bed rest for an extended part of her pregnancy will need a gentle exercise program to avoid fatigue (Figure 11-2).

Pelvic Floor Restoration (Goals- continence, strength, endurance):
- Stop test- once a week stop and start urine flow on toilet to check on integrity of pelvic floor strength:
- Quick contractions- 3 second holds:
- Long contractions- 15 second holds:
- Increasing the frequency and repetitions according to the mother's strength.

Abdominal muscles (Goals-strengthen and eliminate diastasis recti):
- Evaluate for strength and diastasis recti:
- Use a sheet that is crossed across the mother's abdomen to approximate a small diastasis recti and strengthen with curl-ups to front, left and right sides. Incorporate pelvic floor contractions with curl-ups.
- Leg slides while using sheet for approximation of abdominals.

Posture (Goals- restore and strengthen upper back muscles, balance abdominal and back-strength):
- Strengthen upper, mid, low back and buttock muscles

Hip muscles (Goals- stretch and strengthen, improve tone and flexibility):
- Bridging and with abduction and adduction.

ADL Review (Goal- prevent injuries):
- Instruct in proper lifting and carrying of baby;
- Positions for nursing that support mother and baby;
- Avoid overuse injuries of hands.

Bra, Abdominal, Back Supports (Goal- support the mother's spine and abdomen):
- Evaluate mother for supports while she regains muscle tone.

General Aerobic Conditioning (Goal- to promote endurance and general strengthening):
- Mother monitors her pulse and follows guidelines (see Chapter 4).
- Participation in a post-natal exercise class, swimming, walking, bike riding, or any combination of these will help her continue a general conditioning program.

Conscious Relaxation (Goal- increase her ability to cope with all the physical and emotional changes, improve her feeling of well-being):
- Decrease stress with changed lifestyle:
- Practice daily for 20 minutes to increase her overall endurance:
- Practice relaxation during daily tasks:
- Practice slow easy breathing.

Figure 11-2. Exercise and educational program post-uncomplicated delivery (see end of chapter for full program).

POST-CESAREAN DELIVERY

Because of the high Cesarean section rate in the United States, physical therapists should be trained to assist in the recovery of these women. A mother delivering by Cesarean section will have many of the same physical discomforts associated with any major abdominal surgery or with vaginal delivery. Although there will be no episiotomy, the same changes occur in the uterus, pelvic floor, and urinary and gastrointestinal tracts.

Most women will be taken to the recovery room after a Cesarean section, until they have recovered from anesthesia, and will have their vital signs monitored until they are stabilized. While in the recovery room, the parents can bond with their new child, while the mother recovers under supervision. Usually, the intravenous line and catheter remain in overnight, and may be in for as long as 48 hours.

Attention must be given to adequate lung expansion, prevention of wound infection, and a significantly decreased intestinal motility coupled with the residual effects of anesthesia. Clamps or stitches, used to approximate the abdominal wall, are removed around the sixth day, after which, barring any problems, the mother may go home.

The mother who undergoes a Cesarean section will have a longer recovery physically. Common postoperative problems, such as gas, severe pain, and fever, may require medication. For moderate pain, however, the mother might use medications or TENS for pain relief so she can get out of bed and begin walking. TENS applied on the lateral aspects of a low transverse incision has been found to significantly decrease the amount of narcotics needed post-Cesarean.[7] Normal contraindications for TENS use must be followed. Preoperative fitting of electrodes and instruction would be ideal to acclimate the mother to the idea of the apparatus and to gather a baseline for the pain level needed for those who know they will have a Cesarean delivery.

Cesarean support classes are often given in the hospital. Support from her partner, doctor, family, and friends will assist her in her readjustment. She needs to know that that there are many good reasons to have one. She may be relieved that a Cesarean section was done, especially after a long labor or after fetal distress, but she may also feel that she has failed at her own plan or image of giving birth. Here, her self-esteem and confidence may be altered, affecting her parenting and recovery. It is helpful if the mother has been prepared for a Cesarean delivery during her labor and delivery classes.

It is also important for her to know that one Cesarean birth does not always mean another. She will need to adjust her daily activities and conserve her energy. The post-Cesarean mother should have all the time she needs to fully recover before performing household tasks. These mothers are usually not restricted from climbing stairs, but should limit their use. Women should be shown how to contract the pelvic floor and abdominal muscles and use the legs and buttocks to propel the body up the stairs.

Characteristically, post-Cesarean mothers lean forward when walking to protect the incision. This slouching posture will be further emphasized when she carries, changes, or breastfeeds the baby. The mother must begin to ambulate in the first 12 to 18 hours to increase intestinal motility, decrease muscle stiffness, and prevent thrombophlebitis. These mothers should also be started on a physical therapy program the first day in the hospital, and have their exercises monitored and graded throughout their stay.

The mother can be taught to splint the incision by placing one hand on top of the other over the incision with her wrists placed just anterior to the iliac crest. The therapist can also make a splint pillow for her from two towels folded in a square, wrapped, and taped. By holding the incision firmly with this pillow the mother will feel more secure and be better able to walk with good posture. The mother should be told that walking and gentle exercises will not pull apart the incision and that activity stimulates healing by increasing circulation. Sometimes these women will need abdominal supports to enable them to move around with less discomfort. Exercises are the key to successful physical rehabilitation (Figure 11-3).

Breathing exercises (Goal- increase ventilation in lungs post-anesthesia):
- Diaphragmatic breathing-mother splints incision with her hands or a splint pillow while performing deep breathing.
- Mid-chest expansion-mother puts hands along the side of the lateral chest wall while directing air into lungs so that ribs expand into her hands.
- Upper chest expansion-mother places one hand over the sternum, the thumb and fingers are over the clavicle, while she directs the chest expansion into her hand.
- Huffing-mother splints incision and breathes in through the nose and on exhalation, she repeats a forced "Ahhhh."

Abdominals (Goals- increase strength and restore tone, evaluate for diastasis recti)
- Pelvic tilt-side-lying or sitting positions.
- Leg slides-knees bent lying on back, pull stomach in, flatten back, slide one leg up and down, maintaining pelvic control. Do not extend legs down fully.
- Hula-lying supine, legs flat; hike hip up and down.

Pelvic Floor Restoration (Goals- continence, strength, endurance):
- Stop test- once a week stop and start urine flow on toilet to check on integrity of pelvic floor strength:
- Quick contractions- 3 second holds.
- Long contractions- 15 second holds:
- Increasing the frequency and repetitions according to the mother's strength.

Posture (Goals- restore and strengthen upper back muscles, balance abdominal and back strength):
- Strengthen upper, mid, low back and buttock muscles with isotonic exercises in a rest position.
- Practice correct posture during ADL's.

ADL Review (Goal- prevent injuries):
- Instruct in proper lifting and carrying of baby:
- Positions for nursing that support mother and baby:
- Instruct in proper and avoid overuse injuries of hands:
- Instruct in contraction of pelvic floor and abdomen with propelling herself up stairs with use of her legs:
- Instruct in log rolling and huffing with activities.[8]
- Bra, Abdominal, Back Supports; (Goal- support the mother's spine and abdomen):
- Evaluate mother for supports while she regains muscle tone.

General Aerobic Conditioning (Goal- to promote endurance and general strengthening):
- Mother monitors her pulse and follows guidelines (see Chapter 4).
- Participation in a post-natal exercise class, swimming, walking, bike riding, or any combination of these will help her continue a general conditioning program.

Conscious Relaxation (Goal- increase her ability to cope with all the physical and emotional changes, improve her feeling of well-being):
- Decrease stress with changed lifestyle:
- Practice daily for 20 minutes to increase her overall endurance:
- Practice relaxation during daily tasks
- Practice slow easy breathing.

Figure 11-3. Initial exercise and educational program post-Cesarean delivery (see end of chapter for full program and guidelines).

THE FIRST SIX WEEKS AT HOME

Going Home

The health of the mother and infant and the location where delivery occurs often determine when they go home. Traditionally, women recuperated at the hospital for at least 1 week. Now, after an uncomplicated birth, women and their babies leave the hospital in 2 days. At a birthing center, they often leave within a few hours to rest at home.

Once home, fatigue is common, and additional sleep and rest are needed for several days. Early ambulation, whether at home or in the hospital, decreases the chance of thrombophlebitis and improves bowel and bladder functions.[9] New mothers should start pelvic floor and gentle abdominal exercises immediately and continue them at home to increase the tone and supportive functions of these muscles.

Sexuality

Sexual intercourse can be resumed when the bright red bleeding ceases, or at least after 4 to 6 weeks. If another pregnancy is to be avoided, then contraception is necessary. Although the hormones produced by breastfeeding women delay ovulation, it is impossible to tell exactly when ovulation will occur. Breastfeeding is not a substitute for birth control. Low-dose contraceptives have been used in women who are not nursing and who have been screened for contraindications. Diaphragms can be fitted at the post-partum checkup at 6 weeks. In the meantime, condoms can be used, but they are not 100% safe for preventing pregnancy. It is a good idea for women to discuss this with their doctors or nurses prior to delivery.

Post-Partum Checkup

The post-partum checkup is scheduled for 6 weeks after delivery. The physician will check involution of the uterus and vagina and integrity of the cervix, perineum, and pelvic support. The abdominal tone and breasts are assessed as well. Lab work may include examination of cervical cells, assessment of hematocrit level, and a urinalysis. Blood pressure and weight are measured, and the woman's medical and emotional health will be screened.

POST-PARTUM CASE STUDY

Cindy, age 42, following her second pregnancy, comes to physical therapy with the following complaints: aching in her upper back, painful thumbs and feeling unable to cope with all the added responsibilities at home.

Cindy's first child, Erin, is 17 months and her new infant, Jason, is 1 month old. Her pregnancy was complicated by being on bed rest for 5 weeks following pre-term labor. She took trabutaline to stop contractions and medication to increase the lung maturity of the fetus. No other medications were used. Jason was 7 lbs. at delivery and she had a small perineal tear. She is now home and feels overwhelmed with the care of both children. She is nursing the infant for all his feedings and noticed upper back pain in the second week post-delivery. In the last week, she reported that both of her thumbs are painful and it is difficult to pick up either child. During questioning, she complained of leaking urine at least once a day when she coughed, sneezed or occasionally lifted something about 15 lb. Cindy is teary in the interview and reports that she has felt depressed, something she did not have after her first child.

Exam

Posture: Cindy stands with her head in a forward position, rounded shoulders, and protruding abdomen.

Palpation: Spasms noted in bilateral trapezius and rhomboids, marked tenderness to touch at bilateral thumb CMC joints.

Strength: 3/5 strength in the rhomboids and paraspinal muscles, -3/5 abdominals

ROM: Reduced neck rotation-60° left and right and painful, flexion 60°, extension 40°and sore. Shoulder, elbow, wrist are WFL. Hand-full ROM with pain at thumb CMC joints.

ADL: Review of all ADL's reveal that Cindy nurses the infant while holding him in her arms without support, and that she is lifting with her thumbs in wide abduction.

Assessment: Cindy's position during her bed rest added to the decreased strength in her upper back, abdominals and poor posture. Her repeated lifting of both children strained the CMC joints bilaterally. She has some mild incontinence. Additionally it was noted that Cindy was excessively teary and having difficulty adjusting to care of two children while she was in pain.

Goals:
- Increase strength in trapezius, abdominals, and paraspinal muscles to 4+/5
- Increase ROM in her neck to full
- Stabilize both CMC joints. Refer to Occupational Therapist for fabrication of functional splints.
- Eliminate pain, tenderness of her neck
- Eliminate pain at CMC joints
- Improve posture so she is using postural muscles for trunk support
- Instruct in body mechanics, and proper posture
- Increase strength in pelvic floor muscle so she is fully continent
- Problem solve with patient in ways to incorporate exercise regime into her daily routine
- Improve relaxation for stress reduction and refer her to counselor for a consultation

Treatment:
- Physical therapy treatment of Cindy's neck with ultrasound, myofascial release techniques
- Stretching and strengthening of neck, paravertebral and rhomboids. Strengthen abdominals
- CMC-Treat with bilateral iontophoresis set up, massage and ROM
- Instruct in pelvic floor exercises and lifting of pelvic floor muscles for lifting, coughing, sneezing and laughing. Complete a bladder diary and make recommendations accordingly.
- ADL training -alter nursing positions so that the weight of the baby is supported by pillows or the bed, while Cindy can sit or lie in a supportive restful position. Have her demonstrate proper lifting techniques. Reinforce with back care video to view at home several times.
- Home program- encourage Cindy purchase a well-fitting bra with wide straps to support the increased breast tissue. Stretch tight neck muscles, and strengthen upper back muscles, abdominal and pelvic floor muscles. Home treatment of CMC joints includes: heat or ice, controlled ROM and strengthening when indicated.
- Posture correction instruction.

INSTRUCTING POST-PARTUM CLASSES

The physical therapist has an excellent opportunity to assist the mother recovering from birth by instructing classes in post-partum care. Physical changes of the mother have been detailed here, but it is important in childbirth preparation classes to remind couples that the uterus may be sensitive after delivery and after fundal massage. In the days that follow delivery, the bleeding will be heavy and gradually diminish, but if a mother physically overexerts herself, she may have a period of red flow, and she should slow down. The perineum will also feel sore from stretching, even if an episiotomy was not done. The mother may find some comfort from applying ice packs to the perineum to decrease swelling. Early pelvic floor exercises should help decrease discomfort while urinating. These exercises can be started immediately upon delivery and should be done every hour after that. This will promote an increase in circulation, which will decrease stiffness and edema. Sitz baths may help reduce perineal pain and promote healing. On the third day post-partum, the abdominals should be checked for diastasis recti abdominis. Gentle abdominal exercises, leg slides, pelvic rocking in sitting and on all fours, and diagonal curl-ups may be started.

Advice should also be given regarding the restoration of normal voiding. The bladder and urethra may undergo trauma. As a result, the mother may have some loss in sensitivity to pressure build-up in the bladder. She should be reminded to frequently empty the bladder, especially during the first week post-partum, when there is considerable natural diuresis. There is also a slowing of intestinal peristalsis after delivery. The abdominal muscles are lax, and the mother may be constipated. If she has not had a bowel movement by the third day after delivery, she may need an enema to stimulate peristalsis. Roughage in the diet, plenty of fluids, and mild exercise help relieve constipation. If hemorrhoids develop from pushing efforts, sitz baths, pelvic floor exercises, and avoiding constipation may help relieve the discomfort.

Mothers may look to the post-partum instructor for advice on when to return to work after delivery. This choice really rests with the couple and depends on how they plan to raise their child, their lifestyle, and their family situation. They should be encouraged to seek their own answers. Some women arrange day, or live-in care, immediately for their newborn so they can return to work quickly, either because of finances or preference. Other families will pick a number of months for mother or father to stay home with the child or will wait and see, deciding as time passes when to return to work The mother who wants to continue breastfeeding and working, may express and freeze the milk.

Bonding between parents and child takes time. It is important as a physical therapist to dispel the notion that instant parenting happens with delivery of the child. Over time, the family will sort out priorities, and the feeling of being a parent will develop. Physical closeness and caring can encourage the bonding process and should be started as soon as possible. If keeping the baby warm is a concern, a warming light can be placed over the baby, mother, and partner immediately after delivery, so the baby and parents will not be separated. Separation during this critical time is discouraged unless medically indicated for the mother or infant. During this bonding period, the infant is encouraged to suckle. (This helps stimulate uterine contractions.) If the mother has not received medication, the infant will be responsive during the first 1 to 2 hours after delivery and may attempt to focus on his parent's faces. The baby will then most likely become drowsy and sleep.

Integrating the new baby into the family will involve changes in all relationships, whether it is the first child or the last. Usually, by the end of 6 weeks, the post-partum adjustments have been resolved, and the family has made its adjustments and prioritized family, home, and baby care.[10]

Post-Natal Exercise Program

Post-natal exercise contraindications and guidelines are the same as with prenatal exercises, except supine lying and abdominal compression (unless post-Cesarean section) are not restricted after delivery mothers will need to be checked for diastasis recti. To restore maximal overall strength post-natally, exercises should concentrate on pelvic floor toning, abdominal muscles, posture realignment, strengthening of upper back, upper body, and lower extremities to increase strength and circulation.[10] The challenge to the physical therapist is to create an exercise regime that will meet the needs of the mother, avoid contraindications, and be fun to do. Some programs have been developed using the baby as part of the exercise.[10] Designing two programs that can be alternated every other day helps to prevent boredom. Additionally, music and a class format will assist in motivating the mothers. See Table 11-1 as a sample of a post-natal program. It is not meant to be inclusive, and physical therapists should use this only as a guideline for developing a program that best suits the needs of their client and their own teaching style.

Post-Cesarean Exercise Program

Exercises are the key to successful physical rehabilitation after a cesarean section and breathing exercises should be first on the list. Because general anesthesia is used, the mucus may pool in the lungs. Therefore, the mother should be encouraged to breathe completely, so that the lung is totally ventilated. Additional exercises may be started in the hospital before discharge, focusing on abdominals, pelvic floor, and general conditioning. Table 11-2 shows is a sample exercise list for the first week post-Cesarean.

The physical therapist can help the post-Cesarean section mother correct her posture. A Polaroid picture of the mother can show her postural problems, and instruction in proper body mechanics can aid her recovery from surgery. The physical therapist may also wish to provide written guidelines for body mechanics to patients (Figure 11-4).

Using these guidelines, the mother is taught to adjust daily activities. Huffing gently will discourage her from holding her breath. Household tasks should be done with the weight evenly distributed over each leg and can incorporate pelvic floor and pelvic tilt exercises. When completing repetitive rotational activities (sweeping, mopping, vacuuming, and raking), she can put one foot in front of the other and lunge forward and back while shifting weight, decreasing the full arc of trunk rotation.

Table 11-1

Sample Post-Natal Exercise Program

1. Pelvic floor toning- supine, contract-relax exercises. Hold the contractions for 5 seconds, 10 repetitions.

2. Single straight leg raise- supine, alternate knee bent, raise leg straight up and down, stretching the hamstring in the back of the leg, hold at maximal stretch for 5 seconds, lower with control, switch legs left and right, 10 repetitions each.

3. Pelvic tilt exercise- knees bent, flat on back, hold stomach in, flatten back against the floor simultaneously doing a pelvic floor contraction, 10 repetitions.

4. Knee drop- knees together and bent, flat on back, drop knees side to side, allowing hips to come up, shoulders remain flat, head turns in opposite direction of knees, 10 repetitions.

5. Single knee to chest- on back, knees bent, pelvic tilt, pull knee towards chest, lift head, head returns to flat position, lower leg to knee bent position and alternate with other leg, 10 repetitions each leg in an alternating fashion.

6. Hula- in supine, legs straight, hike hip up straight and down, keeping legs straight, alternate side to side 10 times each side. Use hip muscles. Do not lift up buttock.

7. Gluteal set- in supine position, legs straight, squeeze buttocks and hold 10 seconds, relax, repeat 10 times.

8. Ankle pumps- legs straight, flat on back or sitting, pump ankles up and down together 10 times, then circle both feet together 10 times in one direction, 10 times in the other direction.

9. Leg slides- towel under feet, knees bent, flat on back, maintain a pelvic tilt while sliding legs almost to a fully-extended position and bring them back up to a knee bent position without losing the pelvic tilt, 10 times.

10. Curl-ups- on back, pelvic tilt, arms out straight, knees bent, lift head, chest and shoulders up 45 degrees and down, repeat 20 times. Breathe out as head lifts.

11. Sit-backs- (avoid if diastasis recti) in sitting position, knees bent, hands touching knees, lean back at a 45 degree angle and hold 5 seconds, return upright, rest and repeat 10 times.

12. Cat exercise- on hands and knees, drop head down, raise back up, return to neutral, repeat 10 times.

13. Modified buddha- on knees, sit back on heels, lean forward with arms extended and back stretched, drop head. Hold 10 seconds and return to knee sitting position. Repeat 10 times. (Do not raise buttocks above head level.)

14. Knee standing side stretch- on knees, pillow under knees, maintain upright position, bend side to side, trying to touch fingertips to either side. Do not lean forward.

15. Neck stretches- sitting comfortably, stretch neck side to side, holding 5 seconds each way. Also, rotate neck left and right, holding 5 seconds each way, up and down without holding. Repeat the series 5 times.

16. Shoulder series exercises- sitting upright, shrug shoulders up, pull shoulders down, pull shoulders forward, pull shoulders backwards, rotate shoulders forward 5 times, rotate shoulders backward 5 times each, repeat the series 5 times in all.

17. Upper back lifts- prone lying, a) arms out straight overhead, lift head, neck, and chest up and down; b) arms straight out at shoulder level, lift head, neck, chest and arms up and down; c) arms out to sides, elbows bent, lift head, chest, upper back up and down. Repeat series 10 times.

18. Head retraction- sitting, hand on chin, pull chin in and swallow. Repeat 5 times.

19. Posture correction exercise at wall- standing, feet 6 inches from wall, back against wall, bend knees, do a pelvic tilt, shoulders back, arms out at the side, palms up, head back and retracted, drag arms up the wall until there is a stretch in the upper back, hold 5 seconds, stand up slowly, maintaining a pelvic tilt, lower arms, relax and repeat 5 times.

20. Hamstring stretch- long siting, lean over legs and hold 10 seconds, feel gradual stretch, come up to a brig sitting position, repeat 10 times.

21. Pelvic floor exercises- repeat as in Number 1.

Table 11-2

Post-Cesarean Exercise Program

[Adapted from Frahm J: Hutzel Hospital Physical Therapy Department. Post- Cesarean Exercise Program.[8]]

Day 1

1. Diaphragmatic breathing-mother splints incision with her hands or a splint pillow while performing deep breathing.

2. Mid-chest expansion-mother puts hands along the side of the lateral chest wall while directing air into lungs so that ribs expand into her hands.

3. Upper chest expansion-mother places one hand over the sternum, the thumb and fingers are over the clavicle, while she directs the chest expansion into her hand.

4. Huffing-mother splints incision and breathes in through the nose and on exhalation, she repeats a forced "Ahhhh."

5. Pelvic floor exercises.

Day 2 and 3

All of the Day 1 exercises should be done plus:

1. Pelvic tilt-side-lying or sitting positions.

2. Leg slides-knees bent lying on back, pull stomach in, flatten back, slide one leg up and down, maintaining pelvic control. Do not extend legs down fully.

3. Hula-lying supine, legs flat; hike hip up and down.

Day 4 and 5

If mother is up and about easily, discontinue breathing exercises.

1. Check for diastasis recti abdominis and do corrective exercises, if needed; mother crisscrosses hands across abdomen, approximating the rectus abdominis and lifts head up.

2. Partial lower trunk rotation-on back, knees bent, shoulders flat, knees drop together from side to side, head turns in opposite direction of the knees.

Day 6

Do all exercises as previously listed, plus:

1. Pelvic tilt-on all fours, then gradually add more challenging abdominal exercises, including the oblique muscles.

Body Mechanics Guidelines for Post-Cesarean Patients*:

1. Getting up from a lying down position: Do not sit up straight (jackknife). Go slowly. Roll to the side. Swing legs over the edge. Push with the elbow of the side you were lying on and the other hand.

2. When sitting, avoid soft chairs. They are hard to get up from and have poor back support. Avoid extremes of rounded or arched back. Use a cushion or roll in the small of the back for support. Sit on a firm straight chair.

3. Stand with chin in and contract abdominal muscles.

4. Climb stairs slowly, one at a time, to avoid exhaustion. Propel the body up the stairs, using the thigh and buttock muscles, keeping the weight over the feet.

5. When bending over, keep a curve in the low back, and one foot in front of the other. Bend the knees and lower the trunk. Legs should take most of the weight, back maintains a vertical position.

6. To lift, maintain one foot in front of the other, bringing the object close to the body at waist level. Make frequent trips to decrease the weight of heavy loads.

7. When reaching, use a stool for overhead objects. Do not over-extend when reaching. Put frequently used objects closer to shoulder level.

*Adapted from Frahm J: Hutzel Hospital Physical Therapy Department Post-Cesarean Section Program.[8]

Figure 11-4. Body mechanics guidelines for post-Cesarean patients. Adapted from Frahm J. *Hutzel Hospital Physical Therapy Department.* Post-Cesarean Exercise Program.[8]

SELF-ASSESSMENT REVIEW

1. What are the primary uterine changes post-delivery?
2. The _____ is made of serum leukocytes, sloughing endometrial tissue, and blood.
3. Increased urinary production post-delivery is due to _____.
4. Cardiac output returns to prepregnant level by _____ post-partum.
5. Instructions for stair climbing for post-Cesarean mothers should be _____.
6. Immediate post-Cesarean exercises include _____ and _____.
7. _____ and _____ hormones are necessary for milk production.
8. Tingling around the nipple and ejection of the milk from the breast is called the _____.
9. Name four key areas of muscle restoration following delivery.
10. Name four conditions that may limit or contraindicate exercise following delivery
11. What exercises should be started first to speed recovery after Cesarean section?

Answers

1. Decreases and returns to normal size, decrease in weight, and sheds endometrium. 2. Lochia. 3. Diaphoresis. 4. 2 to 3 weeks. 5. Push with legs and buttocks while contracting the pelvic floor and abdominal muscles. 6. Pelvic floor toning and gentle abdominal exercises. 7. Oxytocin and prolactin. 8. Letdown reflex. 9. Pelvic floor, abdominal muscles, back muscles, buttock muscles, and deep hip muscles. 10. Myocardial disease, congestive heart failure, rheumatic heart disease (class II or above), recent pulmonary embolus, acute infectious disease, uterine hemorrhage, severe hypotensive disease, diabetes mellitus, radicular arm or leg signs, sacroiliac pain, excessive vaginal bleeding, marked rectus diastasis. 11. Breathing and pelvic floor exercises.

REFERENCES

1. Danforth DN, Scott JR, eds. *Obstetrics and Gynecology*. 5th ed. Philadelphia, Pa: JB Lippincott; 1986.

2. Noble E. *Essential Exercises for the Childbearing Year*. 2nd ed. Boston, Mass: Houghton-Mifflin; 1982.

3. Walker M, Driscoll JW. *Breastfeeding Your Baby*. 2nd ed. Wayne, NJ: Avery Publishing; 1981.

4. Brazelton TB. *Infants and Mothers*. New York, NY: Delta; 1969.

5. Artal R, Wiswell R, eds. *Exercise in Pregnancy*. Baltimore, Md: Williams & Wilkins; 1986.

6. Section on Obstetrics and Gynecology, APTA: Perinatal Exercise Guidelines. Alexandria, Va. *Bull Sect Obstet Gynecol*. APTA; 1986.

7. Brown G, Viviano J, Machek O. Management of postoperative pain in obstetrical and gynecological procedures. *Bull Sect Obstet Gynecol*. APTA; 1983;7(3):8-11.

8. Frahm J. *Post-Cesarean Exercise Program*. Detroit, Mich: Hutzel Hospital; 1986.

9. Niswander K. *Manual of Obstetrics*. Boston:, Mass: Little, Brown & Co; 1987.

10. Fienup-Riordan A. *Shape Up with Baby*. Seattle, Wash: Pennypress; 1980.

Conclusion

While many parts of this book have been designed for use as a clinical reference and self-study guide, others are limited in scope to meet the needs of the clinician and student just starting in OB/GYN. For the continuing student of OB/GYN, additional questions will eventually come to mind that were not answered in this introductory text. As the field of OB/GYN physical therapy expands, the practitioner will need to know more about the nuances of obstetric patient care. These answers lie within past, present, and future literature directed at OB/GYN physician specialists. In addition, other unpublished and invaluable information will be gleaned from interactions with the various members of the female client's health care team.

As time passes, the physical therapist will become recognized as a specialist in female care. Only the professional who is able to interweave all the factors contributing to the current condition of a female client may effectively and efficiently evaluate and treat. Knowledge of symptomatology related to reproductive dysfunction or the biomechanical results of bearing children can provide answers where there seem to be none. No specialist in another field of physical therapy can boast an awareness of the interactions of every bodily system, from menarche through menopause, when examining a client, when communicating with physicians, and when servicing the client as part of the family unit.

With the vast impact of reproductive events on lifestyle, family dynamics, and psychological well-being, it is no wonder that caregivers are part of a health care team that depends heavily on each and every member. The physical therapist plays an indispensable role in educating other team members and the client about maintaining or attaining a state of fitness, comfort, and health prior to, during, and after pregnancy. In many parts of the country, it is an exciting time for the physical therapist to unveil various aspects of treatment available for women in all stages of life. The only limitations are the imagination of practitioners and the strength of their belief in the part they play in providing total patient care.

Suggested Reading
by Topic

BREASTFEEDING

Eiger M, Olds, SW. *The Complete Book of Breastfeeding*. New York, NY: Workman Press; 1972.

La Leche League International. *The Womanly Art of Breastfeeding*. Franklin, Ill: La Leche League; 1963.

Walker M, Driscoll JW. *Breastfeeding Your Baby*. 2nd ed. Wayne, NJ: Avery Publishing; 1981.

BREAST REHABILITATION

Love S. *Dr. Susan Love's Breast Book*. Reading, Mass: Addison-Wesley Publishing Co; 1990.

Robinson RI. The new back school prescription stabilization training part 1. *Spine*. 1991:5(3):341-353.

Wells SA, Young LV, Andriole DA. *Atlas of Breast Surgery*. St. Louis, Mo: Mosby Year Book, Inc; 1994.

CHILDBIRTH

Kitzinger S. *Giving Birth: The Parent's Experience of Childbirth*. New York, NY: Traplinger; 1971.

Kitzinger S. *Your Baby Your Way: Making Pregnancy Decisions and Birth Plans*. New York, NY: Pantheon Books; 1987.

Simkin P. *The Birth Partner: Everything You Need to Know to Help a Woman Through Childbirth*. Boston, Mass: Harrand Common Press; 1989.

EXERCISE

Artal R, Wiswell RA, eds. *Exercise in Pregnancy*. Baltimore, Md: Williams & Wilkins; 1986.

Bing E. *Moving Through Pregnancy*. New York, NY: Bantam Books; 1977.

Carrier B. *The Swiss Ball: Theory, Basic Exercises and Clinical Application*. Germany: Springer-Verlag Berlin Heidelberg; 1998.

Clapp J. Neonatal behavior profile of the offspring of women who continue to exercise regularly through pregnancy. *Am J Obstet and Gynecol*. 1999;180(pt 1):1:91-94.

Fitzhugh ML. *Preparation for Childbirth*. San Rafael: Margaret B Parley, RPT; 1974.

Heardman H. *Physiotherapy and Obstetrics in Gynecology*. Edinburgh, England: E & S Livingstone; 1951 (out of print).

Mittlemark RA, Wiswell RA, Drinkwater BL. *Exercise in Pregnancy*. 2nd ed. Baltimore, Md: Williams and Wilkins; 1990.

Noble E. *Essential Exercises for the Childbearing Year*. 2nd ed. Boston, Mass: Houghton-Mifflin; 1982.

Section on Obstetrics and Gynecology, APTA. *Perinatal Exercise Guidelines*. Alexandria, Va: Section on Obstetrics and Gynecology of the APTA; 1986.

Section on Obstetrics and Gynecology, APTA. *Post-hysterectomy Exercise Program*. Alexandria, Va: Section on Obstetrics and Gynecology of the APTA; 1988.

Simkin P, Whalley J, Keppler A. *Pregnancy, Childbirth, and the Newborn*. New York, NY: Meadowbrook; 1984.

HIGH-RISK PREGNANCY

Cherry SH, Berkowitz RL, Case NG, eds. *Rovinsky and Guttmacher's Medical, Surgical and Gynecologic Complications of Pregnancy*. 3rd ed. Baltimore, Md: Williams & Wilkins; 1985.

Quinine JT, ed. *Management of High-Risk Pregnancy*. 2nd ed. Oradell, NJ: Medical Economics Books; 1985.

INFANT DEVELOPMENT AND PARENTING

Brazelton TB. *Infants and Mothers*. New York, NY: Dell Publishers; 1969.

Brazelton TB. *Toddlers and Parents*. New York, NY: Dell Publishers; 1974.

Caplan F. *The First Twelve Months of Life*. New York, NY: Grosset & Dunlap; 1971.

Gordon T. *Parent Effectiveness Training*. New York, NY: Peter Wyden, 1970.

LABOR AND DELIVERY

Noble E. *Childbirth with Insight*. Boston, Mass: Houghton-Mifflin; 1983.

Oxorn H, Foote WR. *Human Labor and Birth*. 4th ed. New York, NY: Appleton-Century-Crofts; 1980.

MUSCULOSKELETAL

Cyriax J, Cyriax P. *Illustrated Manual of Orthopedic Medicine*. London, England: Butterworth's; 1983.

Hoppenfeld S. *Physical Examination of the Spine and Extremities*. New York, NY: Appleton-Century-Crofts; 1976.

Kendall FP, McCreary EK. *Muscle Testing and Function*. 3rd ed. Baltimore, Md: Williams & Wilkins; 1983.

Konkler CJ, Kisner C. Principles of Exercise for the Obstetric Patient. In Kisner C, Colby LA. *Therapeutic Exercise, Foundations and Techniques*. 3rd ed. Philadelphia, Pa: F.A. Davis; 1990

Saunders HD. *Evaluation, Treatment and Prevention of Musculoskeletal Disorders*. Minneapolis, Minn: Viking Press; 1985.

Nutrition

Brewer GS, Brewer T. *What Every Pregnant Woman Should Know: The Truth About Diet and Drugs in Pregnancy.* Baltimore, Md: Penguin; 1979.

Goldbeck N. *As You Eat, So Your Baby Grows.* Woodstock, NY: Ceres Press; 1980.

Obstetrics and Gynecology

Danforth DN, Scott JR, eds. *Obstetrics and Gynecology.* 5th ed. Philadelphia, Pa: JB Lippincott; 1986.

Niswander KR, ed. *Manual of Obstetrics.* 3rd ed. Boston, Mass: Little, Brown & Co; 1987.

Rayburn WE, Lavin JP. *Obstetrics for the House Officer.* Baltimore, Md: Williams & Wilkins; 1984.

Wallace K, Sandalcidi D. *Urinary Incontinence Step by Step: A Handout Manual for Patients and Practitioners.* Westminster, Colo: Progressive Therapists; 1998.

Wilder E, ed. *The Gynecological Manual.* Alexandria, Va: Section on Women's Health, American Physical Therapy Association; 1997.

Obstetrics and Gynecology
Books and Chapters by Physical Therapists

Adams C, Frahm J. Genitourinary system. In: Myers RS, ed. *Saunders Manual of Physical Therapy Practice.* Philadelphia, Pa: WB Saunders; 1996.

Appel C. Obstetrical considerations. In: Myers RS, ed. *Saunders Manual of Physical Therapy Practice.* Philadelphia, Pa: WB Saunders; 1996.

Ebner M. *Physiotherapy and Obstetrics.* 3rd ed. London, England: Livingstone Publishers; 1967 (out of print).

Herman H, Pirie A. How to Raise Children withour Breaking yourBack; Somerville, Mass: IBS Publications; 1995.

Noble E. *Essential Exercises for the Childbearing Year: A Guide to Health Before and After Your Baby is Born.* 2nd ed. Boston, Mass: Houghton-Mifflin; 1987.

Noble E. *Having Twins-A Guide to Pregnancy, Birth and Early Childhood.* Boston, Mass: Houghton-Mifflin; 1980.

Noble E. *Childbirth With Insight.* Boston, Mass: Houghton-Mifflin; 1983.

Pauls JA. *Therapeutic Approaches to Women's Health: A Program of Exercise and Education.* Frederick, Md: Aspen Publishers; 1996.

Polden M, Mantle J. *Physiotherapy in Obstetrics and Gynecology.* London, England: Butterworth-Heinemann; 1990.

Sapsford R, Bullock-Saxton J, Markwell S. *Women's Health: A Textbook for Physiotherapists.* London, England: WB Saunders Company Ltd; 1998.

Schussler B, Laycock J. *Pelvic Floor Re-Education.* New York, NY: Springer-Verlag; 1994.

Stephenson RG, O'Conner LJ. *Obstetric and Gynecologic Care in Physical Therapy.* Thorofare, NJ: SLACK Incorporated; 1990 (2nd ed, 2000).

Simpkin P. *Pregnancy, Childbirth and the Newborn.* Deephaven, Minn: Meadowbrooks Books; 1984.

Wilder E, ed. Clinics in Physical Therapy, Vol. 20. *Obstetric and Gynecologic Physical Therapy*. New York, NY: Churchill-Livingstone Publishers; 1988.

Wilder E. ed. *The Gynecological Manual*. Alexandria, Va: Section of Women's Health of the American Physical Therapy Association, APTA; 1997.

SEXUAL ABUSE/DOMESTIC VIOLENCE

American Physical Therapy Association (APTA) Guidelines for Recognizing and Providing Care for Victims of Domestic Violence. Publication No. P-138. Alexandria, Va: APTA; 1997.

Bloom S.L. *Creating Sanctuary: Toward the Evolution of Sane Societies*. Routledge, NY; 1997.

Herman J. *Trauma and Recovery*. New York, NY: Basic Books; 1992.

van der Kolk B.A, McFarlane A.C, Weisaith L. eds. *Traumatic Stress: The Effects of Overwhelming Experience on Mind, Body, and Society*. New York, NY: The Guildford Press; 1996.

OTHER

Ashford JI. *The Whole Birth Catalog - A Sourcebook for Choices in Childbirth*. Trumansburg: Crossing Press; 1983 (out of print).

Gaskin IM. *Spiritual Midwifery*. Summertown: The Book Publishing Co; 1978.

B Product Information and Resources

MATERNITY SUPPORTS AND ORTHOSES

Carpal Tunnel Support

Freedom Long Elastic Wrist Support
AliMed
297 High Street
Dedham, MA 02026
Wrist circumference determines patient's size; custom-made splints for wrists that are difficult to size, $17.50.

Hand and Wrist Support

Elastic Wrist Support Tension Strap, flexion support, splint with thumb abductor
Sammons Preston
P.O. Box 5071
Bolingbrook, IL 60440
(800) 323-5547
www.sammonspreston.com
Elastic wrist support tension strap provides support and compression and does not extend beyond palmar crease-$9.95. Wrist flexion support holds wrist in neutral and unrestricted thumb and finger dexterity-$15.50. Wrist splint with thumb abductor holds wrist in neutral plus gives full length flexible thumb abduction stay-$18.50.

Neck and Upper Back Support

Leading Lady Maternity Bra
Dan Howard Industries, Inc.

4245 North Knox Avenue
Chicago, IL 60641
(800) 468-6700
www.dan-howard.com
Leading Lady Maternity Bra, $18. Shoulder Ease-fits any bra with soft shoulder cushion, $6.

Mid-Back Support

Saunders Corset
The Saunders Group
4250 Norex Drive
Chaska, MN 55318
(800) 654-8357
Mid-back support.

Low Back Supports

Baby Hugger
TrennaVentions
131 Hill Street
Dery, PA 15627
(888) 770-0044, (724) 694-5283
Fax: (724) 694-5255
Info@babyhugger.com
http://www.babyhugger.com
Supports low-back, mid-back, and vulvar varicosities by a panty and strap arrangement designed to lift up the gravid uterus. Invented by a physical therapist, $55 wholesale, $70 suggested retail.

Contour-Form Maternity Support-$90
Contour Form Products
38 Stewart Avenue

P.O Box 328
Greenville, PA 16125
(724)-588-4452

Life Lines Medical, Inc.
14 Wood Road
Braintree, MA 02186
(800) 925-2995
Dale Active Lumbosacral Support Phase IV

Mother-to-Be Back and Abdominal Support
CMO, Inc.
PO Box 147
Barberton, OH 44203
(800)344-0011; in Ohio, (800)452-0001
www.cmo-inc.com
Abdominal sling with moldable back insert; order by patient's dress size; S(3 9), M(12-14), L(16-18), XL(18+) $50 plus shipping.

Saunders Corset-$57
The Saunders Group
4250 Norex Drive
Chaska, MN 55318
(800) 654-8357
Full abdominal and back support with stays and reinforcing straps and maternity panel.

Universal Abdominal Binder-$12
E.M. Adams Co. Inc.
7496 Commercial Circle
Kings Highway Industrial Center
Fort Pierce, FL 34951
(800) 225-4788

Warm 'n Form
Jerome Medical
305 Harper Drive
Moorestown, NJ 08054
(800) 257-8440
Provides back supports that can be used in pregnancy with a custom-molded insert., $46.

Seating: Back Supports

NADA Chair Back-Up
2448 Larpenteur Avenue
St. Paul, MN 55113

(800) 722-2587
http://www.nadachair.com
Portable back support that works without chairs or additional support in chairs. Color choices are navy, black, red, forest green, camouflage, royal with rainbow straps, $39.95.

Original McKenzie SuperRoll
OPTP
P.O. Box 47009
Minneapolis, MN 55447
(800) 367-7393
http://www.optp.com
Firm back lumbar support that can strap into any chair.

Sacroiliac Support

Maternity Lumbopelvic/Sacroiliac Support
IEM Orthopedics
PO Box 592
Ravenna, OH 44266
(800) 992-6594
iem@bright.net
www.bright.net/~iem/
Leather sacral pad and two Velcro side straps and elastic abdominal panel-available for pregnant and nonpregnant clients; designed by a physical therapist, $55.

SOMA S-I Belt
SOMA, Inc.
3737 Executive Center Drive Suite 158
Austin, TX 78731
(800) 441-7662
Comes in either leather or neoprene; sizes S, M, L. Stabilization force is from anterior anchors via a belt that fastens in back, $38.50.

Perineometers

Perineometer and Vaginal Stimulators
Interactive Medical Technologies
7348 Bellaire
North Hollywood, CA 91605
(800) 999-2657
Gynex™ perineometer (Kegel prototype), and Restore™ vaginal stimulator.

Maternity Pillows, Wedges

Body Cushion
Body Support Systems Inc.
300 East Hersey Street
P.O. Box 337
Ashland, OR 97520
http://www.bodysupport.com
Allows prone positioning for the pregnant client, $279-additional $159 for adjuster caddy, $79 carry bag.

Body Pillow
The Linen Source
5401 Hangar Court
P.O. Box 31151
Tampa, FL 33631-3151
http://www.linensource.com
20" x 60", 78 oz. Goose feathers and down. Two year warranty #P 9821 abdominal and back support, $39.99.

Maternal Cradle
Bodyline
3730 Kori Road
Jacksonville, FL 32257
(800) 874-7715

Maternity Support Pillow
Lossing Orthopedic
PO Box 6224
Minneapolis, MN 55406
(800) 328-5216, (612) 724-2669
Fax: (888) 777-5666, (612) 724-5089
$39.99 retail, professional price $25.

Venous Supports

Gottfried Medical, Inc.
PO Box 8966
Toledo, OH 43623
(800) 537-1968

Medi
76 West Seegers Road
Arlington Heights, IL 60005
(800) 633-6334
Stockings measured by a Medi dealer or physical therapist. Available in beige, black, off-white and gray.

USA Sigvaris and Company
PO Box 570
32 Park Drive East
Branford, CT 06405
Available in four thickness': calf, half-thigh length, thigh-length, and maternity stocking.

Calf Support
Beiersborf-Jobst
P.O. Box 653
Toledo, OH 43694
(800) 537-1063
Custom made; Compriform, Relief, Vairox, Fast Fit, Sheer Maternity, Ultimate. $28.50-$50 per stocking. Precise measuring; cotton dacron with seam. Compression depends on measurement. Compriform is seamless-$165.25 -$180.75. Fast Fit Maternity-ready made with ankle and calf, length, 25-35 mm/hg. Sizes S, M, L short and tall-$119.25. Relief Maternity-measured with height and weight; 16-20 mm/hg; sizes S, M, Tall, Extra Tall, beige in color- $48.75. Sheer Maternity-measured with height and weight. 10-14 mm/hg; sizes A, B, C, D, E, F up to 200 lbs. prior to pregnancy. Nude, suntan taupe, off-black or white in color, $24.75.

Made to Measure Garments and Supports
Gottfried Medical, Inc.
P.O. Box 8966
Toledo, OH 43623
(800) 537-1968, (419) 474-2973
Fax: (419) 474-8822
Gottfriedmed@CompuServe.com
Waist length two legs closed crotch maternity support and ready vasculastic - ready made knee length surgical supports

Post-Partum Supports

Mother to Be Maternity support, post-partum/ Cesarean Binder
C.M.O. Inc.
P.O. Box 147
Baberton, OH 44203-0147
(800) 344-0011, (330) 745-9679
Fax: (330) 745-5913
Support@cmo-inc.com
http://www.cmo-inc.com

Osteoporosis Supports

Posture training supports
CAMP Healthcare
2010 East High Street
P.O. Box 89
Jackson, MI 49204
(800) 492-1088, (517) 787-1600
Fax: (800) 245-3765

Shoe Support

Prenatal Back Savers Shoe insole
1028 112th Avenue NE, #C-8
Bellvue, WA 98004
(425) 957-4500
Fax: (206) 454-8225

Thorpe Shoes
P.O. Box 370
1275 Ritner Highway
Carlisle, PA 17013
(800) 366-7643
O.B. Gees footwear for the mother-to-be.

Publications for Childbirth Educators

American Baby Magazine
249 West 17th Street
New York, NY 10011

American Journal of Obstetrics and
Gynecology
CV Mosby Company
1830 West Line Drive
St. Louis, Mo 63146

Birth: Issues in Perinatal Care and
Education
Blackwell Scientific Publications, Inc.
Commerce Place
350 Main Street
Malden, MA 02148-5018

Childbirth Educator
249 West 17th Street
New York, NY 10011

Journal of the Section on Women's Health
Section on Women's Health, The American
Physical Therapy Association
PO Box 327
Alexandria, Va 22313

Lamaze Parents Magazine
1840 Wilson Boulevard, Suite 204
Arlington, VA 22201

Obstetrics and Gynecology
Elsevier Science Publishing Company, Inc.
52 Vanderbilt Avenue
New York, NY 10017

Maternal-Child Health Organizations

American Academy of Husband Coach
Childbirth (AAHCC)
The Bradley Method
PO Box 5224
Sherman Oaks, CA 91413
(800) 423-2397 outside CA, or (818) 788-6662

American Cancer Society- Indiana Division
Inc.
(800) ACS-2345
*Brochure: Reach to Recovery: What You
Should Know About Lymphedema Risks After
Breast Cancer.*

American College of Nurse-Midwives
(ACNM)
818 Connecticut Avenue SW, Suite 900
Washington, DC 20006
(202) 728-9860
Gives listing of nurse-midwives and nurse-midwifery training programs.

American College of Obstetricians and
Gynecologists (ACOG)
409 12th Street, SW
P.O. Box 96920
Washington, DC 20090
Phone (202) 638-5577
Brochure: Exercise and Fitness: A guide for

Women and Women and Exercise. Technical Bulletins: Women and Exercise, Exercise During Pregnancy and the Post-Partum Period.

American Society for Psychoprophylaxis in Obstetrics (ASPO/Lamaze)
c/o Lamaze International
1200 19th Street NW, Suite 300
Washington, DC 20036-2422
(800) 368-4404 or (202) 857-1128
Offers certification in Lamaze method of childbirth preparation, publishes the Lamaze Parents Magazine and provides information about pregnancy and childbirth-related topics.

Bard Urological Division
(800) 526-2687
Brochures: Profiles of Women with Stress Incontinence
Reference Card: Profiles of Women with Stress Incontinence.

Birthworks
PO Box 2045
Medford, NJ 08055
(888) 862-4784
Offers a holistic approach to childbirth and provides information from a holistic standpoint.

The Confinement Line
c/o Childbirth Education Associates
P.O. Box 1609
Springfield, VA 22151
(703) 941-7183
Support group for women on bed rest in Washington D.C. area.

Cooper Institute
12330 Preston Road
Dallas, TX 75230
(972) 341-3200, (800) 635-7050

Council of Childbirth Education Specialists Inc.
8 Sylvan Glen
East Lyme, CT 06333
(800) 822-4526
Childbirth organization offering certification to nurses, physical therapists; offers introductory and advanced seminars.

Hysterectomy Educational Resources and Services
HERS Foundation
422 Bryn Mawr Ave.
Bala Cynwyd, PA 19004
(215) 667-7757

Intensive Caring Unlimited
P.O. Box 563
Newtown Square, PA 19073
(610) 876-7872
Patient support group for high-risk pregnancy and children with special needs.

International Childbirth Education Association (ICEA)
PO Box 20048
Minneapolis, MN 55420
(612) 854-8660
Certifies childbirth educators, has mail-order book store and offers information about pregnancy and childbirth education.

International Foundation for Bowel Dysfunction (IFBD)
P.O. Box 17864
Milwaukee, WI 53217

La Leche League International
1400 North Meacham Road
Schaumberg IL 60173-4048
(841) 519-7730
Headquarters for the 3000 groups throughout the world offering support for breastfeeding, through individual counseling and education.

National Association for Continence (formally HIP)
P.O. Box 8310
Spartanburg, SC 29305
(800) BLADDER
(803) 579-7900 Resource Directory Info

National Center Institute's Cancer Information Service
(800) 4-CANCER

National Clearinghouse for Alcohol Information
U.S. Department of Health Services

200 Independence Avenue SW
Washington, DC 20201
(877) 696-6775
Offers information on effects of alcohol.

National Domestic Violence Hotline
(800) 799-SAFE
National Family Violence HelpLine
(800) 222-2000

National Institute of Health
U.S. Department of Health and Human Services
Building 31, Room 7A-32
Bethesda, MD 20892
(301) 496-4000
Offers all NIH publications and information on antenatal diagnosis, Cesarean birth, toxoplasmosis, and ultrasound imaging.

National Organization of Mothers of Twins Club
Executive Office
P.O. Box 438
Thompson Sattion, TN 37179-0438
(505) 275-0955 - Lois Gallmeyer

National Vulvodynia Association
P.O. Box 4491
Silver Springs, MD 20914
(301) 299-0775
Fax: (301) 299-3999

Nurses Association of the American College of Obstetrics and Gynecologists (NAA-COG)
409 12th Street SW
Washington, DC 20024
(202) 638-5577
Organization for nurses specializing in obstetric, gynecologic, and neonatal nursing, with many publications related to pregnancy and childbirth; continuing education programs and current maternal and child health information.

Read Natural Childbirth Foundation
13301 Elseo Drive, Suite 102
Greenbrae, CA 94904
Offers preparation in the Grantley Dick-Read method of prepared childbirth.

Resolve
1310 Broadway
Somerville, MA 02144
Helpline on infertility and miscarriage issues: (617) 623-0744
www.resolve.com

SHARE
St. Joseph Health Center
300 First Capitol Drive
St. Charles, MO 63301-2893
(800) 821-6819

The Simon Foundation for Continence
Box 815
Wilmette, IL 60091
(800) 23SIMON - Patient Information
(847) 864-3913 - Foundation Information

Sidelines National Support Network
P.O. Box 1808
Laguna Beach, CA 92652
(714) 497-2265 - Candace Hurley
(602) 941-0176 - Laura Maurer
http://www.sidelines.org
Support for pregnant women on bed rest.

Tokos Medical Corporation
1821 E. Dyer Road, No. 200
Santa Ana, CA 92705
Home uterine monitoring services for women at risk of giving birth prematurely.

The Triplet Connection
P.O. Box 99571
Stockton, CA 95209
(209) 474-0885 or (209) 474-3073

U.S. Department of Agriculture
WIC Supplemental Food Section
3101 Park Center Drive
Alexandria, VA 22302
(703) 305-2746
Offers information on nutrition for pregnant nursing women.

Disability Related Organizations

The Christopher Reeve Paralysis Foundation (previously known as the American

Paralysis Association)
500 Morris Ave.
Springfield, NJ 07081
(800) 225-0295

Avenues
P.O. Box 5192
Aonoea, CA 95370
(209) 928-3688

Lupus Foundation
1300 Piccard Drive, Suite 200
Rockville, MD 20850
(800) 558-0121

Muscular Dystrophy Association
3300 East Sunrise Drive
Tucson, AZ 085718
(800) 572-1717

Myasthenia Gravis Foundation
123 West Madison Blvd., Suite 800
Chicago, IL 60602
(800) 541-5454

National Arthritis and Musculoskeletal and
Skin Diseases Information Clearinghouse
1 AMS Circle
Bethesda, MD 20892
(301) 495-4484

National Spinal Cord Injury Association
8701Georgia Avenue, Suite 500
Silver Spring, MD 20910
(800) 962-9629

Women with Developmental Disabilities
http://www.npi.ucla.edu

Patient Education

American Physical Therapy Association
1111 North Fairfax St.
Alexandria, VA 22314
ASPO/Lamaze
c/o Lamaze International
1200 19th Street NW, Suite 300
Washington, DC 20036-2422
(800) 368-4404 or (202) 857-1128

Childbirth Graphics
WRS Group Inc.

P.O. Box 21207
5045 Franklin Ave.
Waco, TX 76702
www.wrsgroup.com
(800) 299-3366 Ext. 295, (254) 776-6461
*Perinatal education materials company: models,
posters, slides, brochures. Catalog company
with over 1100 products.*

Empi, Inc.
599 Cardigan Road
St. Paul, MN 55126
(800) 328-2536 (Professional Services)
*Clinical Guidelines for TENS, reference arti-
cles on use of TENS in labor and delivery.*

ICEA Bookmarks
International Childbirth Education
Association
P.O. Box 20048
Minneapolis, MN 55420
Charts and books.

International Childbirth Educators Association, Inc. (ICEA)
PO Box 20048
Minneapolis, MN 55420-0048
(612) 854-8660 or (800) 624-4934

Milner-Fenwick Inc.
2125 Greenspring Drive
Timonium, MD 21093

Noble E. Audio and Videotapes
New Life Images
48 Pleasant Lake Avenue
Harwich, MA 02645
(508) 432-8040 fax (508) 432-9685
www.capecod.net/newlife
*"Inside Experiences: From Conception through
Birth", "Channel for a New Life" (water birth),
"BabyJoy", "Exercises and Activities for parents
and Infants", "Pelvic Power".*

Pennypress
1100 23rd Avenue East
Seattle, WA 98112
(206) 325-1419

Phoenix Enterprises
309 SW Higgins Box 8231
Missoula, MT 59807
(800) 549-8371
Pelvic Floor Exercise Video

Polymorph Films, Inc.
118 South Street
Boston, MA 02111
(617) 542-2004

RGS Physical Therapy
Rebecca Gourley Stephenson, PT
335 Main Street
Medfield, MA 02052-2045
Videotape: "Back Care in Pregnancy"

Ross Laboratories
A Division of Abbott Laboratories
625 Cleveland Avenue
Columbus, OH 43215
(614) 227-3333

Suzanne Arms Productions
151 Lytton Avenue
Palo Alto, CA 94301

Urogyn Therapy Bookhouse/Beth Shelly
2721 Westerwood Drive
Baton Rouge, LA 70816
(225) 291-8805
bshelly@mail.challenger.net
Resources for therapists and patients for women's health (Water Works and videos, Progressive Therapeutics handout packet).

Woman's Hospital Attn: PT Dept
9050 Ailine Highway
Baton Rouge, LA 708159
(225) 927-1300
Materials include patient education booklets, community education programs in slides format, pelvic floor evaluation forms, courses and PT referral forms.

Publications for Patient Education

Anatomical Chart Co.
8221 Kimball Avenue

Skokie, IL 60076
(800) 621-7500
Pelvic model #267-A

"As You Eat, So Your Baby Grows: A Guide to Nutrition in Pregnancy"
Ceres Press
Route 212, Bpc 495
Woodstock, NY 12498
(914) 679-5573

"Alcohol in Your Unborn Baby"
U.S. Department of Health, Education and Welfare
National Institute on Alcohol Abuse and Alcoholism
5600 Fisher's Lane
Rockville, MD 20857-78521

"Back Care During Pregnancy and Beyond"
Physical Therapy Services
8710 Choctaw Road
Bon Air, VA 23235

"Better Baby Series"
Pennypress
1100 23rd Avenue East
Seattle, WA 98112
(206) 325-1419
Pamphlets available for childbirth classes relating to Cesarean births, obstetrical tests and technology, teenage childbirth, siblings at birth, exercise and nutrition.

"Brittle with Age: The Unnecessary Tragedy of Osteoporosis", brochure.
Melpomene Institute
1010 University Ave.
St. Paul, MN 55104
(612) 642-1951

"Exercise During Pregnancy"
David J. Milano, PT BHCPT
P.O. Box 1272
Burlington, NJ 08016

"For the Expectant Father"
Maternity Center Association
281 Park Avenue South
New York, NY 10010

(212) 777-5000
Fax: (212) 777-9320

"How to Raise your Children Without Breaking your Back"
Hollis Herman, PT, MS, OCS, and Alex Pirie
IBS Publications Dept DY2
P.O. Box 44-1474
Somerville, MA 02144

Krames Communications
1100 Grundy Lane
San Bruno, CA 94006-3030
(800) 333-3022, (415) 742-0400
Fax: (415) 244-4568
http://www.krames.com

National Osteoporosis Foundation
1232 22nd Street, NW
Washington, DC 20037
(202) 233-2226
U.S. Department of Health and Human Service; Public Health Service, National Institutes of Health; Osteoporosis: Cause, Treatment, Prevention, NIH Publication No. 86-2226; "Pregnant Patient's Bill of Rights" and "Pregnant Patient's Responsibilities"

ICEA, International Childbirth Educ-ation Association
PO Box 20048
Minneapolis, MN 55420
(612) 854-8660
"Shape Up for Pregnancy"
Kathy Tooman, PT
2602 St. Mary's Drive
Midland, MI 48640
"Ultrasound Exam in Obstetrics and Gynecology" and "X-rays, Pregnancy and You"

The American College of Obstetricians and Gynecologists
409 12th Street SW
Washington, DC 20090
(202) 638-5577

U.S. Department of Health and Human Services
Public Health Service: Agency for Health Care Policy and Research

Publications Clearinghouse
P.O. Box 8547
Silver Springs, MD 20907
Clinical Practice Guideline Update on Urinary Incontinence in Adults: Acute and Chronic Management. Understanding Incontinence: Caregiver Guide and Patient Guides (AHCPR Publication No. 96-0683 and 96-0684). (800) 358-9295

Electrical Stimulation, Biofeedback, Ultrasound Equipment

Biocomp Research Institute
3710 S. Robertson Blvd., Suite 216
Culver City, CA 90232
(800) 246-3526
htoomim@packbell.net
Biofeedback equipment

BMR Neurotech
4560 North 19th Avenue
Phoenix, AZ 85015
(800) 267-7846, (602) 371-1234
http://www.bmr.com
Neurotech NT200 - Pelvic Floor E-stim

Empi, Inc.
599 Cardigan Road
St. Paul, MN 55126
(800) 328-2536, (651) 415-9000
Fax: (800) 896-1798, (651) 415-8535
Innova PFS Feminine Incontinence Treatment System, Innova Clinical EMG System, Innocence and Minnova.

Incare Medical Products
2000 Hollister Drive
Libertyville, IL 60048
(800) 548-3482
Contimed II Biofeedback; Hollister Clinical Unit - Electrical stim and biofeedback unit, Microgyn 2 Home Trainer for Hollister Clinical Unit

J and J Engineering
22797 Holgar Court NE
Poulsbo, WA 98370

(888) 550-8300, (360) 779-3853
http://www.jjengineering.com
Biofeedback equipment

Myles Medical Stimtech
5 Northern Boulevard
Amherst, NH 03031
(800) 451-7915 or (603) 880-5050
Fax: (603) 880-0575
http://www.stimtech.com
Femex Stimulator System and Femex Vaginal Electrode (hand held), KegelTone vaginal weight.

Neurodyne Medical
52 New Street
Cambridge, MA 02138
(800) 328-4266
Fax: (508) 663-6133
http://www.newumed.com
Clinical Instruments and Software for Biofeedback, Pelvic Floor EMG

North American Distributors, Inc.
16520 Aston Street
Irvine, CA 92606
(800) 995-0510
http://www.webpt.com/usa/nad
Pelvic Floor Exerciser TM, Peritron 9200 Precision Perineometer

Prometheus Group
1 Washington Street, Suite 303
Dover, NH 03820-3827
(800) 442-2325
http://www.members.aol.com/theprogrp
Single and dual channel LCD and LED portable instruments

SRS Medical
14950 NE 95th, Suite F
Redmond, WA 98052
(800) 345-5642
http://www.srsmedical.com
Biofeedback unit

Thought Technology LTD
8396 Route 9
West Chazy, NY 12992

(800) 361-3651 or (514) 489-8251
http://www.thoughttechnology.com
Biofeedback unit

Utah Medical Products, Inc.
7043 South 300 West
Midvale, UT 84047
(800) 533-4984, (801) 566-1200
Fax: (801) 566-2062
http://www.utahmed.com
U-Control Home Trainer, Liberty System: PFS 100, PFS 200 electrical Stim. Units - Vaginal Exerciser, Extended, Vaginal Exerciser, and Rectal Exerciser

Verimed International, Inc.
A Lettler Electronic Company
11950 NW 39th St., Suite D
Coral Springs, FL 33065
(800) 999-9797, (954) 344-2454
Fax: (954) 340-8812
Myoexerciser II, Myoexerciser III, Portable Clinical EMG System, Veristim (surface EMG/muscle stim), EMG Vaginal Perineometer

Lymphedema Products, Wound Care and Post-Surgery Products

Barton Carey
148 East South Boundary Street
Perrysburg, OH 43551
OR
P.O. Box 421
Perrysburg, OH 43522
(800) 421-0444
Lymphedema sleeves

CAMP Healthcare
2010 East High Street
Jackson, MI 49204
(800) 492-1088, (517) 787-1600
Fax: (800) 245-3765
Prenatal supports, medical support stockings, compression pump, breast care products

ForeTech Medical
1405 Chews Landing Road #19
Laurel Springs, NJ 08021

(800) 699-6031, (609) 374-1999
Lymphedema equipment

Wright Therapy Products
305 High Tech Drive
Oakdale, PA 15071
(800) 631-9535
Gradient lymphedema pump system, gradient lymphedema supports-children and adults

Pelvic Floor, Incontinence, GYN Supplies, Equipment

Best Priced Products
P.O. Box 1174
White Plains, NY 10602
(800) 824-2939
OB/GYN hot pack

ConvaTec (Bristol Myers Squibb Co.)
P.O. Box 5254
Princeton, NJ 08543-5254
(800) 422-8811 or (908) 281-2500
FemTone Vaginal Weights, ProSys Products, Conquest Male Continence System, Ostomy Care Products, and Brochures for Male and Female Patients with Incontinence.

Ferno-Washington Inc.
70 Weil Way
Wilmington, OH 45177
(800) 733-3766
Perineal Whirpool

North American Distributors, Inc.
4482 Barranca Parkway, Suite 180-175
Irvine, CA 92604
(800) 995-0510 or (714) 553-0263
Fax: (714) 376-9765
PFX2 Pelvic Floor Exerciser

Syracuse Medical Devices Inc.
214 Hurlburt Rd.
Syracuse, NY 13224
(315) 449-0657
Fax (315) 449-0756
Vaginal dilators come in 4 sizes.

Timm Research Company
6541 City West Parkway
Eden Prairie, MN 55344
(800) 683-8938 or (612) 947-9410
Fax (612) 947-9411
Step Free vaginal weights with one cone shell and 5 weights.

References

Wilder E. *American Physical Therapy Association Section of Women's Health. Products and Service Guide.* Alexandria, Va: Section on Women's Health of the APTA; 1999

Pauls JA. *Therapeutic Approaches to Women's Health: A Program of Exercise and Education.* Gaithersburg, Md: Aspen Publishers, Inc.; 1995.

Stephenson RG. *Products for Pregnancy.* Lecture notes from Combined Section Meeting, APTA, 1996.

Sidelines National Support Network. www.sidelines.org. (714) 497-2265.

Suggestions for Use of the *Guide to Physical Therapist Practice*

SUGGESTIONS FOR USE OF THE *GUIDE TO PHYSICAL THERAPIST PRACTICE*[1] FOR OBSTETRIC AND GYNECOLOGIC CARE IN PHYSICAL THERAPY

With the publication of the *Guide to Physical Therapist Practice*, clinicians may find it necessary to justify techniques, modalities selected, and number of visits when treating clients with obstetric and gynecologic disorders. Therefore, a very basic overview of suggested uses of the document is included below.

Members of the Section on Women's Health have been working with documentation specialists to clarify further practice patterns that encompass aspects of care for this population. Clinicians are directed to the September 1999 issue of the *Journal of the Section on Women's Health*, which published an article by Julie Pauls and Elizabeth Shelly that detailed description of how the guide might be applied to physical therapy management of pelvic floor muscle impairments.[2] Other practice patterns which may direct care of obstetric or gynecologic clients are listed below.

There are some omissions in the guide. For example, Pattern 4J: *Impaired Joint Mobility, Motor Function, Muscle Performance, and Range of Motion Associated with Bony or Soft Tissue Surgical Procedures* specifically excludes patients with obstetric and gynecological surgical procedures, yet those same patients, eg, post-mastectomy, post-episiotomy, post-hysterectomy, post-Cesarean, have not been included elsewhere. Obviously, the guide is limited in that it cannot present every diagnosis. The clinician, therefore, may need to explore several practice patterns as a basis of care for this population if need for justification arises.

Musculoskeletal

Pattern 4A: *Primary Prevention/Risk Factor Reduction for Skeletal Demineralization*: (osteoporosis, aging women, post-hysterectomy, women on bedrest, female athletes).

Pattern 4B: *Impaired Muscle Performance*: (pelvic floor weakness–see above, aging women, women with high-risk pregnancy on prolonged bedrest, weakness from pain from arthritis/osteoporosis).

Pattern 4E: *Impaired Joint Mobility, Motor Function, Muscle Performance, and Range of Motion Associated with Ligament or Other Connective Tissue Disorders*: (women with pregnancy-related acute musculoskeletal complaints, pubic symphysis separations, diastasis recti).

Neuromuscular

Pattern 5D: *Impaired Motor Function and Sensory Integrity Associated with Peripheral Nerve Injury:* (pregnancy-related peripheral neuropathies).

Integumentary

Pattern 7F: *Impaired Anthropometric Dimensions Secondary to Lymphatic System Disorders:* (post-mastectomy lymphedema, edema of pregnancy).

REFERENCES

1. American Physical Therapy Association. Guide to Physical Therapist Practice. *Phys Ther.* 1997;77:1163-1650.
2. Pauls J, Shelly E. Applying the Guide to Physical Therapist Practice to Women's Health Physical Therapy. *J Section Women's Health.* 1999;23(3):8-12.

Glossary

abortion–any loss of pregnancy before the 28th week, either accidentally or intentionally

abruptio placentae–premature separation of the placenta from the uterine wall after 20 weeks of gestation

active labor–the second phase of the first stage of labor during which the cervix dilates from 4 to 8 cm

activin–hormone releasing factor that assists production of FSH at the pituitary

after pains–contractions of the uterus after the fetus and placenta are delivered

afterbirth–amniotic membranes and placenta, expelled from the uterus during the third stage of labor

allantois–the diverticulum from the hindgut of the embryo which appears around the 16th day of development; forming part of the umbilical cord and placenta

alpha-fetoprotein–nonhormonal plasma constituent in amniotic fluid used as a determinant of neural tube defects

amenorrhea–absence of monthly menstruation

amniocentesis–removal of amniotic fluid by a needle through the abdominal wall and uterus to determine the fetal age and genetic characteristics after 4 months' gestation

amnion–the innermost thin, tough layer of the sac surrounding the fetus (bag of waters)

analgesic–a drug that relieves or reduces pain without causing unconsciousness

anesthetic–a drug that produces loss of sensation with or without loss of consciousness

antenatal–during pregnancy

antepartum– the period from conception to birth (also called prenatal)

antral–relating to a body cavity

Apgar score–evaluation of the infant's condition in terms of heart rate, respiratory effort, muscle tone, reflex irritability, and skin color at 1 and 5 minutes after birth

areola–darkened area around the nipple

atrophic vaginitis–inflammation of the vagina in elderly women which can cause adhesions that obscure the vaginal canal

autocrine–method of intracellular hormonal communication

back labor–pain arising from pressure on the lumbar and sacral nerve roots, experienced in some women as the baby's head descends in the birth canal

bonding–the crucial attachment that develops between a mother, father, and their new baby after delivery

Braxton Hicks contractions–intermittent contractions of the uterus during pregnancy

Brazelton Neonatal Behavioral Assessment Scale–scale developed by Dr. T. Berry Brazelton to assess the newborn infant's ability to adapt to itself and the environment

breech–describes the position of the fetus in which anything but the head is presented first

caudal–a form of regional anesthesia administered below the spinal cord in the canal

cephalopelvic disproportion–a condition in which the infant's head is unable to fit through the pelvic outlet and is an indication for Cesarean delivery

cerclage–a purse string ring suture placed around an incompetent cervix at the level of the os at 12 to 14 weeks of gestation to prevent premature delivery from an incompetent cervix

cervix–the neck of the uterus, which leads into the vagina and thins out and dilates during labor

Cesarean section– delivery of a child by abdominal surgery

chloasma–mask of pregnancy; pigmentation appearing on forehead and cheeks of some pregnant women

chloroform–colorless, heavy liquid-formerly used as a general anesthetic

cholestasis–suppression or arrest of bile flow

chorion–the outermost membrane that encases the fetus

chorionic villus biopsy–biopsy of the chorionic villus that determines chromosomal and metabolic abnormalities of the fetus from 9 to 11 weeks' gestation

circumcision–the surgical removal of foreskin from the male infant's penis. Circumcision in females–removal of the clitoris, practiced in some cultures to decrease sexual sensations.

cleansing breath–the breath taken at the beginning and end of a labor contraction to signal the support person and to begin and end each breathing technique

climacteric–major turning point in a female's life from ability to reproduce to a state of non-reproductivity

clitoris–small, round-shaped organ at the anterior part of the vulva

coccyodynia–painful coccyx usually resulting from an injury, where sitting is difficult.

colostrum–watery-like milk secreted from a woman's breasts during pregnancy and during the first few days postpartum

contractions–shortening and tightening of the uterine muscle fibers during and after labor

corpus luteum–endocrine body that produces progesterone and develops in the ovary at the site of the ruptured ovarian follicle

crowning–indicates the presenting part of the infant visible at the vaginal opening; sometimes refers to the time at which the widest diameter of the presenting part is passing through the vaginal opening

cryptomenorrhea–monthly signs of menstruation without blood flow

cystocele–downward and forward displacement of the bladder towards the vaginal opening, often related to weakness or traumatized muscles from childbirth

decidua–mucus membrane lining the uterus (or endometrium) that changes in preparation for pregnancy and is sloughed off during menstruation and during postpartum

DES (diethylstilbestrol)–drug given to mothers during the 1950s to prevent miscarriage; caused congenital abnormalities in both male and female offspring

detrusor muscle–the muscular component of the bladder wall

diameter–measurements of the pelvic inlet and fetal head; (biparietal–the largest transverse diameter of the fetal skull at term)

dilation (dilatation)–the stretching and enlarging of the cervical opening to 10 cm to allow birth of the infant

dipping–presenting part slightly enters bony pelvis from abdominal cavity

disclosure–revealing something personal. Different levels of disclosure in physical therapy include: task-centered disclosure (can be initiated by the physical therapist at the beginning of the treatment asking about sensitivities such as touch, disrobing and body positions), and relationship-based disclosure (revealing of difficulties, initiated by a client, after experiencing the physical therapist as trustworthy).

ductus arteriosus–the channel between the pulmonary artery and aorta in the fetus, usually closing over soon after birth

dysgenesis–refers to the study of factors that result in flawed or inadequate embryonic development.

dysmenorrhea–pain experienced during menstrual periods

dyspareunia–painful intercourse

dystocia–a difficult childbirth; a fetal dystocia is difficult labor due to abnormalities of the fetus relative to size or position; b) maternal dystocia - difficult labor due to abnormalities of birth canal or uterine inertia

eclampsia–an acute disorder related to pregnant and puerperal women, consisting of convulsions and loss of consciousness associated with hypertension, edema and proteinuria

effacement–thinning and shortening of the cervix, occurring before or during dilation expressed in percentages of 0% to 100%

electronic fetal monitoring–the monitoring of the fetus and uterine contractions through internal and external pressure and sound transducers during labor

embryo–baby from conception to 8 weeks gestation

embryotomy–extraction of a dead fetus by dismemberment

endometriosis–abnormal proliferation of the uterine mucus membrane into the pelvic cavity

engagement–signifies that the fetus hasa firm head-down position within the mother's pelvis, and is no longer floating above the bony pelvis

enuresis–involuntary loss of urine: nocturnal enuresis is loss of urine at night, and is known as bedwetting

enterocele–herniation of the intestine below the cervix associated with congenital weakness or obstetric trauma

epidural–anesthesia injected into the epidural space of the spine which can produce loss of sensation from the abdomen to the toes

episiotomy–refers to the incision through the perinium which allows for less pressure on the fetal head during delivery.

estrogen–the female hormone that is responsible for maintenance of female sex characteristics and is formed in the ovary, placenta, testis, adrenal cortex.

fetal distress–decrease in fetal heart rate with the possibility of meconium-stained amniotic fluid related to jeopardized fetal oxygen supply

fetus–describes the baby from the 8th week after conception until birth

first stage of labor–initial part of labor when the cervix effaces and dilates to 10 cm; includes the early, active and transition phases of labor

fistulas–abnormal passage between two organs, (eg, rectovaginal passage between the rectum and vagina)

floating–refers to the fetus floating within the uterus in the abdomen above the bony pelvis

FSH–abbreviation for the follicle- stimulating hormone

footling breech–presentation where a foot is the presenting part

forceps–locked tong-like obstetrical instruments used to aid in delivery of the fetal presenting part

frank breech–position of the fetus where both legs are flexed against the abdomen and the sacrum is the presenting part

fundus–the top upper portion of the uterus

gestation–total period of time the baby is carried in the uterus, approximately 40 weeks in humans

glycosuria–secretion of excess sugar into the urine: often a sign of diabetes mellitus

grand multipara–a woman who has given birth seven or more times

gravida–a pregnant woman

HCG–abbreviation for human chorionic gonadotropin

high-risk pregnancy–a pregnancy where the mother or fetus is in danger of a compromised outcome

hirsutism–excessive hair growth on cheek, lip, chin or chest especially in women which can start in the perimenopausal period

hydatidiform mole–anomaly of the placenta which forms a nonmalignant mass from cystic swelling of the chorionic villi; no embryo is present

hydroureter–abnormal distention of the ureter with urine that is due to an obstruction

hyperemesis gravidarum–extreme vomiting in pregnancy

hyperventilation of pregnancy–because of an increase in respiratory tidal volume during normal respiration there is an increase in the respiratory minute volume which makes the mother feel like she is hyperventilating

hysterectomy–surgical removal of the uterus

incompetent cervix–cervix that prematurely dilates as pregnancy progresses

involution–the return of the uterus to the non-pregnant size and position

Kegel exercises–pelvic floor strengthening exercises developed by Dr. Arnold Kegel

labia–the external folds surrounding the vagina and urethra

labor–refers to the uterine contractions that produce dilation and effacement of the cervix, assisting in descent of the fetus and delivery through the vaginal opening

lacation–refers to the process by which milk is made in the breasts and secreted for nourishment of the infant

LH–abbreviation for lutenizing hormone

lactiferous–secreting milk

lanugo–fine hair on the body of the fetus after the fourth month in utero

latent phase–early phase of the first stage of labor which ends when the cervix is fully effaced and 3 to 4 cm dilated

letdown reflex–the involuntary release of milk through the nipples that occurs at the beginning of breastfeeding

levator ani syndrome–spasm of the muscles surrounding the anus causing severe rectal pain

luteinizing hormone (LH)–a pituitary hormone responsible for developing a corpus luteum

lie of the fetus–relationship of the long axis of the fetus to the long axis of the mother

lightening–occurs when the fetal head drops into the pelvic inlet, allowing the uterus to descend to a lower level, relieving pressure on the diaphragm and making breathing easier during the last few weeks of pregnancy

linea nigra–pigmented line appearing on the abdomen, from the pubis to the umbilicus in pregnant women

lithotomy position–where the person lies supine with the hips and knees flexed and the feet may be supported

lochia–discharge of blood, mucus, and tissue from the vagina after delivery, often lasting up to 6 weeks after birth, but usually referring to the bright red discharge of the first 2 weeks postpartum

lumbar stabilization–exercises whose object is to strengthen the deep spine muscles as a foundation for good trunk stability

lymphedema–swelling of an extremity caused by obstruction of the lymphatic vessels

malposition–faulty or abnormal position not favoring normal descent of the presenting part

malpresentation–abnormal fetal presenting part

mechanism of labor–describes the five positions that the fetal head assumes through the pelvis: descent, flexion, internal rotation, extension, and external restitution

meconium–fetal bowel movements

menarche–the onset of menstration in a female in puberity and is the onset of possible fertility

menopause–the absence of menstruation in the older female and marks the time that she is no longer fertile

micturition–the act of urinating

midwives–attendants who assist women during labor and delivery

miscarriage–spontaneous abortion of a fetus

molding–the shaping of the fetal head by the overlapping fetal skull bones to adjust to the size and shape of the birth canal

mucus plug–a plug produced by the endocervical glands to seal the cervical canal, which is extruded from the vagina in early labor

multigravida–a woman who has been pregnant more than once

multipara–a woman who has completed two or more pregnancies to the stage of viability

multiparity–refers to a condition of having two or more children

multiparous–refers to having given birth to two or more offspring in separate pregnancies

muscle energy techniques–physical therapy manual exercises that bring about controlled movement of joints and muscle through skilled application

myofascial release techniques–specialized physical therapy techniques that decrease the binding down of the fascia around a muscle

myoma–benign tumor consisting of muscle tissue

myometrium–fixed, smooth muscle forming the middle layer of the uterine wall

neonatal period–represents the first 4 weeks of an infant's life

occipitofrontal–a line from the root of the nose to the most prominent portion of the occipital bone of the fetus at term

occipitomental–diameter from the chin of the fetus to the most prominent portion of the occipital bone; the correct angle for the application of forceps

occiput anterior–fetal occiput to the mother's symphysis pubis

oligomenorrhea–longer intervals between menstrual periods from 38 days to 3 months

oliguria–low excretion of urine

oocyte–a primitive cell in the ovary that after meiosis becomes an ovum

oophoritis–inflammation of one or both ovaries secondary to infection as with mumps

osteoporosis–disease of the bone matrix due to deficiency, occurring in postmenopausal women

oxytocin–hormone stored in the pituitary that causes contraction of the uterus

papilla–a nipple-like protrusion from the surface of an organ

paracervical–refers to anesthesia injected in one or several locations around the uterine cervix

paracrine–method of extracellular hormonal communication

paracyesis–pregnancy that develops outside the uterus in the abdominal cavity

parity–condition of having produced viable offspring

parturient–a woman who is in labor

parturition–the act of giving birth, or childbirth

pelvic contraction–condition in which one or more diameters of the pelvis is narrower than normal, not allowing for normal progression of labor

pelvic floor–sling arrangement of ligaments and muscles that supports the reproductive organs

pelvic pain–pain in the pelvis arising from dysmenorrhea, gynecologic pathologies, growth of cancerous cells, sexually transmitted diseases and anatomic obstructions

pelvimetry–method of obtaining pelvic measurements by x-ray

perineometer–pressure sensitive device inserted vaginally to measure the strength of pelvic floor muscles

perineum–the area bounded by the pubis, coccyx, and the thighs which is between the external genitalia and the anus

pessary–a circular ring device used to hold a prolapsing uterus in place when surgical repair is contraindicated

phases–three periods of uterine activity occuring during the first stage of labor

pica–bizarre appetite

piriformis syndrome–characterized by over activity of the piriformis muscle causing external rotation of the leg and buttock pain

pitocin–synthetic oxytocic hormone administered through intravenous drip to induce or augment uterine contractions

placenta–organ that develops within the uterus from which the fetus derives its nourishment; also serves as a filtering system

placenta previa–condition where the placenta implants in the lower segment of the uterus and partially or completely covers the cervical opening

premenstrual syndrome (PMS)–symptoms that occur monthly after ovulation and usually cease at menstruation or shortly thereafter

podalic version–manipulation of a breech fetus presentation internally or externally

polyhydramnios–excess volume of amniotic fluid greater than 2000 ml

position–relationship of the fetus to the mother's pelvis

post-partum–period following birth

precipitate delivery–unexpected or sudden birth following a very short labor

preeclampsia–condition of hypertension, edema and albuminuria noted in late pregnancy, and possibly leading to serious toxemia

premature rupture of the membranes–rupture of the amniotic sac before the fetus is at full-term

presenting part–the part of the fetus that is first engaged in the pelvis

primigravida–a woman who is in her first pregnancy

primipara–a woman who had delivered a child after 20 weeks of gestation

progesterone–a hormone produced by the ovary responsible for changes in preparing the wall of the uterus for implantation

prolapsed uterus–uterus that has descended into the vaginal canal due to weakness of the supporting structures

prostaglandinsynthetase inhibitors–substances that inhibit the synthesis of prostaglandins

prostaglandins–lipid soluble hormone-like acetic compounds occurring in nearly all tissues, used for inducing labor

pruritus gravidarum–generalized itching not relieved by medication

psychoprophylaxis–psychologic and physical preparation for childbirth as taught in labor and delivery classes

ptyalism–increased saliva production, usually returns to normal by the middle of the second trimester

puerperal–refers to the period of time after labor to when the uterus is of normal size

puerperium–the time from the end of labor to when the uterus returns to its normal size, approximately 6 weeks

quickening–the sensation of fetal movement, usually initially occurring between the 4th and 5th months of pregnancy

rectocele–herniation of the rectum with protrusion into the vaginal canal, or prolapse of the rectum into the perineum

reflex incontinence–form of incontinence caused by inability to inhibit bladder stimulatory reflexes

relaxin–a polypeptide ovarian hormone secreted by the corpus luteum, possibly acts on the ligamentous structures of the body, slackening the ligaments to allow greater opening in the pelvic outlet

Rh factor–hereditary blood factor found in red blood cells determined by specialized blood tests; when absent, a person is Rh negative

ritodrine–drug given to suppress labor

round ligament–pair of ligaments that hold the uterus in place, extending laterally from the fundus between the folds of the broad ligaments to the lateral pelvic wall, terminating in the labia majora

rupture of the membranes–refers to the rupture of the amniotic sac prior to delivery

sacculation–presence or the formation of sacs in the uterus

second stage of labor–includes the time from 10 cm of dilation until birth of the baby

shoulder dystocia–occurs when the presenting part in the pelvic inlet is the fetal shoulder, thereby arresting normal progression of labor

show–refers to the blood and mucus plug that is extruded from the vagina in early labor

speculum–an instrument used to hold open and dilate the vagina during inspection

spinal–an injection of anesthesia into the spinal fluid to produce numbness

stages–refers to the three divisions of labor, delivery of the child and delivery of the placenta

strain counterstrain techniques–physical therapy techniques that assist the elongation of the muscle by using the force of the contracting muscle

station–locates the presenting part of the fetus in relation to the mother's ischial spines

steroidogenesis–the production of steroids

stress incontinence–occurs when intravesicular pressure exceeds urethral resistance, detrusor activity absent

stress test–used at the end of pregnancy to attempt to induce uterine contractions to determine fetal well-being

striae gravidae–stretch marks appearing on the distended skin caused by the rupture of elastic fibers due to excessive distention

stillbirth–refers to the birth of a baby who has died in utero

stoma–refers to any small opening or an artificial opening between two pouches or channels

suboccipitobregmatic–diameter of the fetal skull from middle of the large fontanelle to the undersurface of the occipital bone where it joins the neck

synostosis–fusion of adjacent bones which are normally separate

teratogens–substances which will produce abnormal fetal development if given to the mother in pregnancy through drugs or environmental factors

terbutaline–drug given to mothers to stop premature labor

thalidomide–drug used as a tranquilizer in the 1950s that in pregnant women produced severe limb abnormalities in offspring

theca–the sheath surrounding an ovarian follicle

third stage of labor–birth of the placenta

tocolytic–drug used to arrest labor

transition–the last phase of the first stage of labor when the cervix dilates from 0 to 10 cm

transverse lie–refers to the fetus in a horizontal position across the mother's pelvis

trigonal–relating to a triangular shape

unripe–describes a cervix that is not soft and not ready for labor

urethrocele–prolapse of the urethra with bulging into the vaginal opening

urogenital diaphragm–the perineal membrane, the deep muscle layer of the deep fascial layer which supports the pelvic organs

uterine dysfunction–inability of the uterus to contract and relax in a coordinated fashion

uterus–the pear-shaped organ in which the fetus grows; also called the womb

uterine inversion–when the uterus loses its shape and comes out toward its opening

vacuum extractor–device consisting of a cup, hose, and pump that creates a vacuum against the fetal head and to which traction is then applied to assist in delivery of the fetus through the birth canal

vagina–the 5 to 6 inch long elastic canal from the vulva to the uterus

vaginismus–spasm of the vagina resulting in pain

Valsalva maneuver–when intra-abdominal pressure is increased by breath holding during exertion

varicose veins–refers to the enlargment of veins when the valves in the veins become swollen, are unable to close, and have retrograde flow within them

vulva–external female genitalia

vulvadynia–painful intercourse

vulva vestibulitis–irritation of the vestibule of the external genitalia

Wharton's jelly–connective tissue with jelly-like material within the umbilical cord that supports the umbilical vessels

whey proteins–protein content of mother's milk

yolk sac–the highly-vascularized umbilical vesicle surrounding the yolk of the embryo

Definitions adapted from: Dox I, Melloni BJ, Eisner GM. *Melloni's Illustrated Medical Dictionary.* Baltimore, Md: Williams & Wilkins; 1979; and Thomas CL, ed. *Taber's Cyclopedic Medical Dictionary.* 13th ed. Philadelphia, Pa: FA Davis; 1977.

Index

abdomen, anatomy, 17
abruptio placentae, 230
acetabulum, 17
Addison's disease, 141
alcohol during pregnancy, 120, 122
amenorrhea, 48-49
American Physical Therapy Association (APTA), 6, 7, 9, 39, 40
American Society for Psychoprophylaxis in Obstetrics (ASPO/Lamaze), 10
amniocentesis, 216
amniotic fluid embolus, 144
anesthesia, 5-6, 235
anterior innominate, 187-192
aortic stenosis, 167
aortocaval occlusion, 24
Apgar scale, 219
APTA. See American Physical Therapy Association
arthritis and pregnancy, 170-171
ASPO/Lamaze, 10
asthma, 170

back problems
    herniated disc, 199-200
    low back pain, 192-193, 197, 199
    low back strain, 200-201
    pain and labor, 232
    product information, 291-292
bed rest, 163-165
biofeedback, 68, 299-301
bladder, 30-31, 61
blood pressure
    hypertension, 136-138, 168-169
    and maternal exercise, 109

body mechanics
    post-Caesarean section, 279
    and pregnancy, 123-125
Braxton Hicks contractions, 223, 261
Brazelton Neonatal Behavioral Assessment Scale, 219
breast
    anatomy, 15, 16
    changes with pregnancy, 95-96
    rehabilitation, 70-71, 72
breech presentation, 248-249

Caesarean section
    description, 251-252
    exercise and education following, 271-273, 277, 279
    and fetal weight, 250
    history, 4-5
    and pain relief, 247
    reasons for, 261
    vaginal births following, 252-253
caffeine, 122, 123
calcium, 119
caloric requirement during pregnancy, 120
cancer (gynecological), 59, 60
cardiovascular system
    cardiac output with exercise, 109
    changes with menopause, 74
    changes with pregnancy, 89-90, 92
    chronic disease and pregnancy, 167-168
    conditioning and pregnancy, 109-110
    diseases and disorders, 136, 137
    exercise response during pregnancy, 105-109
carpal tunnel syndrome, 183, 291

center of gravity, and pregnancy, 123-125
cervical spine irritation, 157
childbirth. *See* delivery; labor
childbirth education
    certification, 9-10, 112
    class content, 257-262
    course evaluation, 113
    and first stage labor, 235
    instructional materials, 297-299
    learning phases, 113
    post-partum classes, 276-277
    publications, 294
    role of physical therapist, 112-114
chloroform, 5-6, 231
chromosomal analysis of fetus, 216
circulation
    post-partum changes, 267
    venous support information, 293
coccydnia, 58
coccyx mobilization, 195-196
colostrum, 96
conception, 209-210
congenital anomalies, 208
contraindications during pregnancy, 175
cystic fibrosis, 170

De Quervain's disease, 183
death, vs. mortality, 133
delivery. *See also* labor
    alternative options, 245-256
    complicated, 248-250
        breech presentation, 248-249
        Caesarean section, 251-252
        genital fistulas, 257
        multifetal, 253-254
        pelvic joint injury, 256-257
        perineum injury, 254-255
        perineum repair, 254-255
        shoulder dystocia, 249-250
        uterine support injuries, 255-256
    and forceps use, 250-251
    multifetal, 253-254
    positions for, 248
    vaginal, 249
    vaginal following Caesarean, 252-253
dermatologic changes with pregnancy, 102-104, 149
DES (diethylstilbestrol), 150-151, 206
diabetes, gestational, 140, 142

diaphragm, position during pregnancy, 24
diastasis recti abdominis, 267
domestic violence, recognizing, 40
Douglas pouch, 28
dysmenorrhea, 52-54

early pregnancy classes
    about, 114-115
    body mechanics, 123-125
    center of gravity, 123-125
    emotional changes, 116-117
    fetal changes, 117
    maternal changes, 117
    nutrition, 117-121
    outline, 115
    partner's role, 125-126
    pelvic floor toning, 122-123
    relaxation instruction, 115-116
eclampsia, 138, 169
education. *See* childbirth education
electrical stimulation
    for gynecological conditions, 69-70
    and pelvic floor exercises, 68
    sources of equipment, 299-301
    and stress incontinence, 65
endocrine system
    diseases and disorders, 140-142
    and maternal exercise, 110
    and pregnancy, 97, 100-101
endometriosis, 54-55
episiotomy, 242, 255
exercise
    and body temperature, 110
    circulation and bed rest, 163
    effect on pregnancy outcome, 112
    fetal responses, 111-112
    maternal responses, 105-111
    post-Caesarean section, 277, 279
    post-natal program, 278
    target heart rate for pregnant women, 129
    teaching in early pregnancy classes, 126-128
    weightbearing during pregnancy, 111
external genitalia, 32-34

female anatomy. *See* anatomy
fetal alcohol syndrome, 120
fetal death, 133, 134

fetal health
  and conception, 209-210
  congenital anomalies, 208
  and environmental hazards, 206-207
  fetal distress during labor, 247
  and genetic counseling, 205-206, 207
  molding of head at delivery, 243
  monitoring, 217
  and position, 230
  and teratogens, 206-207
  and umbilical cord prolapse, 230
fetal weight
  influence on blood supply, 23-24
fetus
  assessment, 216-220
  descent during labor, 226
  development, 212, 213-214
  growth, 210-211
  physiology, 212, 216
  response to maternal exercise, 111
fibromyalgia, 58-59
follicle-stimulating hormone (FSH), 46-48
forceps, 250-251
FSH. *See* follicle-stimulating hormone (FSH)

gallbladder, 24
gastrointestinal system, 94-95, 148-149, 266
genetic counseling, 205-206, 207
genital fistulas, 257
gestational diabetes, 140-141
gonadotropins, 46-48

health organizations, 294-297
hebdomadal death, definition, 133
hemorrhoids, and pregnancy, 139
herniated disc, 199-200
  and delivery, 232
high-risk pregnancy, 161-165
hormones
  and dysmenorrhea, 52-53
functions in pregnancy, 101-102
  and maternal exercise, 110
  and normal menstrual cycle, 46-48
  and premenstrual syndrome (PMS), 51
hypertension, pregnancy-induced, 136-138, 168-169
hyperventilation
  during childbirth, 261
  and maternal exercise, 108

hypervolemia, 108
hysterectomy, 59

ICEA. *See* International Childbirth Education Association (ICEA)
incompetent cervix, 229
incontinence, 42, 60-65, 301
infectious diseases, 146-147
inferior vena cava occlusion, 25
innominate bones, 17, 18
internal pelvic exam, and physical therapist, 39
International Childbirth Education Association (ICEA), 10
iron rich foods, 121

joint laxity, 27

Kegel exercises, 65
kidney. *See* renal system

labor
  breathing for, 260
  complicated, 229-231, 234
  first stage, 232-236
  maternal position, 231
  normal, 224-229
  pain relief
    childbirth education, 235
    chloroform, 231
    general anesthesia, 247
    medications, 233-234, 246
    psychprophylaxis, 235, 246
    support person role, 246
    TENS (transcutaneous electrical nerve stimulation), 233, 236, 246
  precipitous, 248
  premature, 229
  presentations, 230
  second stage, 241-244
  third stage, 244-245
lactation, 268-269
lactose intolerance, 95
Lamaze, 235
leg cramps, 157
levator ani syndrome, 56
LH. *See* luteinizing hormone (LH)
live-born infant, definition, 133
low back pain, 192-193
  case study, 197, 199

strain, case study, 200-201
lumbar lordosis, 24-25

MacRobert's maneuver, 250
magnetic resonance imaging (MRI)
    and fetal health, 218
marketing physical therapy services, 8-9, 10, 11
maternal death, 133-135
medications for pain management, 233-234,
    246, 261
menopause, 73-74
menstrual cycle
    abnormal, 48-54
    normal, 46-48
metabolism, 98, 110-111
micturition, 62-63
mitral stenosis, 167
mitral valve prolapse, 168
mortality, 133
multiple pregnancies, 104-105
    and conception, 209-210
    delivery, 253-254
    and weight gain, 97
multiple sclerosis (MS) and pregnancy, 171
musculoskeletal system
    arthritis and pregnancy, 170-171
    diseases and disorders, 151, 157-158
        anterior innominate, 187-192
        back pain, 197, 199
        carpal tunnel syndrome, 183
        coastal rib pain, 184
        coccyx, 195
        De Quervain's disease, 183
        diastasis recti abdominis, 183
        knee and patellar dysfunction, 195-196
        listed, 198-199
        low back pain, 192-193
        muscle and tendon injuries, 196-197
        neck strain, 181
        nerve palsies, 196
        piriformis syndrome, 194
        posterior innominate, 184-187
        sacroiliac joint pain, 184
        symphysis pubis, 192
        temporomandibular joint, 181-182
        thoracic outlet syndrome, 182-183
    evaluation
        muscle testing, 178-180
        posture, 175-178

post-partum changes, 267
myocardial infarction (MI), during pregnan-
    cy, 136

nausea, 94-95
neonatal death, 133-135
neurological system
    central system disorders, 154-156
    changes with pregnancy, 94
    diseases and disorders, 151
    peripheral system disorders, 153
neuromuscular diseases, 156
nutrition, 117-122

OB/GYN. See obstetrics and gynecology
obstetrics and gynecology, history, 3-6
osteogenesis imperfecta, 157
osteoporosis, 74-75
    case study, 77-78
    and pregnancy, 157
    support products, 294
ovaries, 29, 150
oxytocin, 225, 246

pelvic cavity, 28-31
pelvic diaphragm, 31
pelvic dislocation, 58
pelvic floor
    definition, 31
    examination, 41, 43-46
    exercises, 65, 66, 67-68, 70
        handout, 124
        sources of equipment, 301
        teaching, 122-123
pelvic pain, 25, 54-59, 55, 56, 57
pelvic relaxation, 61
pelvis
    abnormalities, 22-23
    anatomy, 17-22, 26, 31
    diameters, 22-23
    fracture prior to pregnancy, 158
    infection and pregnancy, 152
    joint injury during delivery, 256-257
perinatal death, 133, 249
perineometers, 68, 292
perineum, 32-34, 266
physical therapy and women's health
    current role, 7-8
    development, 6-7

instructor guidelines, 112-114
marketing, 8-9, 10, 11
necessity of, 8
research, 11-12
piriformis syndrome, 56, 194
pituitary gland, 24, 142
placenta
　　response to maternal exercise, 112
　　and third stage of labor, 244-245
placenta previa, 229
PMS. *See* premenstrual syndrome (PMS)
pneumonia, 144
post-partum changes, 265-269
　　case study, 274-275
　　exercise for, 270-271
　　and sexuality, 274
　　support products, 293-294
posterior innominate, 184-187
postural changes, 24-25
　　and back pain
　　　　case study, 199
　　case study, 197
　　evaluation, 175-178
preeclampsia, 136, 138
pregnancy
　　breast changes, 95-96
　　cardiovascular system changes, 89-90,
　　　　92-94
　　contraindications during, 175
　　dermatologic changes, 102-104
　　effects of supine position, 91, 92
　　and endocrine system, 97, 100-101
　　gastrointestinal changes, 94-95
　　and genetic counseling, 205-206
　　high-risk. See high-risk pregnancy
　　maternal changes by month, 118
　　metabolic changes, 98
　　neurological changes, 94
　　and nutrition, 205-206
　　post-date, 229
　　prodrome to labor, 223-224
　　renal changes, 89, 91
　　reproductive system changes, 89
　　respiratory system, 97, 99, 100
　　teenagers, 165-166
　　weight gain, 96-97
premature labor, 229
premenstrual syndrome (PMS), 49, 51-52
prostaglandins, and dysmenorrhea, 52

proteinuria, 138
psychoprophylaxis, 10, 235
pulmonary embolism, 138
pulmonary system, maternal response to
　　exercise, 105-106
pyramidalis muscle, 17

quadratus lumborum, 17

relaxin, 27-28
renal system
　　changes with pregnancy, 89, 91
　　diseases and disorders, 142-143
reproductive system, disorders and pregnancy, 145, 150-151
respiratory system
　　disease and pregnancy, 144-145, 170
　　exchange ratio and maternal exercise, 107
　　maternal response to exercise, 107-108
　　and pregnancy, 97, 99, 100
Rh incompatibility, 217
rheumatic heart disease, 167

sacrum, 17-18
　　anatomy, 19
　　sacroiliac joint pain, 184
　　　　product information, 292
seat belts, wearing during pregnancy, 157-158
sexual abuse, recognizing, 40
sexually transmitted diseases and pregnancy, 152
shoulder dystocia, 249-250
smoking during pregnancy, 120, 122
spinal cord injury, and pregnancy, 157, 172
stillbirth, definition, 133
stress incontinence, 64-65
　　case study, 76
　　physical therapy management, 65
stress test, and fetal health, 218-219
supine hypotensive syndrome, 24
symphysis pubis, 192

target heart rate, for pregnant women, 129
teen pregnancy, 165-166
temporomandibular joint disorder, 181-182
TENS (transcutaneous electrical nerve stimulation)
　　and dysmenorrhea, 53
　　and labor pain, 233, 236

teratogens, 206-207, 208, 209
Thiele massage for coccyx mobilization, 195
thoracic outlet syndrome, 182-183
thyroid gland
    changes with pregnancy, 24
    disorders and diseases, 141
transplantation and pregnancy, 171
transversalis fascia, 17
transversus abdominus, 17
tuberculosis, 145

ultrasound
    and fetal health, 217-218
    sources of equipment, 299-301
urinary tract
    disorders, 60-65
    post-partum changes, 266
urogenital triangle, 32
uterine tubes, 29
uterus
    anatomy, 29
    blood flow during exercise, 109
    changes with pregnancy/menstruation, 72-73
    and contractions during labor, 225
    diseases and disorders, 145
    dysfunctions and labor, 230
    injuries to ligaments during delivery, 255-256
    post-partum changes, 265-266
    retrodisplacement, 256

vagina, injury during delivery, 255
varicose veins, 138-139
vascular disease, and pregnancy, 138-139
vena cava syndrome, 91, 92, 163
venous thrombosis, 138
vesicouterine pouch, 28
vulvar vestibulitis, 57, 76-77

weight gain, during pregnancy, 96-97
weighted cones, and pelvic floor exercises, 68